MW01622867

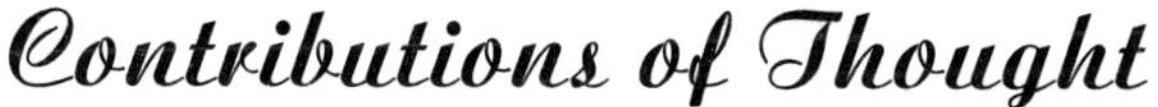
Contributions of Thought

Contributions of Thought

The Collected Writings of
William Garner Sutherland, D.O.

Pertaining to the Art and Science of Osteopathy
Including the Cranial Concept in Osteopathy
Covering the Years 1914–1954.

Edited by
Adah Strand Sutherland and Anne L. Wales, D.O.

Second Edition

The Sutherland Cranial Teaching Foundation, Inc.
1998

Published by Sutherland Cranial Teaching Foundation, Inc.
4116 Hartwood Dr., Fort Worth, Texas 76109
Phone: (817) 926-7705
Fax: (817) 924-9990

First edition 1971
Second edition 1998

Book and jacket design by Lubosh Cech
Jacket photo by Andrew Haltof

Order from Sutherland Cranial Teaching Foundation, Inc.

Originally published by Rudra Press ISBN 0-915801-74-4

Third impression 2002

Printed in the United States of America

ISBN 1-930298-01-3

Dedicated to those who think osteopathy,

practice osteopathy,

and represent it worthily

During my years in practice as an osteopathic physician there never has been one regret for having chosen this field for my life's work. Professional experience daily demonstrates the truth that the science of osteopathy includes the key to the great physiological chemical laboratory, the human body, unlocking the living, potent forces that heal. To the student looking forward to a professional field of scientific research, and with the desire in his or her heart to render beneficial service to humanity, let me truly say: *Osteopathy provides the golden opportunity.*

W.G. Sutherland, D.O.

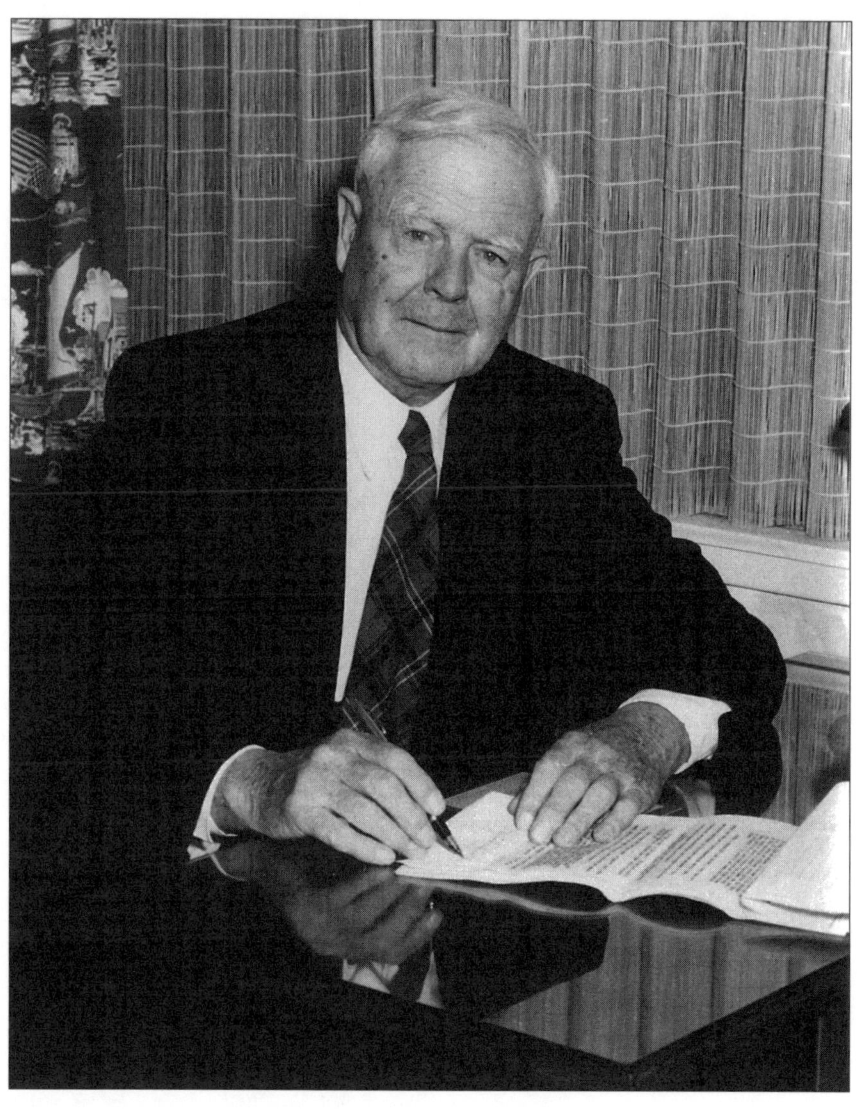

William Garner Sutherland, D.O., D.Sc. (Hon.)
March 27, 1873–September 23, 1954

Contents

Foreword

These works of William G. Sutherland, D.O., which you are privileged to read, illustrate the fundamental principles of osteopathy. There are many principles in the science of osteopathy, just as there are physicians of many different disciplines within the framework of osteopathy: internists, obstetricians, gynecologists, pediatricians, surgeons for all areas of the body, psychiatrists, osteopathic manipulative specialists, and others. Yet the one common denominator for the whole group is the science of osteopathy and the individualized principles as they apply to the work of each group of practitioners.

One of the principles of osteopathy that is so important is the fact that structure and function cannot be separated in the clinical evaluation of the patient. This principle can be divided into two corollaries. It is an accepted dictum that structure determines function, and this requires very little thought or discussion to know that this dictum is true. It is equally true that function determines structure, and this idea calls for a far more searching analysis as to its full understanding in its clinical application.

During the formative time from conception to physical maturity, especially during the early months and years, the growing structural development of the body is going to have considerable influence on the functioning of the growing mind and body. For example, a physical birth strain pattern will influence the entire developing physical and mental pattern for the child throughout life. A scoliotic pelvis, spine, and chest cavity will cause a corresponding displacement of the organs within them and modify the functioning of those structures to meet the needs of the patient. Disease or traumatic conditions in the child's body, such as Legg-Calve-Perthes disease, will modify the functioning of the pelvis and resultant development of the postural mechanism during the rest of the growing period. There are hundreds of clinical applications in this thought.

However, after the body has matured in its physical development, with the modifications caused by of disease or traumatic conditions, then function determining structure becomes the more dominant principles. Function-structure has worked hand in hand with structure-function throughout the formative years from conception onward, but now that the body has matured, it is function-structure that gives a truer insight into the clinical evaluations of the science of osteopathy as they apply to the patient.

The osteopathic physician has to learn to *feel* physiological functioning within, manifesting its ever-changing role in the structural economy of the patient. He needs to observe with his eyes, ears, and touch the differences between the normal and abnormal changes in function within any given area in any given specialty in osteopathy. The science of osteopathy is not confined to the manipulative group of specialists. It is possible for every discipline of specialist to learn the fundamental principles of the total concept of osteopathy and apply them clinically in their respective fields of service.

To learn to *feel* function, to *think* function, and to *know* function within anatomical physiology is not an easy art and skill for the physician to develop. It takes hours, days, weeks, and years to bring this training into the hands, eyes, ears, and mind of the physician. And yet it is fundamental to the total understanding of the science of osteopathy as taught by Andrew Taylor Still.

William G. Sutherland had this understanding and skill. He gave us these principles in his development of the cranial concept, although at no time did he ever separate the head from the rest of the body. He expanded the fundamental principles of osteopathy to create an understanding of the craniosacral mechanism. More importantly, he knew, understood, and used the principles of function and structure in their interrelationships for the whole body.

As you read the material presented in these papers, *feel with* him the functioning of the tissues he is discussing as well as visualize the structures he is describing in his work. Note how, clinically, his work can be a source of basic information and application in all the specialties when appropriate to the subject being discussed. It is necessary to *think* deeply, *feel* deeply, and *know* deeply *with* Dr. Sutherland as one studies his writings.

The principles of the interrelationships of structure-function and function-structure are but two of many that are found in the science of osteopathy, but they serve to give the physician a working tool with which to read and understand the works herein presented. Dr. Sutherland had all the principles of osteopathy in his hands and in his mind in his practice of osteopathy. These principles involve life, sensation, motion, nutrition, and assimilation from the single cell at conception to the total of anatomical physiology in the mature mind and body. They are found in health as well as in disease and traumatic interrelationships within the patient's body. In other words, the science of osteopathy demands a total knowledge of all principles in its application of service to the patient. Dr. William G. Sutherland used these principles in his service to his patients and gave them in his teachings to his physician students.

Rollin E. Becker, D.O.
January, 1968

Preface to the Second Edition

This second edition of *Contributions of Thought* is an effort on the part of the Sutherland Cranial Teaching Foundation to bring the wealth of information contained within its pages to a contemporary osteopathic audience. Modifications and additions have been made to enhance the text, while none of the original content was omitted.

Most of the modifications relate to the book's format and style and were done to improve readability. Minor changes were made in grammar and wording. Great care was taken not to alter meaning, and any ambiguity that existed was left intact. Some of the medical terminology was updated to reflect current usage. The term "circumduction" was changed to "circumrotation" to more accurately describe the normal motion of the sphenoid. The original editor's notes of Mrs. Sutherland are printed in italics; the editor's notes added for the second edition are bracketed in plain type.

Added to the book are a bibliography and a substantial number of footnotes. The purpose of many of the new footnotes is to clarify the things Dr. Sutherland made only passing reference to in his writings and lectures, because he assumed the audience he was addressing understood his allusions. Of these notes, some were added for historical interest, others give deeper meaning to his words. A number of footnotes were also added to provide more complete referencing of quotations, although it was not possible to identify all sources.

The history of the first edition, according to Anne Wales, D.O., is as follows. Dr. Sutherland wished to have his writings compiled into a single text and he and Mrs. Sutherland began the work, but it was largely unfinished at the time of his death in 1954. At a board meeting of the Sutherland Cranial Teaching Foundation in September of 1961, Adah Sutherland and Anne Wales presented a proposal for publication of such a compilation. The board gave its tentative approval for this monumental task, and the work slowly got underway. The death of Dr. Wales' husband, Chester Handy, D.O., in January 1963, delayed the project further until September of that year.

From the fall of 1963 through the fall of 1966, Dr. Wales and Mrs. Sutherland corresponded between their homes in Providence, Rhode Island and Pacific Grove, California. Mrs. Sutherland would gather together each section of material for Dr. Wales to type, and the copies would go back and forth by mail. Harold I. Magoun, Sr., D.O. added his comments to the emerging text, apparently encouraging a somewhat reticent Howard Lippincott, D.O. to compile the index, as the board of the Sutherland Cranial Teaching Foundation gave its final approval for printing. The text was sent to the Journal Printing Company in Kirksville, Missouri but was not printed until 1971 or 1972, when Herb Miller, D.O.–then faculty at the Kirksville College of Osteopathy and Surgery–discovered the manuscript and followed through on its printing.

Descriptions of Dr. Sutherland's early experiments and use of appliances for cranial treatment are included in this text because they represent a phase in his exploration, but the reader is cautioned that he never advocated their use after developing his manual methods. Specific treatment techniques are also described, and again the reader is cautioned that they are intended for use only by those licensed and qualified to use them.

Dr. Sutherland always expressed that his cranial concept resided within the whole of Dr. A.T. Still's science of osteopathy. He often referred to those trained in the use of this concept as "cranial technicians." His use of this term was not meant to imply that this work can be applied as an isolated therapy or by a person trained only in a series of techniques. Instead he was emphasizing the skill required–

that of using thinking-seeing-feeling-knowing fingers trained in the completeness of osteopathy.

Everywhere there is evidence to show that Dr. Sutherland was a most original thinker, and yet he also stressed that there is still more to learn and discover about the human "machine" beyond what he understood and taught. This book is for those who wish to understand more of Dr. Still's and Dr. Sutherland's very original thinking and to forge the possibilities for new discoveries.

M. Tamarin Vick, D.O.
Rachel E. Brooks, M.D.

For more information on the Sutherland Cranial Teaching Foundation see page 355.

William Garner Sutherland
Biographical Information

William Garner Sutherland, D.O., D.Sc. (hon) (1873-1954) was born in Portage County, Wisconsin. He lived with his family in Minnesota, and later moved with them to South Dakota. While in Blunt, South Dakota he became a "printer's devil" for the local newspaper, the *Blunt Advocate*. By 1890 he had worked his way up to being the foreman. In September 1893 he went to Fayette, Iowa to attend Upper Iowa University. After this he returned to newspaper work and eventually became an editor of the *Daily Herald* in Austin, Minnesota. While in this position, in 1898, he heard of Dr. Still and his teaching of osteopathy in Kirskville, Missouri. That year he entered the American School of Osteopathy and graduated with the class of 1900.

Preface to the First Edition

This collection of Dr. Sutherland's osteopathic writings has been assembled in response to requests that such a compilation be available. With but a few exceptions, it includes all the material he himself put in writing regarding the science and practice of osteopathy, as he experienced it and concentrated upon it in practice, cranial research, and in teaching. The only major exception is *The Cranial Bowl,* which was originally published in 1939. This volume of Dr. Sutherland's collected writings–which represents a period of 54 dedicated years, (1900-1954)–has been produced under the auspices of the Sutherland Cranial Teaching Foundation, Inc.

Many of the papers in this collection have been published previously. A few excerpts from correspondence on technical points have also been included. The remainder are prepared manuscripts, transcribed talks taken from records or tapes, and a few that were translated from stenographic notation. Five lectures, produced as phonograph records specifically for distribution, were made in a Pacific Grove, California recording studio in 1953.

Insofar as possible, the papers are arranged in chronological order. Where information was available, notations have been made that relate the circumstances associated with each. Because Dr. Sutherland understood the discipline of saying the same things to different audiences, there was much repetition of some themes. A few of these repetitions have been deleted where their absence did not affect what he had to say in that particular paper. There has been some editing of irrelevant comments and some recasting of sentences in the interest of clarity. In the preparing of this material for publication, I have had the invaluable assistance of Anne L. Wales, D.O. Without her, I could not have accomplished it.

The primary motivation in assembling these writings is, no doubt, that of preservation and accessibility. They depict the progress of an "original thinker." With a steadfast sense of personal responsibility, Dr. Sutherland accepted Dr. Andrew Taylor Still's admonition that D.O. stands not only for Doctor of Osteopathy but for "dig on" as well. His writings convey that he did so, consistently. Digging on and on, at no time did he lose sight of, or deviate from, the fundamental principles of osteopathy as conceived by its founder, Dr. A.T. Still, whom he regarded with appreciation and veneration.

I like to believe that the attentive reader will see revealed in these writings how Dr. Sutherland's self-imposed "digging" heightened his comprehension of osteopathic philosophy and its application in practice. It was through this constructive discipline that he was guided, to his own amazement, into the channel of cranial research. This perseverance culminated in his contribution of the cranial concept to his profession, to "osteopathy in the cranial field," as Dr. Harold I. Magoun has so correctly titled his valuable text.

In assembling and preparing these writings for publication, it has been an incentive to Dr. Wales and myself to realize that they will be available to others in the profession who may desire to become acquainted with, or review their acquaintance with, the ideas of an "original thinker," his utilization of those ideas, and their significance.

This collection is not a complete text, nor is it an organized statement of Dr. Sutherland's concepts, theories, discoveries or technical teaching of osteopathic therapeutics. It is the written output of a completely dedicated osteopathic physician.

Adah Strand Sutherland

1. Early Writings

1. Let's Be Up and Touching!

This highly original article appeared in an early 1914 issue of The Osteopathic Physician.

The admonition, "Touch Not," was not written for the osteopathic physician. God gave to him the instruments with which to feel. Let him touch. Forbid him not. But first instruct him how to feel. His professional task to a great degree is a finger task–that of locating etiological factors beneath as well as throughout all bodily tissues, being as problematic as is the "searching for a needle in a haystack" and requiring fingers with brain cells in their tips. Fingers capable of feeling, thinking, seeing. Therefore, first instruct his fingers how to feel, how to think, how to see, and then let him touch. His fingers should be able to cipher the sensation signal-code found in all tissues along the backbone cable. The finger-feel, the finger-thought, and the finger-sight are the only way to read the diagnostic message. His fingers should be like detectives, skillful in the art of locating things hidden. The mere tracing by fingers up and down, here and there, is not "getting in touch" with things hidden; the "hit and miss" not being the proper osteopathic application of tactile sense.

His fingers should *pause*, here and there, pressing in deeply to the *deeper* things that concern. Sojourning in a city for a day or two affords more opportunity for an acquaintance with the populace than merely driving through. So it is with the sense of touch. The fingers should *tarry*, resting firmly, yet gently, yet deeply, on articulations, on ligaments, on muscles, here and there, and thus form an acquaintance with the "populace" in the "burg." The populace of the spinal-burg is inclined to inform and will tell the fingers many important things. The fingers should not only feel *while diagnosing* but also *feel while treating*. It is requisite to hold the fingers "Johnny-on-the-spot" while treating and follow with their "feel," with their "thought," and with their "sight" throughout the treatment.

Osteopathic technique is *governed by and through* the intelligent application of the cultivated sense of touch. Osteopathic technique cannot be learned by observation–eyesight cannot observe the sense of touch. There must be a finger-feel, a finger-thought, and a finger-sight in order to note *how* the lesion moves, *when* it moved, and the change occurring *after*. To learn this art it is essential to place one's own fingers aside those of the instructor and follow along with him in the *touch*, in the *how*, and in the *after*. Osteopathic technique *includes* the cultivated sense of touch and should be *applied* intelligently both in diagnosis and in treatment. Get the *feeling*! *Let's be up and touching*!

2. "Forearm" Application

The Osteopathic Physician, *May 1914.*

There is a new, yet old, application which I find efficacious. It is the "forearm" application to muscular contractures only. The forearm is a wonderful cushion, in itself composed of muscular fibers that are soft and pliable, and when applied to other muscular tissue quickly rolls out the contractured fibers with great ease and comfort to the patient. It is applicable in the treatment of colds and influenza by rolling contractured fibers in the scalenes and other contractures of the cervical region. It is applicable to contractured fibers found anywhere along the spine.

The forearm application is easily acquired–merely commence using it. The patient lies prone or on the side. Place the cushion area of the forearm over the contractured area. Grasp the forearm with the other hand and apply mild pressure rolling the forearm outward, downward or upward, much in the manner that a pastry cook manipulates a rolling pin. Try it on your next case of inflammatory rheumatism or in some case where the spinal area is especially sensitive to the ten fingers. Keep in mind, however, that you are merely treating muscular contractures, after which one may more readily reach the important bony lesions.

3. Saving Your Own Power

Date and publication unknown.

Utilize the patient's motive power instead of your own in the application of passive elongation to incomplete cervical luxations. Thus: patient reclining on back, physician standing at the head with fingers at desired points on the offending lesion, holding firmly and gently, while the patient raises hands and arms over his head, placing his palms upon the physician's chest and pushing gradually.

This excels any mechanical device for passive elongation of cervical tissues as it is applied to the specific point. No danger either, as the patient is not inclined to utilize too much force upon his own neck!

4. Grandfather's Bootjack Remedy in Flat Feet

Date and publication unknown.

In the early days of his practice Dr. Sutherland was interviewed by a zealous young reporter from the Minneapolis Tribune. The topic was "flat feet." To Dr. Sutherland's astonishment, the interview appeared with this flamboyant heading: "Treat 'Em Rough Says Doctor, Telling How To Cure Flat Feet." The crude report that followed did not squelch the thought, and later, the exact date is not known, it was incorporated in the restrained article which follows.

Exercise Did It

Men who wore the old-time boots and employed the olden-time bootjack were seldom troubled with ailments in their feet. Yet it was not the boots that kept their feet in trim but the daily evening exercise with the bootjack in removal of the boots. You do not need the boots to apply the remedy. Merely apply the bootjack grip to the heel and then follow the same procedure your grandfather exercised in removing his boots.

Heel Forced Backward

Most persons when walking first place the heel in contact with the floor or walkway and then the rest of the foot, thus throwing most of the weight on the heel. This weight has a tendency to force the heel backward and disturb its normal articulations with the bones down in the main arch of the foot, thereby causing the arch to sag down.

High-heeled shoes worn by women aggravate this condition. This backward force on the heel also throws a strain on the long and short plantar ligaments and, in connection with sagging the main arch, constricts the arterial and venous channels beneath the bones, resulting in general weakness and flat feet.

How Grandfather Worked

In employing the bootjack to get his foot out of the narrow bootleg, grandfather pried against the heel, thus forcing the heel bone forward again to its normal position eliminating the constriction to the vascular channels. Consequently his feet rested peacefully, with normal blood supply throughout the night. A little rough treatment with the bootjack type of technique as indicated here is needed–and needed badly–in these days of high heels when feet are bound, otherwise, to go to bed with that "tired feeling" and wake with a cramp.

5. A Suspension Cap in Occipitoatlantal Technique

Journal of the American Osteopathic Association, *Correspondence, January 1915.*

According to "osteological proofs" presented by Dr. Edythe F. Ashmore in the July 1914 issue of the Journal of the American Osteopathic Association, occipitoatlantal articulations are, or should be, especially important to the osteopathic physician. These articulations have experienced, under the cloak of technique, many strenuous pulls, jerks and snaps. Believing that the profession would welcome a successful method wherein such strenuousity becomes impossible, it is a pleasure to present a suspension cap idea.

The chief feature of this method is the adaptation of a fulcrum at the occiput and, at the same time, a fixation of the atlas. With such adaptation the head can easily be rotated posteriorly on the occiput-fulcrum, while the condyles glide anteriorly in the facets of the atlas; or the head may be easily rotated superiorly on the occiput-fulcrum, while the condyles glide posteriorly in the facets of the atlas. Or, sidebending may easily be accomplished without pull or strain, while the occiput rests in the cap-fulcrum allowing the condyles to glide laterally in the facets of the atlas.

The suspension cap is adjustable to the size of the head. It fits snugly around the occiput while supporting straps are so arranged as to give support directly to the occiput. This makes a fulcrum or pivotal point possible at the occiput. Fixation of the atlas is made by the operator's hand or fingers while the free hand is utilized in turning or rotating the head. The operator thus has the advantage of a third hand, so to speak, through the support afforded by the suspension cap at the occiput.

In reducing a bilaterally posterior occiput, the occiput rests comfortably in the cap, the operator makes fixation on the lateral processes of the atlas with the thumb and fingers of one hand while he gently applies pressure on the brow with the free hand, tilting or extending the head backward. Remember that the atlas is fixed and that the occiput, resting snugly in the cap, has become a fulcrum point. As you tilt the brow backwards, the head rotates posteriorly on the fulcrum and the condyles glide anteriorly in the facets of the atlas as adjustment is accomplished. It is a simple, easy method; no pull, no jerk, no snap. The reduction is accomplished providing the diagnosis is correct: a bilaterally posterior occiput.

In reducing a bilaterally anterior occiput, the occiput rests in the cap as before, the same fixation is applied to the lateral processes of the atlas, but in this instance the pressure on the brow is applied in a forward and downward direction; in other words, as flexion of the head rotates anteriorly on the fulcrum point at the occiput, the condyles glide posteriorly in the facets of the atlas as easily and simply as in the previous lesion.

In reducing a lateral occiput, the occiput rests in the cap as before. If the occiput is lateral to the right, the head is flexed, or rotated forward on the occiput-fulcrum, where it rests. One hand then fixes the atlas on the left side while the other hand pushes against the mastoid process on the right side, thus pushing the condyles from right to left in the facets of the atlas. The advantage gained in flexing the head on the occiput-fulcrum in lateral lesions is that the condyles glide posteriorly in the facets of the atlas to the point of widest divergence of the facets. When the occiput is lateral to the left, fixation of the atlas is made on the right side and pushing is applied on the left mastoid process.

In reduction of "rotation" lesions, say a unilateral posterior occiput, the occiput rests in the cap as before. If the occiput is posterior on the right, fixation is made at both lateral processes of the atlas together with fixation of the mastoid process on the left with one hand. The free hand extends the head on the fulcrum at the occiput and turns it from right to left. In this instance, the head rotates upon an axis centered at the left facet of the atlas. In other words, the right condyle glides anteriorly in the right facet while the left condyle remains stationary in the left facet. The supporting straps pass through a pulley, making this method of procedure possible. If the occiput be unilaterally posterior on the left, merely reverse the process. Unilateral anterior occiputs are reduced in the same manner.

In reducing a right posterior occiput plus a left anterior occiput, the occiput rests in the cap as before; fixation is applied at both lateral processes of the atlas, and the head is rotated from right to left on the pivotal point lying midway between the facets of the atlas.

Although the suspension cap is particularly adaptable to

occipitoatlantal lesions, it is also helpful in the reduction of any cervical lesions.

Editor's Note: The apparent varieties of positional relations between the condyles of the occiput and the facets of the atlas, other than those characteristics of flexion and extension, were otherwise explained in Dr. Sutherland's later thinking. He came to realize that the nodding motion was the only motion permitted by the anterior convergence-posterior divergence and the inferior convergence-superior divergence of the facets of the atlas. Apparent lateral and rotation effects are to be seen resulting from compression of the condylar parts of the occiput with deformation of the foramen magnum.

6. Reaching the Ascending Colon Without the Use of High Enemas

Journal of the American Osteopathic Association, *September 1915.*

Among many valuable points carried home from the recent annual meeting of the Minnesota State Osteopathic Association was that presented by Dayton B. Holcombe of Chicago, in reference to the importance of the ascending colon as a factor to be carefully considered in auto-intoxication.

Dr. Holcombe, like many others, advocates the use of the high enema, which is an excellent and reliable method in reaching the ascending colon. Yet there may be a few in the profession like myself who feel timid in using high enemas because of a possible puncture when inserting the tube. The method is all very well and proper to experienced fingers, for specialists like Dr. Holcombe, Dr. C.W. Young, and others. But for the inexperienced, like myself, it is well to exercise a degree of caution. This necessity mothered a little technique which is here presented.

The patient lies on the right side. A well-padded belt, about six inches in width and twenty-three inches in length, is passed beneath the ninth, tenth, eleventh and twelfth ribs. The belt is then fastened to a suspension strap and this region of the body is raised a few degrees from the table and allowed to rest in this position for a period of three to four minutes, perhaps longer if necessary, depending upon the results and the comfort of the patient.

One case wherein the ascending colon was impacted from the cecum to the hepatic flexure and almost as hard as a rock may be of special interest in testimony of the technique. The patient was suspended in the above manner for three minutes. The result was manifested by a rapid fire of gas from the rectum continuously for ten minutes. The odor was frightful, and the patient, losing his false modesty, added to his apology a profound gratitude for his relief.

An hour later a voluminous defecation occurred followed later by mucous and the thread-like material to which Dr. Holcombe called attention. In this case there was no manipulation of the spine nor reduction of a lesion, no massaging of the colon, no enema, merely the three minute suspension.

If anyone interested in the technique will try it upon himself before experimenting on the patient, he will most likely find that the belt, when suspended, lies snugly around the costals and seems to spring them inward from the side. Whether the springing inward of the costals in this manner brings about a peristalsis by stimulation of the ganglia near the heads of the costals, or whether the inward position of the costals changes the position of the ascending colon or removes a possible kink of the hepatic flexure, I am not prepared to say. Yet it brings results without the high enema.

Charles Hazzard, in his *Practice and Applied Therapeutics of Osteopathy*, cites several reasonable theories that may explain the excellent results obtained through use of the above technique. I refer to the chapter in the first edition entitled "An Osteopathic Study of the Diaphragm, Its Relation to Abdominal Disease," page 196.

This technique is an excellent aid in treating appendicitis and "sick headaches."

7. Occiput Posterior Lesion

Journal of the American Osteopathic Association, *March 1916.*

The patient, a man 50 years of age, consulted me for headaches which I diagnosed as due to a posterior occiput. From the history, the lesion was produced at about the age of ten. At that time he attempted a somersault over a rail fence and lost his balance. With his head caught between the rails, and the rest of his body continuing the somersault, he so hung until released by a boy chum.

He had the X-ray taken because he was not satisfied with my diagnosis. We both were convinced by the negative that the diagnosis was correct.

8. X-ray of a Wry Neck

Journal of the American Osteopathic Association, *May 1916.*

The accompanying radiograph shows clearly a malposition of the first ribs. [The accompanying plates were not reproducible.] Note the equal distances between the second, third and fourth ribs and then compare with the distance between the first and second ribs. Pass a thread all along the line of vertebral spines and note the apparent rotation of the sixth and seventh cervical and first dorsal. Note also the position of the anterior ends of the clavicles as shown in the region of the shadows of the third and fourth ribs. The X-ray specialist who prepared the plate stated that all articulations were normal and advised massage. The patient was cured by corrective flexion, rotation and extension, thus "massaging" into place the first ribs, clavicle and a markedly posterior seventh cervical and first dorsal.

This was a case of so-called "wry neck" of seven weeks duration up to the time I saw him, coming on after a severe fall wherein the patient struck his head. The seven weeks of treatment, according to the patient's statement, had included "thrusts" in the upper dorsal and lower cervical and "jabs" beneath the ear by another operator. Aside from a rigid neck, no other neck symptoms were manifest, but the patient complained of an oppressive feeling through the upper chest.

At my examination before the X-ray was taken, I found the first ribs to be depressed at the sternal end and the left clavicle inward and downward at the sternal end. The picture confirmed this part of the diagnosis and also convinced the patient.

How an expert X-ray diagnostician could overlook this evidence and advise "massage" seems strange. Yet stranger still, in nearly every case where this M.D. specialist has done X-ray work for me he has advised massage.

9. Pouring Water Onto the Fire

Journal of the American Osteopathic Association,
Current Comment, February 1921.

The older osteopaths in the field will remember an axillary method presented by the Old Doctor[1] which he described as "pouring water onto the fire"–this axillary method being similar to the axillary technique offered by Dr. C.E. Miller in the treatment of acute infections through the lymphatics. While it may require ages of scientific research to settle the interesting discussion between Drs. Miller, Millard and Tasker, we all know that results usually follow the application of technique presented by Dr. Andrew Taylor Still.[2] There is satisfactory proof in my own practice as testimony of the Old Doctor's axillary method. Yet I am inclined to think that the results have not been in response to local manipulation of the axillary region or local "milking" of lymph

---

1. In his later years, Dr. A. T. Still was respectfully referred to as the Old Doctor.

2. C. Earl Miller, D.O. , Frederick P. Millard, D.O., and Dain L. Tasker, D.O. apparently had differing opinions regarding the lymphatic system. The specifics of this discussion are unknown, but may perhaps be elucidated from a text written by Dr. Millard, *Lymphatics: The Third Circulation; A Brief Popular Discussion of the Circulation Involved in All Disease Conditions.*

channels. Instead, they were due to vasomotor action taking place at the second dorsal, or thereabout, brought about indirectly through leverage exercised upon the first and second ribs.

In describing his technique, Dr. Miller says, "Place the four fingers of the hands in the axillae and the thumbs just below the clavicles over the points where the thoracic duct and the lymphatic duct empty into the venous circulation. By an upward lift of the fingers in the axillae followed by a downward pressure with the thumbs just below the clavicles...." If I am not mistaken, this upward lift with the fingers in the axillae and the downward pressure with the thumbs just below the clavicles exert a marked leverage upon the first and the second ribs, thereby elevating them at their sternal ends and forcing them downward at their vertebral ends, establishing a strong leverage point at the second dorsal.

Try the method out for yourself by having an osteopath follow out Dr. Miller's technique upon your own axillae, and see whether I am mistaken. You will probably note the leverage taking place in the first and second ribs and feel the effects therefrom by a vasomotor change, noticeable in the head and other channels of the blood stream. In this connection let us keep in mind that lesions in the vicinity of the second dorsal are as common as elsewhere and that this area is always found tense and rigid in influenza, pneumonia, and various acute complaints.

I believe that application of proper technique at the second dorsal area is bound to bring satisfactory results, whether applied by indirect leverage of the first and second ribs, or directly. Good results are accomplished by merely getting my fingers or thumbs as far beneath the scapula as possible and exerting a downward pressure upon the angle of the second rib, holding it in this position firmly and gently for a few minutes. I have seen rigid cervical tissues relax without any local treatment following this pressure upon the second ribs. "Tell me the moment when the blood flow is altered and I will tell you the moment when disease begins," said Dr. Still. The second dorsal area is proving to be a great vasomotor center, in my practice at least.

10. X-ray Proof of Osteopathic Lesions

Journal of the American Osteopathic Association, *July 1921.*

From a paper read before the Southern Minnesota District convention at Stillwater, Minnesota, February 7, 1920.

The custom of having X-ray exposures made in all lesions wherein the history was of a forcible or violent nature has unexpectedly provided negatives revealing osteopathic lesions previously diagnosed by the tactile sense.

Of course there are a few difficulties present in the X-ray proof. Among them we find the possibility of imitation...the X-ray negative or radiogram is no more and no less that a mere shadow of the bones and other bodily tissues cast by the invisible ray upon a photographic plate. Well do I remember how my uncle, with the tallow-candle light, made various shadow imitations–first the rabbit, then the monkey, then the mule, and so forth. It is possible for the expert radiographer to reflect these very same rabbit-monkey-donkey shadow faces upon a photographic plate with the finger bones and the invisible ray.

Within his specialty it is likewise possible to imitate almost any shadow negative which might be presented as proof of an osteopathic lesion–but not all. I present an occiput-lateral lesion shadow as proof evidence.

In such a lesion the condyle of the occiput on one side rises high up on the edge of the saucer-like facet of the atlas, while on the other side the condyle sinks down into the facet. This X-ray shadow shows this side-tilt plainly. Note the outline of the foramen magnum, then note the tip of the odontoid process of the axis, faintly appearing just above the arch of the atlas. Then note its position markedly to one side in the outline of the foramen magnum...this shadow is an anterior-posterior exposure through the mouth, with the mouth wide open so that the inferior maxillary will not obstruct the shadow of the odontoid process of the axis and the upper cervical vertebrae.

Note the perfect alignment of the upper cervical in the shadow, then compare the space between the rami of the inferior mandible, maxillary and the vertebrae. Note how one ramus lies closer to the vertebrae than does the ramus on the other side. This is what would occur were one to open the mouth in an occiput-lateral lesion.

This is the point in the shadow which the expert could not imitate. In the imitation shadow, the vertebrae would not show this perfect alignment. Were he to attempt the imitation by tipping the occiput to one side, without the condyles being in the lateral lesion in the facets of the atlas, to show the closeness of one ramus to the vertebrae, he would be confronted with a curve in the upper cervical which would immediately differentiate between the lesion and the imitation.

The patient in this case is a young man whose complaint had been diagnosed as epilepsy. Learning that the "spells," as he called them, began to appear soon after a severe bump upon the head (tripping and falling forward, striking the right parietal bone against a cement wall) an exposure was made to clear up the possibility of a hidden fracture of the odontoid process of the axis. The exposure failed to show a fracture but pictured the occiput-lateral lesion which had been previously diagnosed by the tactile sense. Reduction of the lesion cleared away the "spells." We entertain considerable doubt as to the diagnosis of epilepsy.

The next two shadows presented as evidence concern an interesting case. The patient, a foreman in a tile factory, grasped an electrical cord feeding juice to an automatic cement scale, at a point in the cord where the insulation had become defective, the right hand grasping the cord and the left hand resting on the cement scale. The upper thorax was violently pulled forward toward the cement scale and at the same time rotated somewhat to the left. At the same instant, an iron rod supporting a sand bin in the immediate vicinity caught him across the left ramus of the inferior maxillary and the left mastoid process, sidetilting the head to the right and forcibly twisting the entire cervical region in the same direction. It is a wonder the patient lived to tell the story. He did not even lose consciousness.

Twelve hours later he walked in with his head in a sidetilted-rotation position, twisted way around to the right, with immobility throughout the entire cervical region.

Tactile examination located a sidetilting-rotation at the second and third cervical and a slight crepitus in the same region, also a general torsion from the occiput down to the first or second dorsal with a possible indication of a specific lesion at the sixth and seventh cervical.

Aside from sensitiveness to touch at the left lateral border of the second and third cervical, the immobility and slight crepitus, there were no apparent complications. Three exposures were made to clear up possible hidden fractures but none appeared on the negatives. Two of the negatives plainly revealed the sidetilting-rotation at the second and third cervical and the general torsion, as had previously been diagnosed by the tactile sense. After one treatment he returned to his daily labor with a normal neck.

Now view the pictures of the lesion pertaining to the case. The first is an anterior-posterior exposure of the cervical region and upper dorsal. Note how the spine of each vertebra from the first dorsal up to the third cervical gradually appears farther and farther to the left as you follow upward. Note the general twist or torsion of the entire cervical region.

The second is an anterior-posterior exposure through the mouth, wide open. Beginning at the extreme bottom edge of the print, trace the outline of the cervical vertebrae as their shadow lines pass upward past the shadow of the inferior mandible maxillary to the occiput[3]–convincing evidence to anyone of a general torsion. Note the outline of the foramen magnum. Note the position of the odontoid process of the axis, located a little to one side in the atlas. Note the same sidetilt at the second and third cervical, pictured the same here as in the first picture–proof additional of the sidetilting-rotation.

The next shadow concerns a young man who thought he might enjoy a dive in shallow water. He came to a sudden stop with his head

---

3. The "inferior maxilla" is an older term for the mandible.

forced either forward or backward and his neck forcibly twisted to one side. Partial paralysis of both upper extremities soon followed. Three months later a tactile osteopathic examination gave a diagnosis of a rotation lesion between the fourth and fifth cervical. Exposures were made to clear up a possible hidden fracture. None being found, the lesion was immediately reduced and normal condition returned to the upper extremities.

This picture shows the lesion between the fourth and fifth cervical as had been previously diagnosed by tactile sense. Note the light area between the fourth and fifth cervical. Note that it is wider at the left.

The cervical region is more susceptible to hidden fractures than other areas. These exposures being specifically made to clear up fracture indications and not to reveal lesions are confined to the cervical vicinity. However, it is possible to find X-ray proof in other areas.

2. Thinking Versus Tinkering

Journal of the American Osteopathic Association, *February 1925, March 1925, and June 1925. Reprinted in the 1952* Year Book *of the Academy of Applied Osteopathy.*

Part I: February 1925

Osteopathic technique, when considered in relation to osseous alignment, is an intelligent application of the tactile sense, not possible of acquisition through observation of the other fellow's manipulation. The osteopath is a thinker, not a tinker–his fingers, when properly trained, possess the art of thinking intelligently at their digital tips. Therefore, technique cannot be taught through demonstration of a series of manipulations.

This can be acquired only by the student having his fingers there "Johnny-on-the-spot" alongside those of the instructor, following intelligently, with tactility, feeling, seeing, thinking at those finger tips, as the tissue is being guided carefully, gently, firmly and scientifically into normal relationship. Manipulations, various routine movements, thrusts, pulls and jerks lacking in intelligent tactility at the desired area of movement might well be called tinkering. These are frequently advanced as technique, but they are not osteopathic technique–that skilled art, when considered in relation to osseous alignment, that is the intelligent application of tactility beneath muscular tissue. Time now occupied in demonstrating manipulations to students could be devoted more advantageously to the training of tactility. Tactility is embedded among the fundamental principles of osteopathy and more stress should be laid thereon in instruction. Tactility is essential in treatment as well as in diagnosis. Without it, treatment is nonintelligent, savoring of the blind thrust of the imitators.

With students and osteopaths skillfully trained in tactility, there would be less need for others to tour the country teaching manipulations as they are doing today. Any person, even without mechanical experience, can turn a visible nut with a monkey wrench, the manipulation being easy. But when the nut is invisible down beneath the engine, it requires the intelligent application of tactility by an expert machinist to execute assistance properly. The expert machinist, through trained tactile sense, knows whether the bolt is turning in a faulty manner with the nut or whether the bolt is remaining stationary in a proper manner as the nut turns. He also knows when the task is accomplished. He is the expert machinist to the engine. The osteopath is called the expert machinist to the body. He should constantly bear in mind that many of the problems in osseous alignment lie hidden beneath muscular fiber and that mere manipulation, gained through watching the other fellow, will not touch because it is lacking in the intelligent application of touch.

In manipulation without tactility, one is apt to stray into the faulty angle of utilizing unnecessary leverage with neighboring tissues. Examples of this are the sidebending lateral pull in the cervical region while endeavoring to reduce an upper rib lesion and the application of the leg as a lever while correcting a sacroiliac malposition. The leverage method is much like an endeavor to jerk a nut from a bolt when the rust of time has made the turning difficult, the leverage tending to destroy the threads on the bolt. In habitual acquired pathology, time has wrought conditions similar to rusty threads in the articulations. Jerking or leverage endangers the threads and should be avoided.

Mere lifting of the chin, or extension in an occiput lesion, will not accomplish desired results because, in the habitual lesion, we find that the facets of the atlas move forward with the condyles. It is necessary to hold the atlas while the occiput turns, that is, to hold the bolt while the nut turns. Leverage by adjacent tissues is usually greatest on points other than the lesion area. It is not specific in application and it lacks intellectual tactility. That statement can be proved with tactility by placing the fingers upon the lesion area while another applies the leverage or traction. A method of drawing the tissues together with tactility in application, rather than pulling them apart is preferable.

As an illustration of a drawing method, view the situation–sometimes called an occiput posterior lesion–in which the condyles of the occiput are found, in relation to the atlas, at the point of widest divergence of the facets. Associated aspects of this situation include the view of the jugular foramina and other osseous avenues of vascular and lymphatic drainage carried backward, thus causing a crowding upon the drainage system of the head by softer tissues. This important, matter-of-fact obstruction should be considered by all osteopathic physicians. In this situation we are considering the type of occiput posterior that commonly results from occupational routine that necessitates habitual flexing of the head. When this posture has become a habit during childhood, the posterior relation of the occiput to the facets of the atlas may be a common predisposing factor in cases of brain fatigue, eye strain, colds, tonsillitis and other acute diseases. Immediate reduction of this type of occiput posterior is not to be considered an act of wisdom because of the gradual, habitual nature of the events leading to this pathology. Quick cervical jerks or pulls, like the snapping of a finger joint, are contraindicated, and traction, in an effort to lift the occiput forward, merely tightens the tissues in relation thereto and makes reduction difficult. Assuredly, it is possible to make it snap, but pop and snap do not indicate arrival. To repeat: The gradual, habitual nature of the events leading to this pathology indicates gradual, cautious correction, not force or haste. Lesions of recent history and accidental forces, not habitual in initiation, may be evaluated differently.

The drawing-together method, suitable to this pathology, is applied in the following manner. Have the patient lie on a side, clasping the hands over the crown of the head. Then have him draw the head downward, somewhat as a turtle does in crawling into its shell. Hold firmly in this position while tipping the head backward. This movement, entirely by the patient's effort, draws together all neighboring tissues more closely and thus into a state of complete relaxation. While held firmly in this position by the patient, the physician's fingers are applied to the lateral processes of the atlas, gently and firmly pressing upward and backward, practically holding them stationary while the motive force by the patient draws the condyles of the occiput anteriorly in the facets of the atlas. This is a specific procedure in which intelligent tactility is directly in the neighborhood where one expects movement to occur, and where the osteopathic fingers can feel what is taking place in the effort to accomplish a scientific end.

As one progresses in repeated efforts, this being an habitual lesion, he will note the condyles being drawn forward in the facets of the atlas. It will not be the feel of the condyles directly, for like the surgeon with his probe, the movement of the condyles is detected through the trained tactile sense. The difference in the movement of the joint when it is back in normal relationship is particularly noteworthy. Instead of being sunk into the facets of the atlas posteriorly at their widest divergence, the condyles will be found midway between the widest and narrowest parts, a location that is important in the nodding or rocking movement of this articulation. The condyles will be higher, the jugular foramina and other avenues for drainage will be forward. The obstruction caused by crowding of soft tissues will be removed, and the great end towards which we have been endeavoring will begin to manifest itself in less complaint of eye strain, less brain fatigue, less susceptibility to colds and acute diseases. When this improvement has occurred the patient will testify to wakening in the morning feeling refreshed by nature's beauty-parlor method. Who knows but what the neighbors will be able to sleep also because attention to this anatomical phenomenon sometimes overcomes snoring.

We might cite other areas where a pathological situation in osseous alignment develops under habitual and occupational conditions for which a drawing-together method which includes intellectual application of tactility has been devised. An entire chapter could be written about upper ribs.

Part II: March 1925

In the preceding chapter, reference was made to occiput posterior pathology resulting through the habitual routine of head flexion which, in many cases, had its initiation by poring over books during school days and was accentuated later through occupational routine that required constant flexion. Associated with the occiput posterior, we frequently find a compensatory or secondary atlantal-axoid pathology necessitating important considerations; a pathology requiring the thinking-feeling-seeing fingers to diagnose; a pathology to fathom in which the patient has been told and continues to be told, "Nothing ails you but your nerves." Herein we can reason that the posterior position of the condyles of the occiput in the facets of the atlas has gradually forced the inferior articular surfaces of the atlas to glide forward on the superior articular surfaces of the axis, thereby tilting the odontoid process of the axis into close proximity with the ventral area of the spinal cord. Hilton, in that valuable little volume, Rest and Pain [pp. 102-105], cites an interesting experience with the odontoid process that is well worth an osteopathic physician's time to read. It acts as incentive to less tinkering with cervical osseous malalignments and more of the intelligent application of tactility in the treatment of delicate tissues, common in the cervical area. The odontoid process in itself stands as an "Oh Don't" contraindication to neck tinkering.

The spinal cord is a bundle of nerves. Imagine tickling that bundle with a blunt instrument shaped like the odontoid process of the axis. Nothing would ail but the nerves. Nothing ails but the nerve in a tooth when the dentist tickles its fiber with an instrument and how it then commences to wiggle. Take the bones of old Mike[1] from the

---

1. "Mike" was the name of the skeleton in Dr. Sutherland's office in Mankato, Minnesota. When trying to prove to himself that cranial bone movement was impossible, Dr. Sutherland used the skull of Mike, disarticulating the specimen to observe the articular sutures (and using only his fingers and a penknife to remove the temporal bone from the rest of the intact skull). Dr. Sutherland may have named this skeleton after the first cadaver at the American School of Osteopathy, whose name was also "Mike."

closet, place the inferior articular surfaces of the atlas forward on the superior articular surfaces of the axis and note the position of the odontoid process in an immediate tickling vicinity to the ventral area of the spinal cord, to say nothing of the possibility of its crowding heavily upon this area. Possibly the spinal cord is susceptible to wiggles also, and who knows but what its "wiggles" stimulate various contractures through the voluntary muscles of the backbone. But it matters not about the possibility; the fact of atlantal-axoid pathology is present and in need of correction.

Here, as in the occiput posterior pathology, the drawing-together method is utilized in reduction. For instance: The patient, in any position, is instructed to clasp hands over the crown of the head and to draw the head and neck downward in the manner of a turtle crawling into its shell. In the meantime, fixate the lateral processes of the atlas with the fingers of one hand and thus have intelligent tactility directly in the area where movement is desired. The lateral processes are held firmly backward while the fingers of the other hand gently but firmly press the spine of the axis in a downward direction. The "feel" of the tissue during the period of correction reveals the inferior articular surfaces of the atlas moving posteriorly as the superior articular surfaces of the axis glide forward or anteriorly. It is well to remember that this is an habitual pathology, the type that is gradual in development, and that immediate miracles are among the impossibilities.

Lay Explanation of "Feel of the Tissue"

The intelligent feel of the tissue was recently illustrated by a layman in an endeavor to explain the fundamental feature of osteopathic skill to an individual unacquainted with osteopathy. He said, "See that office safe? You can't open it. Jimmy Valentine, the safe-opening expert can, with his educated fingers. That is the way with the osteopath. With his educated tactility, he unlocks the laboratories that feed the body." Would that more osteopaths realized the importance of having such a degree of tactility right there directly on the spot during treatment, to tell when and how the bones are moving, as does the safe-opening expert tell when and how the bolts are turning. The fingers are the thinking-feeling-seeing instruments at our command. Feeling and seeing the tissue as you move it is that skillful art known as osteopathic technique when applied to osseous malalignment.

Upper Rib Pathology

In my opinion, rib malpositions are posterior at their vertebral ends–not up, not down, as most osteopathic diagnosticians contend. The apparent up position of the rib is due to vertebral flexion and the apparent down position to vertebral extension. More correctly speaking, the rib is outward as well as posterior. As the head of the rib glides backward, or posteriorly, from its articular facet with the body of the vertebra the angle glides outward, or laterally, from its articular facet on the transverse process of the vertebra. The first, second, and third ribs appear to be the most troublesome, especially the second rib. In most cases they are found difficult to replace when in malposition because of their relation with the scapulae. Yet, when one understands the pathological position, the task becomes easier. This area of the upper thorax might well be called the great vasomotor center of the entire body. This coincides fairly well with the experimentations of Gaskell relating to the involuntary nervous system.[2] Without question, rib pathology in this area disturbs blood and lymph channels to and from the head, as well as elsewhere. It also affects secretions and excretions and involuntary action pertaining to the viscera.

A malposition of the second rib especially can be counted upon as a disturber of peace to body tissue. Second rib pathology has even been known to have causative connection with a case of ulcer of the stomach wherein all remedies, osteopathic and otherwise, failed to relieve paroxysms of the most severe cramping type. Finally, in desperation, an osteopath tried the avenue of the second right rib. The paroxysm ceased immediately, and later attention to this rib brought

---

2. Gaskell, *Involuntary Nervous System* , 1916.

about what is said to be a cure. However, we keep a framed notice on our wall which states: "Miracles not performed; cures not guaranteed; professional skill to the best of ability our only guarantee."

Attention to the right second rib has also brought about emptying of the gallbladder through its duct and proved a source of comfort in various cases of a biliary nature. The rib has also been found guilty in many heart ailments, functional and pathological. As an illustration of the functional type, reference is made to the man who, while sitting in a chair, threw both arms around the neck thereof and tilted the chair backward. Both right and left second ribs immediately shot out of place posteriorly and the poor fellow suffered untold agony from dyspnea for 45 hours. Osteopathic skill finally replaced the ribs, and the heart began immediately to run away. After a few minutes of high speed, it quieted down to normal action.

As an illustration of the pathological type, we cite the instance where an osteopath was called in on consultation. Upon arrival at the bedside, he found the relatives in an adjoining room awaiting the end, which had been pronounced by heart specialists as quite near–a time when, if anything is to be done, it must be accomplished quickly without time to go over the patient with a stethoscope and the other necessary procedure in making a heart examination. So we do not know to this day whether the lad had a pathological heart condition, nor can we tell anything about its real nature. We believe the condition was pathological. It had been so diagnosed by physicians skilled in the knowledge of heart pathology, including the osteopath in charge of the case. There is no reason for us to disagree. We do know that our fingers were led carefully beneath the patient's thorax to the region of the left second rib and that there they found something wrong. They detected that the offending rib was pulled inward and forward at its vertebral end. That's all. We did not see the patient again but recovery began. He continued treatment under the capable skill of the family osteopath, recovered, and went to work.

I thought of these two cases during a clinic at which one of our leading heart diagnosticians presided recently, and I commend his skill. Among the clinic patients was an osteopath whose heart had recently begun to act up in a peculiar way. He was given the usual heart soundings, measurements and stethoscopic examination, but no spinal examination. The condition was diagnosed as a strain of the heart, if I remember correctly. The history revealed that the osteopath had been sawing with a crosscut saw. The complaint followed that period. With all due respect to the diagnostician, I cannot but feel that the fundamental examination was overlooked. Here was a case history pointing directly to a possibility of second rib pathology due to an unaccustomed tussle with a crosscut saw, each move in the swing of the saw pushing the ribs backward.

As was said in a recent *Journal of the American Osteopathic Association* editorial: "Perhaps some of us might be encouraged and stimulated to a little more definite and deeper digging in our own garden plot by a study of the most advanced medical literature." One might go on illustrating experience, profitable and otherwise, with second rib pathology. Experience, as Dr. Littlejohn used to say, that is "not found in the book."[3] But enough for the present.

Adjusting the Second Rib

Here again we utilize the drawing-together method in reduction. Remembering that the rib is posterior and outward at its vertebral end, it becomes a matter of retracing the step, that of drawing the rib inward and anterior. It is an inward movement of the angle toward its own articular facet on the transverse process of the vertebra. As the

---

3. John Martin Littlejohn, D.O. (1865-1947: American School of Osteopathy, 1900) was born in Glasgow, Scotland. Resigning as president of Amity College in Iowa, he began a series of visits to Dr. A.T. Still for relief of physical ills in the late 1890's. In 1897 he became a lecturer in physiology at the American School of Osteopathy (ASO), enrolled as a student in 1898 and was appointed dean of faculty and professor of physiology shortly thereafter. He graduated in 1900 and established the American College of Osteopathy and Surgery in Chicago, Illinois with his two brothers (also prior faculty members at the ASO) in that same year. In 1913 he returned to England and founded the British School of Osteopathy. See Berchtold, *History of the Chicago College*.

angle travels inward, the head of the rib naturally glides forward or anteriorly to its proper articular facet in the body of the vertebra. Any effort to draw the rib forward, without the inward movement at the angle, would tend to catch the head of the rib just back of its articular facet in the body of the vertebra and hamper progress. It is the inward draw that counts, the forward movement of the head then taking care of itself. It does not require any special position of the patient or any special manipulation to draw the angle inward, except to use your head along with your tactile sense and keep away from leverage by adjacent tissues.

Part III: June 1925

In part two, upper rib pathology had our attention. Osteopathic physicians and osteopathic students being familiar with the etiological relation of this pathology to brachial neuritis, it seems unnecessary to waste valuable space thereon. It is sufficiently established as one of the scientific facts in osteopathic channels. However, our "book of experience" serves as an incentive to mention a pathological condition found in the acromioclavicular arthrodia, which is frequently associated with upper rib pathology. Although not of etiological consideration in brachial neuritis, it has much to do with muscular restriction thereabout. This arthrodia might well be termed the "sacroiliac" of the shoulder, its malpositions in "ups" and "downs" having perhaps as many diverse opinions.

In our opinion, the ups and downs are of minor importance, and we will endeavor to point out a different angle for consideration. Acromioclavicular pathology requires especial skill in tactility to diagnose and is also one of frequent occurrence through habitual, routine etiological avenues, like that of an unnecessarily tight grip on the steering wheel while on a long drive. Frequently it follows fractures of the forearm, possibly as a secondary complication due to the position of the arm while carrying the forearm in the sling. It could occur through the accidental agency which caused the fracture. In this pathology, the articular surface of the acromion process has glided or rotated anteriorly while the articular surface of the outer end of the clavicle has glided posteriorly: one forward, the other backward–not "up" nor "down." The acromial end of the clavicle consequently crowds and retards the activity of the supraspinatus muscle and thus restricts, to some extent, the movement of the arm. As the acromion's articular surface glides forward, the coracoid process also changes its normal position to one involving muscular restriction. This likely accounts for the indication that the long head of the biceps slips from the bicipital groove. Possibly it has. But what profit in replacing it if the acromioclavicular pathology is neglected? Attention to the acromioclavicular malposition usually takes care of the bicipital tendon without local attention, but it is well to lift the tendon of the supraspinatus muscle in all cases.

As to technique: First, be sure of the diagnosis; the rest is easy. Merely draw the acromion articular surface posteriorly while guiding the clavicular articular surface anteriorly. Yet it is well to remember the possibility of hidden fractures and that they occasionally evade the most skillful thinking-feeling-seeing fingers. In all cases where a history of violence is recorded, the Roentgen ray is indicated. It may reveal only a small fragment of osseous tissue at the acromion end of the clavicle, yet that small end is a great end in the consideration of normal movement; and, of course, the coracoid process has fracture possibilities. As a general rule, the shoulder cases are of several weeks duration before consulting osteopathy, and by this time little "knits" become negative indications to the reduction of a subluxation. Fractures in close approximation to articular areas are always of serious consideration to normal movement. Furthermore, they do not necessarily have to be in close proximity in some instances. A recent experience in limitation of supination in the forearm gave testimony to this.

The fracture had occurred at the lower third of the radius and had been set and reset some six weeks previous and had probably been considered a good task well done under peculiar circumstances. An

X-ray, taken just before removal of the cast, showed a slight deviation or lapping at the fracture union. There was also a slight shortening of the radial bone itself which brought the semilunar and cuneiform bones of the wrist into an uncomfortable nearness to the ulna, which in itself was sufficient to hinder supination. The slight deviation at the fracture union also played a prominent part in limiting supination. For instance, imagine driving your car in a case where the driving rod had broken and been welded together in this unshapely manner. Every time the driving rod made a revolution, you would hear a grinding in the gear. In this case every attempt at supination met with a grinding in the inferior radio-ulnar articulation.

Give Heed to Eleventh and Twelfth Ribs

All ribs of the thorax can be handled in much the same manner as the upper three, to which mention was made in a previous article. But the eleventh and twelfth ribs have a pathological association with sacroiliac malpositions, and it is wise to give heed whenever the floating ribs appear in luxation. Much has been said, pro and con, regarding sacroiliac pathology by leading diagnosticians, so perhaps the less others say, the better, although one might write a volume or two. However, these are a few words from the book of experience concerning points not to be overlooked in connection with sacroiliac strains whether diagnosed up or down, or posterior or anterior. For the time being, it is sufficient to know that all osteopaths recognize the sacroiliac malposition, that it has had acceptance by our medical friends, and that osteopaths as a rule are very successful in reducing the malposition.

In association with the malposition, we find a muscular strain as well–in many instances, although not all–especially of the psoas major muscle. The strain of the psoas major muscles extends into the lumbar area and is manifested by marked lumbar rigidity, wherein any amount of so-called "loosening up" methods applied to the spine or lumbar muscles will never prove effective in relaxation. Loosening up methods never did appeal as a scientific osteopathic procedure. If the tissues are rigid, it is well to hunt for the cause of the rigidity, devoting the time spent in loosening up to searching with intelligent tactile sense. It pays to hunt with the feel of the tissue. It is the only hunting that I enjoy. Here we find the strain to the psoas major muscle as the cause of lumbar rigidity. Following reduction of the sacroiliac malposition, it will prove advantageous to lift the tendon of this muscle near its insertion at the lesser trochanter and thus provide it an opportunity to spring back through its own tractility into normal line. In many cases this small lift will overcome the lumbar rigidity and assist in the prevention of recurrence of the sacroiliac malposition. Thinking-feeling-seeing fingers should understand the muscular as well as the osseous tissue. As one seeks osseous malalignment down through the softer tissues, the fingers are bound to become cognizant of the feel of the tissue in the muscular. Hence the lesson to keep in practice with tactile sense. There is another muscular tendon that sometimes gets into trouble through association with the sacroiliac strain, the obturator internus. Here again, lifting of the tendon allows the muscle to spring back into line and assist in eliminating a false indication of the sciatic nerve caught by the trochanter.

While dwelling on the subject of muscular tissue in the neighborhood of the pelvis, it may be profitable to recall the wonderful contractile nature of various muscular tissues and how self-adjusting such tissues become when given an opportunity. In the early days of osteopathy, there was a familiar saying: "The tendency is always toward the normal." Let us view this "tendency toward the normal" from an unusual angle, e.g., in the instance where the abdominal viscera, in a downward descent, are in possible danger of becoming pelvic viscera. You know the condition. This is no idle dream but a condition that is common in this age of faulty sitting posture. The viscera consist of muscular tissue of contractile nature and will spring back into normal position if given an opportunity. The technique of the opportunity is best illustrated with a bowl of water. Tip the edge of the bowl and the water seeks its level near the tipped edge. One can tip the pelvic bowl at the pubes and the viscera naturally will seek their level near the tipped edge. When thus released, the opportunity is afforded for the natural contractility of muscular tissue to draw the viscera back into its natural position. Try it out upon your own pelvic bowl.

Assume a position on the back, reach down with the fingers and push the pubes in a downward direction toward the feet. Note the viscera beginning to rise. Be careful to get the right push in your technique. Catch a little posterior to the pubes as you push, and be gentle in that push. This is not a forcing method, just a gentle assistance to normal muscular contractility. Having learned through experience upon one's own anatomy, then try it on the next case of such nature needing attention.

But this is but a small beginning to the possibilities through tilting the pelvic bowl. One may assume the prone position with better effect. Or seek other advantageous postures: that of semi-prone, tilting the edge near the junction of the iliopectineal line; or that of directly on the side, tilting the edge near the junction of the iliopectineal line with the auricular surface of the ilium, the last of these two positions being farthest reaching in beneficial effects.

If the edge of the pelvic bowl is tipped to the right laterally, then the ascending colon, including the offending cecum and its little appendix, are found assuming a normal position. If tipped to the left, then the sigmoid flexure is given assistance. In either side, the drag to the lumbocostal arches of the diaphragm muscle is given relief, and then we find, as a natural consequence, the tension in cervical fascia becoming relaxed. Relaxation of cervical fascia signifies relaxation of cervical muscular tissues also, which is of much importance. The technique opens up the channels of the lymphatic system, and pelvic congestions and those found elsewhere are provided a normal avenue of escape. No pumping of the lymphatics is necessary. Local treatment by way of rectal and vaginal routes becomes less indicated. Likewise local attention to hemorrhoids and various complaints peculiar to both sexes has less significance. However, we advise caution in application. The feel of the tissue is essential at every moment. One must know the condition with which one is dealing, must be gentle in the tipping of the pelvic bowl, and at the same time keep tactility there directly in the neighborhood of the softer tissues and be watchful and alert to the least indication of a strain.

Osteopathic technique, when considered in relation to osseous, muscular, and other bodily tissues, is the intelligent application of the tactile sense. Thinking, feeling, and seeing with intelligent fingers, not tinkering blindly, opens up the avenues to many possibilities in the osteopathic field.

3. Bedside Technique

In September 1929 Dr. Sutherland presented this paper in Redwood Falls at a district meeting of the Minnesota State Osteopathic Association. Aside from its technical value in the care of several specific conditions, it has historical value also. In it the first public reference was made to what he called "his personal hobby"–the theory of cranial articular mobility. This might be called a "trial balloon" before a segment of his profession. The paper was sent subsequently to the chairman of the Bureau of Professional Development of the American Osteopathic Association upon the request of the late Dr. John A. MacDonald of Boston, who was then president of the association. It was then sent to five members of the committee, who remained unidentified, for their evaluation and consideration. They found the cranial phase, which was their main concern, so new and so surprising that no conclusions were expressed specifically, pro or con. Although Dr. Sutherland had already arrived at conclusions relative to the cranium which he found stimulating and convincing and wished to share with his colleagues, he realized he must be conservative and disciplined and not make the error of stating them prematurely.

"Bedside Technique" was reviewed and the technique presented at the annual meeting of the Osteopathic Cranial Association in Washington, D.C. in July 1958.

The osteopathic physician is a thinker, not a tinker. His fingers, when properly trained, possess the skillful art of thinking intelligently at their digital tips. Therefore his technique cannot be taught through class demonstration of a series of manipulations. It can be acquired only by the student having his fingers "Johnny-on-the-spot" alongside those of the instructor, following intelligently, with tactility–feeling, seeing, thinking at the digital tips–as the tissue is guided carefully, gently, firmly and scientifically back into normal relationship.

Manipulation, various movements, thrusts, pulls and jerks lacking in tactility at the desired area of movement might well be called "tinkering." My endeavor today lies in the presenting of methods adaptable to application in bedside cases.

Bedside patients, especially, require delicacy in the application of the anatomical-physiological touch. In presenting our method of attaining this, it is well to picture the type of lesion commonly found in most acute diseases. We are told that "barbers were the first surgeons." One of these aged tonsorial artists still resides in Mankato, Minnesota conducting a foot clinic in connection with his barber shop. He tells his patients that "flat foot" is due to a "slipped vertebra in the foot." In picturing the type of lesion we have in mind, we shall place the "vertebra of the foot" back into the spinal column and call your attention to "flat foot" in the back.

We have heard it said from the platform and have read in print: "I looked for a lesion but found none," and then Argyrol or its like was used.[1] Flat foot lesions in the spine exist without any apparent osseous luxation. A flat foot lesion may be only that of spinal hyperextension causing tensity anteriorly in ligamentous and other tissues. An osteopathic lesion of this type, apparently existing only as tensity in anterior ligamentous and other tissues, is frequently of graver importance as an etiological factor to secondary pathology than that of osseous luxation. Flat foot spinal hyperextension lesions obstruct the blood and lymph channels specifically in relation to the spinal cord through anterior ligamentous and other tissue tensity. Such anterior ligamentous and other tissue tensity also has a specific reflex tendency in relation with the sympathetic ganglia. This type of lesion is found in the cervical, upper middorsal and lumbar areas, even as far north on the human map above the occiput as the falx cerebri And as

---

1. Argyrol was a compound of silver nitrate which contained a mild silver protein and used topically for its antimicrobial properties. It found particular favor in inflammatory eye, ear, nose and throat conditions, but was also used in rectal, urethral and vaginal applications.

far to the south as the ganglion impar. It is especially active as a predisposing factor to complications arising in acute diseases which require specific bedside technique.

The flat foot hyperextension spinal lesion, with its ever present anterior ligamentous and other tissue tensity in acute diseases, is especially emphasized in influenza, the anterior ligamentous and other tissue tensity in influenza apparently being similar in rigidity to that found in the cadaver. In influenza, the pathological picture includes the rigidity of the crura of the diaphragm and the ligamenta arcuata [lumbocostal arches] as well.

This understanding of the type of lesion apparently present in bedside ailments indicates a constructive criticism of some methods of treatment in spinal hypertension. The contraindications to the application of hyperextension are the additional tensities of anterior ligamentous and other tissues which are specifically in opposition to the relaxation of anterior ligamentous and other tissues that is desired in all cases. No matter whether the hyperextension be applied specifically or not, there is bound to be additional anterior ligamentous and other tissue tensity at other and undesired areas along the spine. Personal experience with hyperextension treatment on our own spine coupled with personal experience in the application of hyperextension treatment of others has led us to view all hyperextension methods as detrimental in application, whether given by an osteopathic physician on an osteopathic table or otherwise.

Apparently we have found a better way: that of the application of tactility with the patient lying on the side in flexion posture. This affords the "drawing of the lesion posteriorly" while in flexion rather than forcing anteriorly. As an illustration of what we mean by "drawing posteriorly" in flexion, let us mentally place the patient in a "hammock suspension" position. That is, we will suspend him with the hammock, in a supine position between two tables, with fixation points on the edge of the tables, at the lower cervical and pelvis. In this manner we will expect the law of gravity to draw the spine posteriorly while in flexion. Should you care to experiment personally with your own spinal column, you will find the law of gravity active in drawing posteriorly. You will also note relaxation occurring in tissues anterior to the spine. Likewise you will find the experiment refreshing in relief from fatigue following a heavy day's work. But suspension in this manner when lying prone has the opposite effect–that of fatigue. With this picture in mind, we will visit the bedside and give further illustration of the application with the patient lying on the side in flexion posture.

We will draw a rocking chair to the bedside and fill the seat with cushions up to the level of the rocker's arms. We then place the "upper dorsal half" of the patient onto the arms of the rocker, the patient lying lateral. Placing the rockers in diagonal position to the side of the bed brings the patient into flexion posture and provides a pendulum-like swing either forward or backward. We now apply our anatomical-physiological touch in guidance, drawing the lesion in a tripod manner into reduction. The picture includes the privilege of reversing the "pelvic lower half" to the rocker, as bedside patients require professional service at both ends. Although we now have an especially equipped rocker in use in connection with our office table, the bedside flexion posture pendulum method may be accomplished without the rocker. We merely present the rocker here to illustrate the method of application. However, if a rocker is available, you will find it advantageous in many ways.

As one might expect, relaxation of spinal anterior ligamentous and other tissue tensity effected in this way usually secures relaxation of spinal posterior tissues as well, indicating that the "breaking up" methods known as "general treatments" are unnecessary. General treatments are contraindicated in bedside ailments because they are on the one hand unnecessary and on the other not osteopathic in anatomical-physiological touch–lacking in tactility. Rendering osteopathic service in acute ailments requires the utmost skill in the "feel of the tissue" in every move. The special goal is the relaxation of spinal anterior ligamentous and other tissue tensity to insure normal blood and lymph channels in relation to the spinal cord, as well as the removal of disturbing reflex influences through the avenue of the sympathetic ganglia.

Relaxation of spinal anterior tissue tensity may be accomplished through other avenues than central application to the spine. In illustrating other avenues of approach, attention is called to the importance of the diaphragm. That is, its normal activity is important in control of acute diseases. The diaphragm is the "piston" to the big "combustion cylinder" of the body. Its crura are the "legs" that lead down from the piston to the "crankshaft" in the lumbar vertebrae. Its ligamenta arcuata are the "piston rings." The lungs might represent the big "combustion chamber" to the cylinder with the nasal region the "carburetor," while the "ignition" and "self-starter" might be found somewhere within the "cranial bowl." When there is a tight bearing down in the lumbar crankshaft, or the ligamenta arcuata piston rings are sprung in tension, then the big compression cylinder loses its motive activity.

In our thinking, this is what happens as a secondary complication when the "air" of influenza "chokes the carburetor." Inactivity of the diaphragm apparently is present in influenza and in many acute diseases, the crura being on tension in anterior relation to the spine and likewise the ligamenta arcuata. Again the picture is one of spinal anterior tissue tensity.

We endeavor specifically to reach this tissue tensity with the "feel," and the "feel" is exemplified through relaxation of the ligamenta arcuata. This method finds the anatomical-physiological touch in a finger or thumb traveling gently around under the twelfth rib, holding firmly while the patient inhales, gradually working farther upward and posteriorly as the patient exhales. From this application surprising results have occurred in relief of secondary complications of influenza such as spasmodic diaphragmatic coughs, heart fluctuations, slight heart murmurs, downward pulls on the fascia surrounding the cervical muscles, difficult breathing and, in addition, a better elimination through the kidneys has occurred including the passing of renal calculi the size of peas and one the size of a bean.

The diaphragm area, from our viewpoint, is as important as the dorsal upper half and should not be overlooked in bedside ailments. Your own anatomical-physiological osteopathic intelligence understands well the significance of relaxation to crural tensity as a scientific therapeutic measure in securing relief in many pathological or functional conditions above or below the diaphragm. The diaphragm is as important as is the heart in the physiological control of the blood and lymph streams wherein "the moment of alteration" means the initiation of disease.[2] Its normal activity is a more reliable "lymphatic pump" than the widely heralded "hand pump." Frankly, the hand pump is wearisome to the patient and strenuous work for the "pumper." It is contraindicated in bedside cases. Now that we have allowed our tongue to bluntly go that far, we will add, contraindicated in office cases as well. We are not saying that the hand pump is ineffectual but that it is not osteopathic in technique, lacking the anatomical-physiological touch in guidance. A blind series of rapid up and down movements incurs the possibility of irritation to some hidden gastric ulcer causing it to erupt suddenly like the belching forth of a volcano–a hemorrhage, if you please, securing an immediate passport for a silent ride by way of the "house boat on the river Styx." Having been present at one of these volcanic eruptions the lesson has left a deep impression, the lesson signifying "careful driving" in all local abdominal treatments.

Careful driving has a relation with motors. The dorsal upper half carries a motor as interesting as the motor in your car, the vasomotor, which controls the physiological circulation of the lymph. This vasomotor, like the motor in your car, is subject to occasional misbehavior because of "high tension" leakage through loose wire (or nerve) connections. It is more scientific to regulate the vasomotor controlling the lymph channels by attention to the osseous "terminals" found

2. Reference is being made to the statement ascribed to Dr. Still: "Tell me the moment when the blood flow is altered and I will tell you the moment when disease begins."

in the dorsal upper half. Such attention saves tearing the motor to pieces unnecessarily in search of "engine trouble" which in so many cases is not there.

We avoid abdominal local treatment wherever opportunity affords another way, finding the central avenue of approach with the rocking-chair-pendulum method in drawing posteriorly more scientific. It is decidedly advantageous in securing relaxation to the tensity of the crura, the ligamenta arcuata, and other tissues in anterior relation to the spine. However, we do give local abdominal treatment when found necessary. But the application is gentle, as in the holding and lifting of the sigmoid flexure, or the raising of the ascending colon up out of the pelvic bowl, with the anatomical-physiological touch guiding our movements. We also find a central avenue of approach to abdominal viscera by catching the eleventh rib and holding it down in limitation of movement for a few seconds at a period, which apparently is very effective in securing intestinal activity. In fact, the false ribs as well as the floating can be handled in this manner. On one occasion the holding of the right tenth rib in limitation of movement apparently resulted in the passage of gall stones painlessly in a few minutes in a case where, on previous occasions, there were hours of discomfort while under the hypodermic.

In some instances where the history includes a strain, like that sustained while pulling a post up out of the ground, thereby bringing anterior spinal hyperextension muscular tensity along the psoas major and iliacus muscles, lifting on the tendon [*of the psoas*] near its insertion on the femur has resulted in relief to a case with a false diagnosis of renal calculus, the history in this case being the differential diagnostic point between the false and the true. The same lift on other occasions has cleared up bedside cases of sciatica that have remained stubborn following sacroiliac reduction. Where indications signify caution in appendicitis, acute or chronic, we confine abdominal treatment to the avenue between the rectum and obturator membrane, two intelligent fingers traveling upward, intent on a gentle lifting of tissues out of the pelvic bowl.

Certain types of rib lesions, wherein the head of the rib recedes posteriorly into the depression back of the demifacet, augment spinal hyperextension anterior tissue tensity. In such cases, attention to the rib lesion is the first step in treatment. Fixation in the head of the rib in the depression back of the demifacet holds the spinal area in hyperextension. This type of rib lesion, because of fixation, is difficult to handle, especially so when in relation to the dorsal upper half.

Our method of application pictures the rib in the shape of a horseshoe or a quoit. For illustration, we will place one leg of the horseshoe in malarticulation in the depression back of the demifacet, resting its tubercle near the neighboring transverse process. We now catch the other leg of the horseshoe and draw in a posterior direction, finding that at the same time the vertebral leg of the horseshoe moves outward from the depression and forward to its normal location in the demifacet. Ribs are similar in shape to the horseshoe, one leg being longer, and one especially shorter. With the head of the rib in malfixation in the depression back of the demifacet, our movement must be like that with the horseshoe.

With the patient lying on the side in flexion posture, we cling firmly with a finger, or two fingers, on the rib near its sternal end and draw posteriorly, while at the same time, intelligent fingers lift laterally below two spinous processes of the vertebrae in relation to the rib articulation. This lifting upward laterally on the spinous processes rotates the bodies of the vertebrae involved away from the head of the rib, carrying the depression forward as the head of the rib glides outward, the feel of the tissue guiding.

Experience in handling rib lesions of this type, through the horseshoe method, evolved a bedside method effective in securing relaxation in the upper dorsal half in cases of pneumonia. The bedsheet is brought up around the dorsal upper half and snug pressure applied in the manner of a tourniquet, providing no rib lesions are present. The tourniquet pressure draws the ribs posteriorly in the horseshoe angle way, causing the heads of the ribs to move outward and forward at their vertebral articulations, thereby securing desired relaxation of spinal anterior tensity in the tissues of the upper dorsal half ganglia. We also use the tourniquet as an efficient "handle" in drawing the upper dorsal half into desired flexion to secure as much relaxation as possible to the spinal anterior ligamentous and other tissue tensity so apparently present in acute ailments. It has been found beneficial in application around the dorsal lower half in pleurisy. It will be found useful as a handy handle around the pelvis, also.

In the cervical region, the patient is asked to render assistance because of the importance in limiting to the smallest degree all unnecessary strain to delicate tissues, both osseous and muscular. For instance, have the patient elongate the neck while the physician holds the tissue, osseous or muscular. The patient is instructed to stretch out the neck in the manner of a turtle and to leave the body "shell" behind in the stretch, being careful not to lift the chin or hyperextend the occiput. That is, the patient elongates the neck only in a semiflexed position while tactile sense, without jerk or pull, feels out the proper avenue of reduction and holds firmly in that direction as the patient relaxes from elongation. When afforded the opportunity, osseous malalignment has the natural habit of springing back into normalcy through its own motive power. The utmost delicacy is indicated in the care of all cervical tissues. In some cases we have the patient sit on the edge of the bed, place both hands upon the physician's shoulders, flex the body forward, with the weight of the body resting solely on the arms, and hang the head in flexion, also. We then place both thumbs as low down as possible on each side of the trachea, or tissues in relation and apparently in tensity, and then hold firmly with the thumbs while the patient bends back to sitting posture with the head remaining in flexion. The endeavor is aimed to relieve spinal anterior tissue tensity common in this region in acute diseases.

Clavicular-acromial-sternal luxations, under the false diagnosis of brachial neuritis, occasionally require bedside professional service. The clavicular-acromial-sternal luxation is perhaps better known as "acromioclavicular," but apparently the lesion includes luxation at the sternoclavicular articulation as well. The clavicle is in luxation at both articulations. The method of reduction requires tactile sense simultaneously in application at both articulations. We accomplish this by having the patient sit on the edge of the bed with both hands on our shoulders and bend forward in flexion. If, for example, the lesion is in relation to the right clavicle, our left fingers catch at the acromial end and the right fingers at the sternal end. The patient then rotates the body slowly to the left which brings about a desired separation at both clavicular articulations. Reduction occurs simultaneously at both articulations under the guidance of the anatomical-physiological touch.

This same bedside sitting posture, with arms resting on the physician's shoulders, is adaptable in upper rib reduction also. The physician fixates the sternal end with his fingers while the patient rotates the body to the left, if the rib lesion is on the right side. This rotates the body of the vertebra in relation away from the head of the rib, thus freeing it from the malposition in the depression back of the demifacet. Perhaps one might call this simultaneous separation of both end articulations and simultaneous reduction, as has been exemplified in the clavicular-acromial-sternal luxation. Yet, the method lacks tactile sense in guidance at both articulations.

Sacroiliac luxations have been known to regain normal articular position while riding horseback with a saddle. When occasion indicates sacroiliac reduction with the patient lying supine, as frequently occurs in bedside cases, the nurse may render assistance by abducting the patient's lower extremities in the manner of the horseback straddle. That is, the nurse renders such assistance after we have fixated our hands in the manner of a saddle. This is accomplished by passing one hand down beneath the sacrum and the other over the pubic arch, hands clasping; the palm of the under hand is in fixation on the sacrum in the manner of the saddle back and pressing anteriorly, while the wrist of the upper hand fixates over the pubic arch drawing upward and posteriorly. The nurse then abducts and pushes upward. In the actual horseback ride occurrence that secured a reduction, apparently the back of the saddle was in fixation at the sacrum while the curved front of the saddle, near the base of the pommel, was in fixation at the pubic arch, making possible posterior and anterior pressure simultaneously during the gallop, while abduction through the straddle with the aid of the stirrups pushed upward. As testimony, a severe case of uterine hemorrhage has been allayed through this "saddle method." In another case where catheter insertion was contraindicated, it was instrumental in bringing benefit. The method, however, lacks tactile sense in application and is recommended only in supine bedside emergency cases.

We are inclined to think that the tissue tensity effects so markedly present in influenza have their initiation through the falx cerebri and tentorium cerebelli, with resultant restriction of drainage channels at the jugular foramen and in the postnasal region, and that other spinal anterior tissue tensity follows secondarily. Consequently, we endeavor to seek out a specific application in rendering service to the initiatory tissue tensity. Now please consider the next paragraph or two as being related to a personal hobby in the line of experimentation.

With thumb and fingers of one hand in fixation on the frontal bone, a little to the right and left of the orbits, and with thumb and fingers of the other hand in fixation at the mastoid processes of the temporal bones, the patient assists by pushing upward with the neck. Then, if one is capable of stretching the imagination that far, the mental picture is provided by lifting the frontal bone forward and the mastoid processes backward with the squamous portions of the temporal bones opening laterally, like the gills of a fish, while the basilar process of the occipital bone pushes the sphenoid bone upward and forward. This would free one of the most important drainage channels in the human system, that of the jugular foramina and neighboring tissues of the postnasal area. In one instance, the voluntary appearance of two large-sized nasal polyps followed this experimental anatomical-physiological application.

Again, grasping the mastoid processes of the temporal bones with the palms and pressing inward and downward while the patient elongates the neck apparently swings open the door to the "cuckoo clock" (the squamous portion of the temporal bones), causing our imagination to visualize the petrous portions of the temporal bones as swinging away from the basilar process of the occipital bone, thereby freeing blood and lymph channels and indicating great possibilities in handling psychological cases. In testimony, it has been gratifying to note a return to normal expression in the eyes and face and a change occurring in the heart rhythm.

On other occasions, we have pushed outward laterally on the mastoid processes of the temporal bones and upward on the zygomatic arches while formulating the mental picture of the squamous portions of the temporal bones as gliding in their bevel-like articulations, instead of opening laterally like the gills of a fish, and at the same time viewing the basilar process of the occipital bone as receding posteriorly and downward, the dorsum sella of the sphenoid bone following, this movement having the material effect of widening the jugular foramina while the pterygoid processes of the sphenoid wiggled, securing relaxation of tissue tensity in the postnasal region. Thus far, from experimentation, we believe this application to be most favorable in securing results. There has been beneficial testimony in cases relating to the eye, ear, and nose indicating possibilities of an osteopathic specialty.

In connection with these experiments, one might venture a few words concerning possible physiological movement in the cranial articulations, were it not for the probability of finding my audience as skeptical as were the M.D.'s concerning physiological movement in the sacroiliac articulations. We might picture the falx cerebri and the tentorium cerebelli as cooperating with the cranial articulations in physiological movement rhythmical with that of the diaphragm. In the movement, one might see the mastoid processes of the temporal bones expanding or rotating laterally outward while exhaling and then returning inward while inhaling, with other cranial articulations cooperating and all in accommodation to blood and lymph flow. The dovetail cranial sutures, in some instances, and the bevel-like articulations in others, coupled with testimonial anatomical-physiological experience, lead one further and further into the possibility of discovering more of the "tail" of the Old Doctor's "squirrel in the hole in the tree" through "digging on" and on into the "holes" and articulations of the cranial bowl.[3]

Thus far we have been applying methods of treatment mainly to the effects in influenza, such as spinal anterior ligamentous and other tissue tensity. When we know more about the falx cerebri and the tentorium cerebelli in relation to the cranial articulations, perhaps we may be able to deal with tissue tensity effects more efficiently and specifically. Perhaps the falx cerebri and tentorium cerebelli have other physiological functions than that of being mere partition walls to keep the cargo of brains from shifting. At any rate, it is an interesting avenue for research.

According to a reliable authority, the membranous cranial sutures commence to ossify at the age of forty. If interested in keeping them in physiological movement while in the stage of ossification (until the age of 80 according to Davis, *Applied Anatomy*), you might find the following exercise in research experimentation of value. At any rate, the exercise will be beneficial in affording clean arterial refreshment to the brain cells if nothing more:

Get out into the open air and exhale deeply and slowly. As the diaphragm rises upward, draw the head downward and force the mastoid processes of the temporal bones laterally simultaneously. Pause a moment or two. Then inhale slowly and as the diaphragm sinks downward, elongate the neck and draw the mastoid processes simultaneously inward.

According to my viewpoint, tensity in the falx cerebri and the tentorium cerebelli with restriction of the physiological movement at

---

3. Dr. A.T. Still (respectfully referred to as the Old Doctor) presented osteopathy as a science, a philosophy and an art whose potential was not fully realized, much as a squirrel only partially seen within a hole in a tree would not be fully visualized. He stated that only the tail of the squirrel was currently in view.

The phrase "digging on" represents Dr. Sutherland's own approach to his study and the approach he encouraged others to follow. For his telling of the boyhood story that inspired this, see article 26, "Philosophy of Osteopathy and Its Application," note 1.

the jugular foramen and in postnasal tissues signifies incomplete drainage of the brain and facial regions. Complete drainage of the brain area before adding pure arterial blood is as essential as is complete drainage of old oil from the crank case of an automobile motor before adding pure oil. Adding a quart of pure oil to four quarts of old carbonated oil does not help the lubrication in the motor. So with the brain. Adding a lesser amount of pure blood to a larger amount of the deteriorated venous blood only means poor lubrication to the brain cells–therefore, the importance of a pause after exhaling to allow the venous blood to drain thoroughly before filling up the "think tank" with pure unadulterated arterial lubrication. The pause holds the jugular foramen "wide open," the postnasal tissues in relaxation, and allows complete drainage.

When the Great Architect planned the osseous jugular canal "fifty-fifty" in osseous formation between the temporal and occipital bones, He likely made provision for physiological expansion service separation through a rotation movement of their articulations, the jugular foramen being like the spinal foramina in articular formation. Apparently, restriction in the rotation-articular-expansion service at the jugular foramen indicates osteopathic consideration equal to that of an occipitoatlantal osseous luxation. In our viewpoint, the jugular foramen restriction is of greater importance than the occipitoatlantal in so far as restriction of the venous drainage from the internal cranial region is concerned.

There also are osteopathic research possibilities through the articulations of the facial bones that might render beneficial professional service on behalf of hay fever and other local effects. It is likely that Lon Chaney, once the facial contortionist of the movies, was able to wiggle his zygomatic bones with ease. As an experiment, one can catch beneath the junction of the zygomatic and maxillary articulation and lift both bones gently forward and upward in beneficial service to lacrimal ducts, nasal and postnasal regions. We might add, in connection with our remarks concerning lateral rotation expansion of the mastoid processes of the temporal bones while exhaling, that the zygomatic arches, at the same time, will tilt the zygomatic bones and the zygomatic bones in turn rotate the maxillae, while corresponding movement occurs in relation with the wing of the sphenoid bone. The indicated physiological facial bone movement while exhaling is essential to normal drainage of the blood and lymph channels in relation to the orbital, nasal, and postnasal areas. In acute diseases, there are indications of restriction to such normal articular movement.

In closing, realize that we have frequently used the word "apparently." Our main endeavor lies in stimulating thought concerning tissues in anterior relation to the spinal column as they apparently exist in acute diseases, especially influenza. Also, to initiate a closer cultivation of the feel of the tissue in technique. The feel of the tissue offers a specialty rare in competition. It is as essential in major and minor surgery as it is in the application to muscular and osseous tissue. It is the rendering of service through the intelligent application of the cultivated anatomical-physiological touch in diagnosis and treatment rather than mere "blind treatment." Rendering service osteopathically signifies more of the anatomical-physiological touch in diagnosis, more of the same anatomical-physiological touch in treatment and less and less of blind manipulation.

Flat foot lesions in the spinal column are common. Flat foot lesions, not osseous luxations, but in the nature of hyperextension strains, are frequently overlooked in osteopathic examination. Flat foot lesions include ligamentous and other tissue tensity anteriorly in relation to the spine and therefore are of graver importance as etiological factors than osseous luxations. Although in many instances sustained through occupational routine, the ligamentous and other tissue tensity follows in the wake of acute diseases, especially that of influenza. In acute ailments we are confined to the treatment of effects only, that is, to the securing of relaxation of tissue tensity in anterior relation to the spine.

It is possible that these tissue tensity effects, apparently indicated in the wake of acute ailments, may have their initiation in the falx cerebri and tentorium cerebelli, other tissue tensity effects in anterior relation to the spine being secondary thereto. A deeper understanding of the apparent functioning of the falx cerebri and the tentorium cerebelli, in coordination with cranial articular movement rhythmical with that of the diaphragm, may bring forth an effective and specific treatment of such tissue tensity effects in acute diseases.

Experimental treatment with the cranial articulations indicates possibilities. The housewife's old-time bandage remedy for headaches, coordinated with mild tourniquet pressure around the frontal and occipital bones, and the mastoid processes of the temporal bones, pulled downward and upward in the manner of pulling a tight hat on and off alternately, provides interesting indications of specific therapeutic value. Flexion posture methods in technique are advocated; extension posture methods tend to increase tissue tensity. Drawing the flat foot area posteriorly in flexion position is specific. General and breaking-up methods are nonspecific and unnecessary.

4. Possibilities in Relation to the Basilar Articulations of the "Cranial Bowl"

In 1929, while the late Dr. John A. MacDonald of Boston, Massachusetts was president of the American Osteopathic Association, he advised Dr. Sutherland to submit the following paper to the chairman of the Bureau of Professional Development for a reading by the five unidentified members of the Bureau. The manuscript had been submitted to the Journal of Osteopathy earlier but was not accepted. Dr. MacDonald's desire was to stimulate interest, curiosity, and critical discussion, for mutual benefit. His personal attitude was one of genuine interest. The response of the five bureau members, when it came in a year and a half later, ranged from exceedingly frank skepticism to "it invites study." This presentation of Dr. Sutherland's cranial thinking was his first written expression to have contact in any way with the national organization.

The discussion appearing in one of our oldest periodicals indicates that the subject of pharmacology has a close kinship with prohibition, that of endless discussion and disagreement.... The writer is inclined to think that the valuable space is being wasted toward a fruitless end–disagreement. Why not devote this valuable space to the study and discussion of the minutiae of the tissues in relation to the vertebral and cranial articulations? If osteopathic physicians are to succeed in gaining a firmer grip on the "tail" of the Old Doctor's "squirrel in the hole in the tree," there is need for everlastingly "digging on."[1] The articles on the subject of "Vertebral Mechanics" by

---

1. Dr. A.T. Still (respectfully referred to as the Old Doctor) presented osteopathy as a science, a philosophy and an art whose potential was not fully realized, much as a squirrel only partially seen within a hole in a tree would not be fully visualized. He stated that only the tail of the squirrel was currently in view.

The phrase "digging on" represents Dr. Sutherland's own approach to his study

Dr. Albert E. Guy of Paris, France that are appearing in the American Osteopathic Association's journal present interesting avenues for a venture into the holes of the Old Doctor's tree.[2]

To stimulate activity in the study and discussion, the writer calls attention to the numerous osseous holes in relation to the basilar articulations of the cranial bones. And to make the study and discussion more inviting, he will say that he can demonstrate mobility in these basilar articulations. Further, in such a demonstration, there will follow relaxation of muscular contractions and ligamentous tensity in cervical tissues–a demonstration entirely specific to basilar articular mobility, with no attention whatever, nor with any manipulation applied, to occipitoatlantal or other cervical tissues. The demonstration will also give evidence of normal change in the nourishment to physiological centers within the medulla oblongata. We are too prone to accept the version of authorized texts and reason from the cold cadaver. Dr. Still reasoned through evidence on the living structure and demonstrated mobility of the sacroiliac.

Someone has written, "To the dreamer who can work, and the worker who can dream, life surrenders all things." In our study of the life forces of the body, it becomes necessary to dream and to stretch the imagination.

Very little is known about the falx cerebri and the tentorium cerebelli except as texts have pointed out: "...partitions to keep the cargo of brains from shifting." Of course, these tissues are known to be the continuation of the dura mater, to assist in the dural vascular chan-

---

and the approach he encouraged others to follow. For his telling of the boyhood story that inspired this, see article 26, "Philosophy of Osteopathy and Its Application," note 1.

2. The articles appeared in the *JAOA* from July 1930 through March 1931. Dr. Guy was originally from Paris, France. Following World War I, he visited his son at the American School of Osteopathy and apparently was quite impressed during his visit. He subsequently immigrated to the United States and enrolled at the school himself.

nels, and so forth. But why does the falx cerebri have attachment to the crista galli of the ethmoid? One might imagine, as an initiative for the dream, that the falx acts much in the same manner as does a locomotive bell rope, swinging the ethmoid forward and backward. Then, imagine the falx and the tentorium working automatically in cooperation with the basilar cranial articulations in a physiologic movement rhythmical with that of the diaphragm. In that instance, one might visualize influenza entering through the nasal region and beginning its tense effect upon bodily tissue, first, in the falx, causing tensity thereof, and continuing on down to the dura mater to cause immobility in the basilar articulations–such tensity of falx and dural tissues, and immobility of basilar articulations obstructing vascular drainage channels, thereby disturbing normal physiologic centers of the medulla oblongata. In that consideration, specific attention to the reestablishment of mobility to the basilar articulations would mean more specific treatment in influenza, and perhaps many more of the acute ailments.

Faulty teeth and pathological tonsil indications to the contrary, we are inclined to believe that most cervical muscular contractions and tensities of ligamentous tissues have their initiation somewhere within the skull, and that specific treatment should be applied accordingly.

We have testimony in a severe case of acute torticollis that was relieved in one specific treatment through the endeavor to reestablish mobility at the basilar articulations. In fact, the case was so acute that cervical or upper dorsal treatment seemed to be contraindicated. Nor were there indications of tonsil, mastoid or teeth pathology. We believe this case of acute torticollis had its initiation within the skull, perhaps through the agency of influenza. We might cite other instances, but perhaps enough has been said to stimulate thought and discussion along an avenue which presents promising possibilities.

5. Skull Notions

By "Blunt Bone Bill, D.O.," an "Old-timer" in Minnesota.

The following six papers were first published in the July, August, September, October, November, and December 1931 issues of The Northwest Bulletin, *a monthly publication of the Minnesota State Osteopathic Association which was sent to members of the osteopathic profession in several midwest states.*

"Skull Notions" appeared as a column in response to a request that Dr. Sutherland contribute regularly to the Bulletin. *This he agreed to do with the understanding that his contributions retain anonymity by his use of the pseudonym "Blunt Bone Bill." His identity was not revealed until the editor insisted, due to the mail which arrived at his desk with questions that necessitated more direct communication than anonymity permitted.*

The inquiries were not many, but they led to substantial interest in the subject matter of the column. This in turn led to lectures in several states and to further demonstrations of interest.

1. July 1931

In the main, "Skull Notions" are visionary through having both foresight and hindsight.

The saddle of the sphenoid was not intended for a straddle, though in line with vision, 'tis a fine site for a drive. But, why the wonderful arrangement in the tentorium's attachment?

The crista galli does not indicate permission for man to crow, but *why* the falx and its peculiar attachment? Is it the locomotive bell rope that swings the ethmoid outward in a sneeze?

Why the falx and the tentorium anyway? 'Tis well not to stop with the text. 'Tis wise to launch a small research craft through the vascular channels.

❧

...the wrestler's headlock, through dire effects, may indicate reasoning higher than the occipitoatlantal for articular strains.

❧

According to unskilled infantile skull contact with forceps, in contrast to the skillful technique demonstrated by many obstetricians, there is testimony of articular strain higher than the occipitoatlantal. More properly, articular-membranous strains that may continue as predisposing factors.

❧

According to an impacted tooth in contact with "frozen" anesthetic and skillful dental surgery, there may be found additional testimony of articular strain higher than the occipitoatlantal. Severe and painful complications of two weeks duration were immediately relieved through a gentle one-finger application between the maxilla and the pterygoid process of the sphenoid.

❧

According to an intimate mandibular contact with concrete pavement, there is testimony of articular strain higher than the occipitoatlantal.

❧

Can articular strains higher than the occipitoatlantal be given osteopathic attention?

❧

'Nuff said. More if you wish. But please so indicate by dropping a postal to the editor. Otherwise, there shall be silence.

❧

"Believe it or not," visionary though they may seem, "Skull Notions" present a *few* fundamental truths.

2. August 1931

Were it possible to visualize a rotation, or twist, of the occipital bone–anteriorly on one side and posteriorly on the other–between the temporal bones, we would quite likely find a restriction in function, or faulty position, in the articular relationship of the petrous portion of the temporal bones with that of the basilar process of the occiput. Investigation throughout the skull of the inanimate cadaver concludes with *impossibility.* Observation of the animate model indicates *possibility.* Experimentation therewith encourages further investigation.

The exit known by anatomists as the jugular foramen possesses a fifty-fifty osseous articular cooperation between the petrous portion and the basilar process, similar to the fifty-fifty osseous articular cooperation found in the construction of the vertebral foramina. Granting the possibility of a restriction in function, or faulty position, in the articular relation of the petrous portion with the basilar process, we might picture a disturbance to venous drainage and the initiation of intra-cranial pathology.

A case picture, for example: dull occipital ache which could not be classed as suboccipital; osseous articular lesions: upper cervical, upper dorsal and right first rib; marked tensity of ligamentous tissue in relation to osseous articular lesion; and muscular rigidity from occiput to upper dorsal on right side–the ligamentous tensity and muscular rigidity very stubborn in resistance to all local attempts for relaxation; and osseous articular lesions subject to frequent recurrence.

Same case picture, visualized skull-notionally: a history of forcible contact of the head with a stone wall (more specifically speaking, contact on right parietal bone somewhat posteriorly). Observation located what seemed to be a rotation, or twist, of the occipital between the two temporal bones, apparently anterior on the right side, and posterior on the left. Drawing posteriorly on the occiput and anteriorly on the parietal, right side, somehow relieved the dull occipital ache.

Furthermore, same case picture viewed skull-notionally: The ligamentous tissue and muscular rigidity from occiput to upper dorsal *readily responded to relaxation without further treatment.* The cervical and upper dorsal osseous articular lesions were then locally reduced and, *what is more*, lost the tendency to frequent recurrences.

A fish story? No! A demonstrable fact indicating osseous articular strains that occur higher than the occipitoatlantal.

Much is written concerning the physiology and pathology in relation to the pituitary body but very little about possible etiological factors that might disturb its normal functioning. The contact of the gluteus maximus with a saddle fastened to a bucking bronco provides a cue: The pituitary body has contact with a "saddle." In the animate skull, the sella turcica area of the sphenoid possesses flexibility, and as with the bronco, there might be occasion for springing up and down.

Visionary? Yes! Also, NO! With enough "no" and "know" to encourage "digging on" to learn all there is to *know concerning* the various "holes" found within the basilar area of the skull, *wherein* we may grasp with firmer grip the "tail" of the Old Doctor's "squirrel in the hole of the tree."[1]

Do osseous articular strains occur higher than the occipitoatlantal? Yes! "Dig On!"

---

1. Dr. A. T. Still (respectfully referred to as the Old Doctor) presented osteopathy as a science, a philosophy and an art whose potential was not fully realized, much as a squirrel only partially seen within a hole in a tree would not be fully visualized. He stated that only the tail of the squirrel was currently in view.

3. September 1931

More favorable comments pour into the editor's office. One physician writes: "...Dr. Blunt Bone Bill's articles have opened up some new avenues of thought, which may revolutionize technique above the occiput. Don't let him 'go off the air.'"

A notion, within the skull of Christopher Columbus, finally materialized into that historical voyage across the Atlantic. The world *is* round.

Another notion, inside the skull of Colonel Lindbergh, *grew* and *flew* in the exemplification of an airway across this same Atlantic. A later flight encircled the globe. The world *is* spherical.

A notion, nourished in the fertility of probabilities beneath the writer's skull, is assuming material growth through experimental cultivation. He is hoping to aver: that cranial membranous articular strains occur frequently in conjunction with *influenza*; that they also happen occasionally as secondary effects from traumatic factors; and, in either occurrence, inactivity of the cerebrospinal fluid, lymph and blood follows, and "at that moment disease begins."[2]

Hence, a case picture taken at random from his "experimental garden" which relates to the *influenza* type: male, age 67; severe frontal and temporal headache; indications of frontal sinus infection; inability to blow the nose, or to secure secretion of any nature therefrom; bronchial cough, following a severe attack of influenza; tonsillectomy and medicinal treatment unsuccessful; no apparent cervical nor upper dorsal osseous articular lesions; marked muscular rigidity and ligamentous tensity on right side.

---

2. Reference is being made to the statement ascribed to Dr. Still: "Tell me the moment when the blood flow is altered and I will tell you the moment when disease begins."

Same case picture viewed skull-notionally: veins standing out prominently in right frontal and temporal areas, indicating circulatory blockage; mastoid process on right bulging outward; prominence of right squamous portion of the temporal bone at its articulation with the parietal; similar prominence of the greater wing of the sphenoid. Reasoned: a plain case of membranous-articular expansion at the cranial articulation in conjunction with, or as a sequela to, influenza.

Same case picture treated skull-notionally–an instance wherein Jones submitted voluntarily to the experimental garden through the testimony of another Jones and as a consequence: cerebrospinal fluid, lymph and blood activity was reestablished; prominence of veins disappeared; headache departed; the nose was successfully blown; and cervical muscular rigidity and ligamentous tensity relaxed without local attention.

Now a case picture of cranial membranous-articular strain as secondary to a traumatic factor, one chosen from several of similar type in relation to teeth extractions: male, age 58; dull occipital ache and pain throughout right maxilla for several days following extraction of two live upper molar teeth; also a peculiar pressure sensation under right parietal; no abscess on either tooth, free bleeding; no dry socket to indicate cause of pain and other phenomena.

Same case picture reasoned skull-notionally: in the extraction of these two live upper molars, with their large and curved roots under novocaine anesthesia, the skilled dentist finds it necessary to loosen their solid foundation in a "frozen" area by a strenuous torsional and lateral shaking before pulling. Consequently, as the dentist applies forces laterally, torsionally and downward in an anterior direction, the occiput is in contact with the headrest of the dental chair and is pulling posteriorly in the opposite direction. Thereat, the entire basilar cranial area from the pterygoid process of the sphenoid to the lambdoidal undergoes a tense, elongative membranous-articular strain. Thereabouts arise membranous-articular lesions higher and more seriously important than that of the occipitoatlantal.

Same case picture skull-notionally prescribed: Adductive compression with specific contact at right lambdoidal suture and frontal area reduced the membranous-articular strain; cerebrospinal fluid, lymph and blood activity was thereby reestablished and recovery followed. Wherein the writer testifies, "This concerns my own experience in the dental chair."

4. October 1931

In the following "Skull Notions" column, reference is made to a "helmet-bandage" mechanism which Dr. Sutherland first devised for research purposes in determining articular mobility within his own skull. Through his meticulous and intelligent use of the arrangement, coupled with his microscopic anatomical visualization, it proved of value, also, in the reduction of cranial membranous-articular strains, or lesions. The helmet-bandage mechanism was utilized for a brief time only and then was replaced by the more desirable manual techniques which he developed, employing tactile sense. It is of interest now only because it was part of a transitional background. For that reason, mention of it has not been deleted from the context of this "Skull Notions" column.

An Iowa D.O. writes to this column: "I would like to see you state how you determine motion between various cranial bones, a 'lesion' and the way you correct it. So please carry on your writings along this line."

Although this request could be accomplished more explicitly through a demonstration on the living model, we will endeavor to comply with the Iowan's wishes.

Normal motion between the cranial bones is determined through the intelligent application of the *cultivated* tactile sense at the junction of the zygomatic process of the temporal bone with the temporal process of the zygomatic bone, also at the junction of the squamous portion of the temporal bone with the parietal. Normally, these two articulations have a slight movement during inhalation and exhalation.

Recognition of motion at these two points indicates movement at other articulations of the temporal bone. Movement in one could not be had without movement in all others.

"Lesions," which we prefer to call *membranous-articular strains*, are expansile in type, that is, the articulation is found in a state of extreme expansion.

Diagnosis: As one views the position of the body of a vertebra through the application of tactile sense posteriorly at the transverse processes, so we likewise and necessarily view the petrous portion of the temporal bone at the basilar articular area through the application of tactility at the temperozygomatic and squamoparietal articulations. In some cases, especially in association with migraine, hay fever and sinus pathology, expansion is found at the articulations of the facial bones, this expansile feature being readily recognized through observation alone. The expansion sometimes is quite apparent at the squamoparietal junction and at the lambdoidal suture. Occasionally, one mastoid process of the temporal bone projects outwardly. There are many other features in diagnosis, including all those usually considered in the vertebral lesions.

Reduction: The type of membranous-articular strain being that of *expansion,* the reduction must be that of *compression.* This is accomplished through a helmet-bandage mechanism. [*In the original column, a cut of the arrangement was shown.*] It consists of a specially designed moleskin bandage passing around the head with four appendages running up over the vault. The four appendages pass through a leather helmet which is lined with resilient rubber. A *mild* uplift compression is thereby secured through a tourniquet application over the helmet. Compression can be applied bilaterally, unilaterally, anteriorly or posteriorly according to the *specific* needs of the case. In applying the method, one must exercise the same technical skill as that employed in the reduction of a vertebral lesion. One must have a perfect picture in mind of all the cranial and facial bone articulations, as well as the intracranial tissues–the brain, falx cerebri, tentorium cerebelli, cerebrospinal fluid, lymph and blood channels. In fact, application of the technique requires special skill. Compression can also be applied to the zygomatic bones in connection with cranial technique. Compression of the zygomatic bones through connection with the maxillae reaches all other facial bone articulations. As in all cases, the technique should be seen and demonstrated to be fully appreciated.

We expect our Iowan colleague to reason along with Gerrish and other anatomical authorities that: "The bones of the skull are *immovably* joined together by sutures.[3] Yet Davis, in *Applied Anatomy*, tells a different story: "The bones of the base of the skull originate in cartilage, while those of the vault originate in membrane...the sutures of the vault *begin* to ossify at about the age of forty years and continue to fuse until about the *eightieth* year."

Applied anatomy upon the *animate* skull is quite different from that found in relation to the inanimate cadaver. The writer, through experimentation with *applied anatomy* upon the animate skull, contends that in the vault we find *expansile and contractile articular service* provided through the dovetail sutures and that *these sutures do not completely ossify while life remains.*

Now, a few *whys* about other cranial articulations, found so differentiated from the dovetail suture arrangement in the vault, wherein all may gain by reasoning for themselves:

Why: the bevel juncture between the squamous portion of the temporal bone with the parietal? Its striking resemblance to the gill of a fish indicates–mechanical facility for gliding movement.

Why: the semioblique overlapping of the zygomatic process of the temporal bone with the temporal process of the zygomatic bone?

---

3. Gerrish, *Textbook of Anatomy*; emphasis added.

Quite likely—so arranged as a rockshaft bearing to accommodate articular action elsewhere.

Why: the special arrangement in the articular surface of the mastoid portion in its contact with the parietal and the occipital? We can reason—a combined rockshaft pivot-bearing providing rotation and undulation of the petrous portion.[4]

Why: the unique design for rotation and undulation in the articular surface of the petrous portion at its contact with the basilar process? It can be assumed—a door-hinge device affording a rotary and undulatory movement.

Then, if these be true, we might formulate this idea: The falx cerebri and tentorium cerebelli cooperate with the cranial basilar area in articular functioning, the rotary-undulatory movement thereof being rhythmical with that of the diaphragm.

Then, granting the above probability: Restriction of such functioning alters cerebrospinal fluid, lymph and blood circulation, and at "that moment intracranial pathology had initiation."

NOW, consider facial and cranial articulations as a *whole*. Because of the fact that both the facial and cranial articulations take part in this functioning, one may reason that expansion of the facial articulations is primary to the basilar restrictions and, on the other hand, that basilar or cranial articular expansion is primary to facial restrictions, if we consider the whole. For instance, the maxilla articulates with its fellow and with the zygoma, nasal, frontal, lacrimal, ethmoid, palatine, vomer, inferior turbinate, and sometimes with the sphenoid bones. In fact, movement of the temporal bone, via the zygomatic process, would wiggle the entire facial bone articulation.

Roots of the mighty oak buckle in their longitudinal growth, crowd

---

4. Mechanically speaking, a rockshaft is an oscillating rod used to transmit motion, as in the connection between an engine and a wheel. The end of the shaft rests and turns in a bearing that functions as a pivot—the area around which the rod rotates or oscillates. Dr. Sutherland viewed the occiput as the pivot-bearing part and the temporoparietal mechanism as the rockshaft.

one another and thus heave up the earth.

Roots of the incisor and canine teeth buckle in their longitudinal growth. They have been known to reach the extraordinary length of one and one sixteenth inches. Thus they crowd one another and heave up the maxillae.

The writer infers: Live dental roots in some instances are greater trouble makers than dead ones. They have been known to initiate membranous-articular strains throughout the articulations of the facial bones. Such irregularities are of graver importance than those of the turbinate bones.

5. November 1931

Commenting on our skull notion, a leading osteopathic surgeon wrote: "It strikes me that you have something that is worthy of investigation. The proposition is an interesting one and personally I would like to know more about it. It is not one to be passed upon lightly."

The articular *surfaces* of the cranial and facial bones present mysteries as deep as those of the sea. These *mechanical articular surfaces* were designed for a specific purpose. They possess articular features necessitating a mechanical interpretation which cannot be grasped by passing upon lightly. Interpretation requires a deep mechanical-detail study of the articular *surfaces* on the *disarticulated skull.* The human body has been termed a "machine" and the osteopathic physician the "mechanic."[5] He must *know his anatomy*, and this knowledge should include the articular mechanism of the skull.

The ethmoid bone with its turbinates provides thought for extended study, to say nothing of others in relation to it. The ethmoid breathes.

---

5. Dr. A. T. Still frequently referred to the body as a machine and to the osteopathic physician as a mechanic, stressing that knowledge of this machine (i.e. anatomy) was essential. Cf. Still, *Autobiography*, pp. 287, 304.

A little bone, yet it has articular relationship with 13 others. Why? It might be the "bell sheep" of the entire flock of cranial and facial bones, leading them in membranous-articular mobility. It could be the "air propeller" that lifts the sphenoid. The sphenoid bone with its greater and lesser wings could be called the "airship." Its front end ascends during expiration and makes a "nose dive" in association with inspiration. In relation therewith the superior and middle turbinates of the ethmoid swing bell-like anteriorly as the ship ascends and posteriorly during the nose dive. In the meantime the falx cerebri, acting in the capacity of the "bell rope" through its attachment at the crista galli, functionally cooperates in the bell-like movement. As the front end ascends, the rear end descends, thus assisting in the undulatory-rotary articular mobility of the petrobasilar articulation. The tentorium cerebelli, having attachment to the clinoid processes, provides a functional cooperation with the falx cerebri.

Furthermore, as the sphenoid ascends, its pterygoid processes glide upward in the articulation with the palatine:maxillae, and the palatine:maxillae in turn glide downward. In the meantime, the temporozygomatic articular rockshaft bearing rocks downward and outward to accommodate the undulatory-rotary movement at the petrobasilar articulation. The brain quite possibly officiates as the pilot of the ship, and the small "undergrowth" beneath the third ventricle known as the pituitary body rides and rocks in the "cockpit" called the sella turcica. Therein lies a thought that should stimulate the "brain shovels." Dr. Still said: "Nothing I tell you about osteopathy is a little thing." The skull notion is osteopathic and requires study. It is "not to be passed upon lightly."

We commend the manner in which osteopathic editors exercise their wisdom in rejecting manuscripts pertaining to the unusual and seemingly impossible. One editor of a leading publication very courteously writes:

> I have gone over your article very carefully and discussed it with members of the faculty but find we are unable to follow

> you in your theories. Before complete ossification of the skull, it is obvious at the lines of the sutures that one could secure slight movement, hence possible displacements. However, when ossification is complete, there is no joint structure whatever at the sutures. Our anatomist tells us that it is impossible to pry apart the bones of an adult with a lever. Dislocation is usually accomplished by filling the cranium with corn and beans and soaking them so that by expansion the bones are separated. True, this would indicate that the articulations were weaker than the solid bone, but X-rays of the skull fracture indicate that the various bones will fracture before the articulations separate. To us this would indicate that it is unreasonable to expect "lesions" at these articulations. We admit the probability that you know more about this matter than we do, as you have experimented with the idea.

Allow us to repeat the assertion made last month: *The sutures of the vault do not completely ossify while life remains.* Animate skulls posses a potent life force that promotes normal membranous-articular expansion and contraction at the dovetail sutures of the vault, unlike the inanimate skull. Even the trunk of the mighty oak possesses a certain degree of flexibility until it becomes a sapless log. X-rays have also indicated that fractures occur in the vertebrae and in the long lever bones without separation of their articulations. The vault is convex in shape which largely accounts for fracture without separation at the suture. The dovetail sutures were not designed for separation but to protect from separation while, at the same time, affording articular expansion and contraction to accommodate mobility at other articulations of the cranial and facial bones.

A leading osteopathic anatomist writes:

> The matter of the mobility of the cranial bones is not a new idea altogether. The idea that the falx and tentorium may have some bearing on any possible movement is a new idea as far as I know. Some time ago we took a preserved specimen and put the skull under pressure and observed the possible variations

> at the jugular foramen. We found the lateral pressure forced some fluid out of the vein but that the anterior-posterior pressure did not. Proving that the bones in the region of the pterion were slightly flexible but not so in the sagittal plane. This we anticipated for the reason that the skull is very thin in this region.

This pressure experiment upon the "preserved specimen," coupled with our skull notion experimentation in association with the animate "specimen," strengthens one's endeavors.

We were especially pleased with the attention given our talk and demonstration at the convention in Red Wing, Minnesota. A few "echoes" follow:

At a volunteer "clinic," a D.O. remarked, "That's the first time since World War I that a pressure sensation back of my eyes has been relieved." That remark, "first time since the World War," indicated the possibility of shell shock being an initiatory etiological factor to cranial membranous-articular strains.

Another D.O. after having spent a sleepless night because of pain due to sinusitis, tried the skull notion method. Hence this "echo:" "No question about it, that relieved me. I am going out of here feeling a great deal better than when I came in."

A third D.O. sought advice concerning a patient who had a lot of worry about a pressure in his head. His blood pressure was normal. He was very studious and his mind was always overactive. She wrote me later of relief she had been able to give him with a compression method. Take note that the patient was a "very studious man and his mind always overactive." One may reason here that cranial membranous-articular strains occasionally have their initiation through mental activity as well as through elemental and traumatic forces.

Skull notion compression, as advocated here, should be mild and specific in its application.

6. December 1931

Publication of The Northwest Bulletin *was discontinued with the issue in which this column appeared. This was a circumstance due to an economic situation, not from choice.*

Writing for publication is like broadcasting. One never knows whether the attitude of the listener or of the reader indicates a receptive mood, or otherwise. Therefore comments both favorable and unfavorable are appreciated.

A criticism from the pen of a highly esteemed counselor, which we appreciate, came to our desk lately. It is not written concerning the material appearing in *The Northwest Bulletin*, but it relates to an unpublished article written several months previous to the *Bulletin's* initial issue. Doubtless many of our readers have views that coincide with those of the counselor, hence the following quotation:

> The writer makes some assertions and offers theoretical possibilities without any case histories nor descriptions of experiments to substantiate those assertions. To mention a case or two showing certain subjective symptoms that were relieved following an undescribed technique that is asserted to have produced motion in the basilar articulations is not valid evidence. It is too much like the removal of warts by drawing a thread of red yarn across the wart and tying a knot in the thread for each wart. There are many persons ready to testify that as a child they had all the warts upon the backs of their hands removed by some old grandmother this way. Osteopathy is suffering in professional advancement because of too many instances of the adoption by its members of things that are spectacular in its therapy. Regular medicine is suffering from the research complex and the attention of its workers to things spectacular in medicine. But osteopathy is suffering even more because without research we are seeking and adopting the spectacular.

This straight-from-the-shoulder comment nearly tore the backbone out of our "Notion" column. In fact we wrote our editor that we were "signing off." However, he wrote back: "Please carry on, Bill. We need just such basic osteopathy."

We admit that our notion is rather unusual, and possibly even "spectacular," yet the profession is not expected to adopt it without sufficient investigation. Our stub-pen endeavors thus far were merely intended to stimulate thought and study, and even research activity. At present our "child-notion" is not old enough for professional adoption.

For the benefit of the counselor and others, allow us to say that the notion might be called *one* of the "old grandmother's." That is, grandmother's olden-time bandage remedy around the head, to relieve migraine attacks, provided the incentive for our own investigation and experimentation. This good old grandmother was one who did not advocate the yarn remedy for warts, but some of her olden-time remedies are still in successful use today. Her experience, gained when physicians were not available, taught her much that was valuable and practical.

Although we lack experience in the yarn remedy for warts, we have applied a rubber band tourniquet around the middle finger of a patient and noted the consequent congestion and discoloration in the finger. We have then applied skull compression before the removal of the tourniquet and noted a marked change occurring in the congestion and discoloration. That sounds like a "red yarn," yet it is a demonstrable fact. A fact not stated to be spectacular, but to stimulate research in order to fathom *why* and *how* the change occurred. We have also applied a tourniquet above the ankle in a case of ankylosis which followed a severe attack of inflammatory rheumatism, and then applied skull compression before removing the tourniquet. We have been agreeably surprised at the change occurring in the texture of the tissue throughout the foot and ankle. We have applied skull compression occasionally in a case of stiff fingers covered with large nodules, during a period of four weeks. The patient will testify that the stiffness departed, as did the nodules, without the use of yarn.

We have endeavored to be modest in our statements and cautious in our claims without presenting case histories or case reports. We have merely presented case histories occasionally that seem to manifest promising growth in our "experimental garden." Case reports at this stage might appear too much like the patent medicine testimonials. We might present a few so-called "cures" in sinusitis and migraine, with the written affidavits of the patients, but ethical modesty in the interest and for the advancement of the basic principles of osteopathy holds all that in check. Description of the technique is rather difficult to put into words. Like all osteopathic technique, it should be seen through demonstration in order to be comprehended. Demonstration is also requisite in determining cranial mobility and in the diagnosis of what we term cranial membranous-articular strains.

Our first experimentations were personally applied to our own skull, wherein we were vividly impressed by a change occurring in the texture of tissue of the fingers and toes, with the accompanying sensation of being stripped or "milked." That in itself was sufficient to keep us "digging on" to fathom the reason *why*. A stretch of the imagination? If so, then the stretch was a rather extended one wherein we became convinced that our lymph stream had undergone a very noticeable change. That experience was not made in an effort to compete with the Miller pump.[6] It just happened. Later it was repeated with similar results. Then followed other experiments upon the skulls of patients with their full understanding that the method was of an experimental nature. Results in sinusitis and migraine kept us "digging." We are still digging. There is much to learn about the mechanism of the skull, and of the intracranial membranous tissue in relation.

Skull compression relaxes spinal muscular contractions and the tensity of ligamentous tissue. One might say also that it is serviceable in the differentiation and diagnosis of spinal osseous articular lesions needing local attention.

---

6. C. Earl Miller, D.O. taught a method in about 1920 for gently springing the upper rib cage with the intent of facilitating the movement of lymph.

We have demonstrated to the satisfaction of a few that skull compression changes the rhythm of the diaphragm. We now call your attention to the importance of the normal activity of the diaphragm by quoting Dr. Still, from his *Philosophy and Mechanical Principles* [p. 145]:

> We will draw the attention of the reader to the fact that the diaphragm can contract and suspend the passage of blood and produce all the stagnant changes from the beginning to the completed tubercle, the cancer, the wen, glandular thickening of the neck, face, scalp and fascia... This diaphragm says: "By me you live and by me you die."

If we are able to demonstrate change in the diaphragmatic rhythm as stated above, why not give some consideration to the possible presence of cranial membranous-articular strains that might be disturbing this important muscular structure that can "contract and suspend the blood" and even obstruct the thoracic duct, as Dr. Still has also pointed out in another paragraph.[7] Now is a good time to look for the cranial membranous-articular strains in the influenza cases.

After closing our column for this issue, an interesting comment came from a distinguished member of the profession, a one-time president of the American Osteopathic Association. We quote in part:

I have carefully read your articles and am mighty glad to find someone who has worked out an idea I have had for some time. I have been subject to headaches all my life and they nearly always followed any period of excitement, worry or nervous strain. Several years ago I told my wife that my headaches were not due to neck lesions, or to toxic poisoning, but to intracranial pressure from an excess of blood into the brain from mental stress. Or possibly, to an *unyielding skull structure*...I have avoided activities that cause such stress and have gotten along better in the last few years. If there is some way to fix the bones of my skull so that I can get away from such headaches I surely

---

7. See Still, *Philosophy and Mechanical Principles* , chapter 7, "The Diaphragm," specifically, p. 140.

want to know...I am going to clean up the head of a dissecting specimen and see if I can get some notions about the bony structure. Let me hear from you about this.

That's fine: "Cleaning up the skull of a dissecting specimen" to "get some skull notions." Others can do likewise and profit thereby. Please note that he has been troubled with headaches all his life, and that they follow periods of "excitement, worry or nervous strain." Doubtless we have a feature here that coincides with that of the patient mentioned in our last issue, the exciting cause being that of mental stress. One might reason that a predisposing membranous-articular strain was sustained by a bump on the head during childhood or boyhood days. We would expect to find a limitation in cranial membranous-articular mobility occurring during the ascension of the sphenoid. We would look for expansion at the greater wings of the sphenoid.

As a tryout in long-distance treatment, we have advised him to have his wife, who also is a distinguished D.O., look for such expansion and try, gently and cautiously, pushing downward on the greater wing and upward on the frontal bone and also upward on the greater wing and downward on the frontal bone, likewise upward on the zygomatic process of the temporal bone at its juncture with the temporal process of the zygomatic bone and downward on the same process. Keep in mind that this is merely long-distance advice, without a diagnosis. Get out the disarticulated skull or the head of a dissecting specimen and *dig*. There really is something about this membranous-articular mechanism worthy of investigation. But each must *dig* into its fundamental depth.

6. Cranial Membranous-Articular Strains

In 1932 Dr. Sutherland was invited to demonstrate general techniques at the annual convention of the American Osteopathic Association in Detroit, Michigan. More important in his estimation, however, was an additional request that he discuss some of his cranial thoughts and suppositions. The advance program announcement read:

> Dr. W.G. Sutherland describes the anatomy and physiology underlying his principle of cranial joint lesions which he says closely resemble osteopathic lesions elsewhere and are equally amenable to treatment. Discussion by Dr. John A. MacDonald.[1]

For this first presentation of the subject under official auspices, an article entitled "Cranial Membranous-Articular Strains" that had appeared in the December 1931 issue of The Western Osteopath. *was revised and augmented. This more comprehensive version is presented here rather than the earlier published paper.*

Because of its timely content, the discussion by Dr. MacDonald is also included. It was subsequently printed in the March 1933 issue of The Western Osteopath.

It is my belief that the articular surfaces of the cranial and facial bones were designed for articular mobility. These articular surfaces, in their mechanical characteristics, present a study as deep as the mysteries of the sea. Osteopathic "machinists" of the body's articular mechanisms should be equally familiar with the mechanical mobile-articulative construction of the skull because the cranial mechanism is subject to expansive membranous-articular strains that alter intracranial vascular channels.

---

1. Dr. MacDonald was president of the American Osteopathic Association in 1929 and had an early interest in Dr. Sutherland's ideas.

Until otherwise demonstrated, we expect the profession in general to reason along with Gerrish and other anatomical authorities that: "The bones of the skull are immovably joined together by sutures." Yet Davis, in his *Applied Anatomy*, provides a thought wherewith all may reason otherwise. He says: "The bones of the base of the skull originate in cartilage, while those of the vault originate in membrane...the sutures of the vault *begin* to ossify at about the age of *forty years*, and *continue* to *fuse* until the *eightieth year*."[2] These authorities base their conclusions upon experiments with the *inanimate* skull.

Joyce Kilmer wrote, "Only God can make a tree."[3] The beautiful, tall Norway pine flexes and sways to the wind. A dead Norway pine standing ten feet away, of the same diameter and height, is as rigid and inflexible as a telephone pole. Like the live oak and the pine, the human skull possesses flexibility to a certain degree until the life-giving stream ceases. Applied anatomy and the *animate* skull indicate a wide differentiation between the texture of living cranial membranous-articular tissues and those found in the *inanimate* cadaver.

I contend that: In the living skull, normal mobility occurs throughout the articulations of the basilar area and in the facial bones. This mobility is compensated for by accommodative expansile and contractile articulative service provided in the vault sutures through their specially designed serrated or dovetail arrangement; and I contend that these sutures do not completely ossify while life remains.

This contention is based on personal study and experimental results. The first experiment was conducted upon my own skull. A linen bandage was fastened snugly around the head. Two lateral appendages were then pinned to the bandage and tied together over the vault. The appendages then were twisted with a small stick much in the manner of a tourniquet. This increased the bandage compression and, at the same time, lifted upward laterally. The effect upon the blood

---

2. Gerrish, *Textbook of Anatomy*. Davis, *Applied Anatomy*; emphasis added.

3. Alfred Joyce Kilmer (1886-1918) was an American poet.

and lymph activity was surprising. The change in blood activity was manifested by a comfortable warmth which occurred first in the intracranial area of the cerebellum and then throughout the facial and postnasal areas. This was followed by a general relaxation of spinal muscles, from the occiput down. The change in the lymph activity became very noticeable in the fingers and toes, hands and feet, accompanied by a vivid sensation of being stripped, or milked. There was a marked change in respiration also, and I heard the gurgle of bile and felt it emptying into the duodenum.

Several months later this same experiment, by consent, was tried upon a patient. The case was that of ankylosis in the right foot and ankle, following a severe siege of inflammatory rheumatism. My contact began when the case was at the ankylosis stage. There was considerable hyperplasia throughout the foot and ankle. A tourniquet was applied above the ankle in order to confine the experiment to the lymph channel. Head bandage compression was then given. An almost immediate change occurred in the tissue texture of the foot and ankle, manifested by reduction of the hyperplasia. Another experiment, also a case of inflammatory rheumatism nearing a stage of ankylosis, reduced the hyperplasia and relieved the pain.

Still another experiment concerns a personal visit to a dentist and the extraction of upper molar teeth under novocaine anesthesia. With my maxilla apparently "frozen" in sensation and my occiput resting firmly on the headrest of the dental chair, I could feel the articulations in the basilar area separate as each upper molar was being extracted. A dull occipital ache and severe pain in the maxilla followed. This continued for several days. There was no abscess on either molar, nor was there a dry socket to indicate the cause of continued ache and pain. Seeking relief, I applied the head bandage compression and again noticed movement occurring in the articulations of the basilar area. There was immediate relief. In three other cases of trouble of a similar nature following the extraction of teeth, this same experiment was used and was followed by immediate relief. Also, a case of torticollis responded without manipulation of cervical tissues. Thus one might continue on with numerous examples of experiments that kept me "digging on" into the articular surfaces of the facial and cranial bones.[4] But these are enough for illustration.

As an introductory study of the cranial membranous-articular functioning, we shall liken the sphenoid bone, with its greater and lesser wings, to an airship, the frontal end ascending during expiration and then changing to a "nose dive" as it descends in association with inspiration. In conjunction with the basilar process of the occipital bone, the sella turcica area undergoes an undulatory downward movement as the frontal end ascends and changes to an undulatory movement upward as the frontal end descends. In relation to this undulatory basilar functioning, the vault dovetail sutures function in accommodative contractile and expansile service, the sutures being in contractile accommodation as the basilar area undulates downward in expiration, and being in expansile accommodation as the basilar area undulates upward during inspiration. Contractile and expansile accommodation sutural service may be exemplified by interlacing the fingers without clasping the palms, then pushing the fingers closely together for contractile service and relaxing the fingers for expansile service.

Mobility in the basilar area includes the petrous portions of the temporal bones, which mobility is rotary as well as undulatory in type. It is accommodative through a combined rockshaft and pivot-bearing articulation of the mastoid articular surface with the occipital and parietal bones, as well as a rockshaft bearing in the semi-oblique articulation of the zygomatic process with the temporal process of the zygomatic bone.[5] This articular functioning also includes gliding mobility at the beveled articulation of the squamous portion with the

---

4. The phrase "digging on" represents Dr. Sutherland's own approach to his study and the approach he encouraged others to follow. For his telling of the boyhood story that inspired this, see article 26, "Philosophy of Osteopathy and Its Application," note 1.

5. Mechanically speaking, a rockshaft is an oscillating rod used to transmit motion, as in the connection between an engine and a wheel. The end of the shaft rests and

parietal and the greater wing of the sphenoid. During expiration, the petrous portion rotates internally and undulates downward. During inspiration, it rotates externally and undulates upward.

The maxilla articulates with its fellow, with the zygoma, nasal, frontal, lacrimal, ethmoid, palatine, vomer, inferior turbinate and sometimes with the sphenoid bones. Movement of the temporal bone moves the entire facial articulation via the zygomatic process.

Through its articulation with the frontal, the zygoma swings somewhat like a pendulum, the momentum being in conjunction with the zygomatic process of the temporal. During expiration, it pushes on the antrum of the maxillary sinus through the maxillary articulation and apparently forces the air outward. During inspiration, it pulls backward at the maxillary articulation and apparently pumps the air inward.

The ethmoid, with its superior and middle turbinates–the little bone that breathes–might be said to possess a bell-like movement during expiration and inspiration. The attachment of the falx cerebri to the crista galli likely functions therewith in the manner of a locomotive bell rope. It also has a small jigger articulation with the spine of the sphenoid.

The vomer plows forward by a thrust in a universal-joint articulation from the rostrum of the sphenoid.

The palatine bones oscillate with the maxillae and glide in conjunction with the pterygoid processes of the sphenoid.

The lacrimal and inferior turbinate bones likewise perform an important duty in the movement.

The falx cerebri and tentorium cerebelli, lacking in muscular and elastic fibers, are, to a certain extent, taut or tense in texture. They form a balance-band of membranous tissue affording reciprocal, or alternating forward and backward, movement between the various

---

turns in a bearing that functions as a pivot–the area around which the rod rotates or oscillates. Dr. Sutherland viewed the occiput as the pivot-bearing part and the temporoparietal mechanism as the rockshaft.

articular poles. We have chosen to call this falx-tentorium band of tissue: the *balance-reciprocant.* It cooperates with articular functioning in a movement rhythmical with that of the diaphragm. This balance-reciprocant's functional activity may be illustrated by placing two flexible poles upright in the ground some distance apart and then attaching a taut wire from the top of one pole to the top of the other. Bending one pole in the longitudinal direction of the wire flexes the other pole in the same direction and with the same degree of flexion. Allowing the first pole to spring back allows the second pole to do likewise. We would call this taut wire which affords reciprocal, or backward and forward, movement of the two poles, the wire *balance-reciprocant.*

In relation to the falx-tentorium balance-reciprocant, we have various articular poles of attachment. We have an anterior superior pole at the crista galli, lateral poles along the lateral sinuses and petrous portions of the temporal bones, and an anterior-inferior pole at the clinoid processes of the body of the sphenoid. In addition, there is a central intersection of the tentorium cerebelli with the falx cerebri. Consequently, the falx-tentorium balance-reciprocant functions in a backward-upward-forward circular manner and alternates in a backward-downward-forward circular manner.

The question naturally arises: What actuates the falx-tentorium balance-reciprocant in its functioning? For the time being, suffice it to say: Some latent pulsatory or *rhythmical* agency provides the actuation. However, we have various cognizable convolutions and fissures in relation to the cerebrum that provide workable avenues for a scientific venture. We also recognize *rhythm* as an important characteristic in relation to life's material manifestation. We know that the piano tuner detects inharmony by listening to the rhythms emanating from the strings and that the automobile mechanic locates motor trouble by listening to the hum or rhythm.

As osteopathic membranous-articulative mechanics, we can gather additional knowledge relative to all bodily activity through the study of life's material fundamental *rhythmical* principle. The cerebrum is the primary agency governing all bodily activity external to the cranium. Therefore one can hypothesize that, possibly, the cerebral convolutions and fissures were designed to accommodate pulsatory or rhythmical activity of the brain itself, that is, that the brain functions automatically in rhythmic actuation through its various convolutions. It governs its own intracranial rhythmic actuation and thereby actuates secondary rhythmic impulsion of the pituitary body that rides in the sella turcica of the sphenoid. Thus it becomes instrumental in initiating cranial membranous-articulative rhythmical mobility.

One might visualize the cerebral convolutions as recoiling during inspiration and, in conjunction with the pituitary body, actuating the sella turcica and basilar area into upward undulation, that is, the pituitary body operates in the manner of a fulcrum and shifts the membranous-articular "gears" into upward undulation. On the other hand, during expiration, the convolutions *dilate* or uncoil and the pituitary body shifts the gears into downward undulation. In conjunction with our *hypothesis*, we have the material anatomical evidence of the attachment of the tentorium to the clinoid processes. In addition, Gerrish says [*Textbook of Anatomy,* emphasis added]:

> [Going] Under the names of the diaphragm-of-the-sella and tentorium of the pituitary body, a small fold of dura extends inward from all sides over the sella turcica, covering the pituitary body, and leaving a small opening for the infundibulum. The presence of the fold accounts for the fact that the pituitary body is usually torn away when the brain is removed.

In other words, the pituitary body is suitably anchored in the sella turcica of the sphenoid by this fold of dural membrane. In connection with the falx-tentorium *balance-reciprocant* and cranial articulations, it typifies the silent synchromesh transmission of an automobile in its functioning. Just a hypothetical skull notion. Not a theory.

Osteopathy recognizes vertebral ligamentous-articular strains. We likewise have "cranial membranous-articular strains." These are expansive in type and cause *restriction of the normal membranous-articular functioning.* Such restriction *alters cerebrospinal fluid, lymph and blood activity*. And, "at that moment intracranial pathology has initiation."[6]

Cranial membranous-articular strains occur frequently in respiratory influenza and may be considered as secondary effects of that disease. They are found in association with hay fever and sinus pathology and might be considered as both initiatory and secondary thereto. They are present in migraine and in eye and ear complaints. They occur occasionally as secondary effects of trauma, such as tooth extraction under novocaine anesthesia. They may occur through falls, blows, shell shock, mental stress, and in connection with the improper application of obstetrical forceps. They may occur in a normal occipital presentation, the occiput being crowded upward and forward while the head of the babe is passing through the pelvis–a possibility that presents an opportunity for study in child development. One may reason that expansion of the facial articulation is primary to restriction in the cranial or basilar articulative functioning, or that cranial or basilar expansion is primary to restriction in the facial region.

Cranial or basilar membranous-articular strains can be expiratory or inspiratory in type. The inspiratory type is the most frequent. They are found unilaterally with a side-dip to the sphenoidal "ship," in which instance the tentorium portion of the *balance-reciprocant* on the side affected has become intensified in its tensity. They are present also bilaterally, wherein the balance-reciprocant as a whole has become intensified in its tensity.

In expiratory expansive strains, the greater wings of the sphenoid will be upward and prominent and can be easily diagnosed along their narrow external surfaces between the frontal and temporal bones. In inspiratory expansive strains, the wings are downward and in closer approximation with the temporozygomatic rockshaft junction. In hay fever and sinus pathology, expansion in the facial articulations is easily diagnosed by observation alone. As one views the position of the

---

6. Reference is being made to the statement ascribed to Dr. Still: "Tell me the moment when the blood flow is altered and I will tell you the moment when disease begins."

body of a vertebra through the application of tactile sense posteriorly at the transverse processes, so we likewise and necessarily view the basilar area through palpation at the greater wings of the sphenoid, the temporozygomatic junction and the squamoparietal articulation. The expansion is sometimes quite apparent at the lambdoidal suture. There are many other features in diagnosis, including those usually considered in vertebral lesions.

Treatment is a specific treatment that *requires an adequate working knowledge of the mechanical articular surfaces of all the cranial and facial bones and their mode of action.* Without this knowledge, it is wiser to leave it alone. The "skull notion" is my contribution to the science of osteopathy. To the earnest investigator, it is an opportunity to gain a firmer grip on "the tail" of the Old Doctor's "squirrel in the hole in the tree."[7] It is a demonstrable skull notion.

A Discussion of "Cranial Membranous-Articular Strains"

By John A. MacDonald, D.O.

I believe we should consider carefully the theory and demonstrations of Dr. Sutherland's idea of cranial membranous-articular strains. Too often we are ready to accept without question the findings of the older school of medicine. We realize that the older school, for the most part, meets severe tests of research; that the ideas advanced by its exponents are likely to be of an authoritative character; and that they are entitled to reasonable acceptance from the old school viewpoint. But we are exponents of a new idea in therapeutics and our direction of thought and investigation leads us to a new interpretation of the facts of anatomy and physiology.

I am unable to say from trial and use that Dr. Sutherland's idea of cranial

---

7. Dr. A. T. Still (respectfully referred to as the Old Doctor in his later years) presented osteopathy as a science, a philosophy and an art whose potential was not fully realized, much as a squirrel only partially seen within a hole in a tree would not be fully visualized. He stated that only the tail of the squirrel was currently in view.

membranous-articular strains is positively more than theory, but there are many scattered evidences...which make me believe we may find in this theory an answer to some obscure questions.

Osteopathic ideas come slowly. We do right to scrutinize carefully the new ideas advanced by members of our profession that we may avoid accepting anything footless or fantastic. On the other hand, *our* latitude for the entertainment of a new theory or interpretation is great because we are exploring a field new even to us–a field given scant consideration by "regular" therapeutic investigators. We need not fear giving full consideration to new ideas advanced by our colleagues. I believe it is true that we have a hard time getting even ordinary consideration of osteopathic ideas, while many dicta of the old school are too frequently accepted by D.O.'s without question. For myself, it is enough if an osteopathic proposal seems sane enough to attract my attention–and if I find that I have seen scattered evidences seemingly related to the idea, I feel urged to do what I can to have our profession investigate.

Embryologists and anatomists refer to the skull bones as modified vertebrae. Dr. Sutherland's quotation from Davis' *Applied Anatomy* is rather startling: "The bones of the base of the skull originate in cartilage while those of the vault originate in membrane...the sutures of the vault *begin* to ossify at about the age of *forty years*, and *continue to fuse* until about the *eightieth year*." [Emphasis added.]

Consider the origin of these osseous plates, the foregoing statements regarding the age at which the sutures fuse should give us something to think about.

Dr. Sutherland points out the great difference in the evidence offered by the animate and the inanimate skull.... This is not new to us. It may be recalled that the sacroiliac joint was formerly believed to be immovable–a belief which was considered proved by the exhibition of a cadaver in a court trial about thirty years ago. It may also be recalled that an osteopathic physician called for a fresh preparation and insisted that a sacroiliac joint in the recent state was movable. I believe he proved his contention.

These data may prove nothing, but it is interesting to consider the scattered clinical evidences of effects due to incidental approximation, separation, or any kind of movement in the sutures of the skull. The most common effect is seen in patients suffering from severe headache who are relieved by placing a tight band around the skull over the frontal and *above* the occipital base.

Again, I believe I can demonstrate that pressure on the nasal bones will reduce congestion in the upper respiratory membranes. Pressure on the frontal bone with the palmar surface of the hand probably has the same result, but both effects are unmistakable.

And further: In cases of cerebral palsy, in which at some time the question of surgical interference usually comes up, brain surgeons are guided by what they consider the state of the falx. If they find evidence that the falx is torn, or badly injured, they consider it useless to operate. In every surgical inquiry that I have made in birth palsy cases, one surgeon or another has always made some such statement regarding the falx.

It seems reasonable that some mechanical change may take place in the falx upon manipulation of the skull plates. Dr. Sutherland believes that tension in the falx does change and is influenced by the procedure he describes. If this is so, it should be the basis of a procedure from which far-reaching results may be expected in obscure and difficult cases–such as migraine, projectile vomiting and cerebral congestion–to say nothing of obscure conditions more remotely related.

I was first attracted to Dr. Sutherland's idea by the knowledge he had of the parts he was investigating. Two years ago I asked him about the falx, and he replied that he could not answer on the basis of what he then knew but that he believed that two more years of study on the falx should give him the lead he expected. I was gratified thus to discover his scientific attitude.

Dr. Sutherland is to prove his case and gather such adherents as he may. I am not writing a testimonial. I simply say I have seen enough to make me believe his idea should be carefully considered by every one of us and tried and used if we feel it is effective for good.

When I think of the time and the study Dr. Sutherland has spent, and the experience he has had with this idea, I am in no mood to outline and present a critical discussion at this time. I am impressed with his idea. I urge you to investigate it carefully.

7. Recognition of Cranial Membranous-Articular Strains

Part I

The Western Osteopath, *March 1933.*

The formation of a mental picture of the articular *surfaces* of the cranial and facial bones is the first necessity in the recognition of cranial membranous-articular strains and in their successful treatment. It is just as essential as is the mental picture of the sacroiliac articular surfaces.

The fertile field of cranial *surfaces* covers a more extended and intricate area than does that of the sacroiliac joint, that is, there are *many* separate articular surfaces in the cranial field, while in the sacroiliac there are but two. Nevertheless, the separate articular surfaces must be considered as a whole in the mental picture of the cranial articular mechanism. The picture should be like that of the watchmaker in his mechanical knowledge concerning the intricate works of a lady's small wristwatch. Without this detailed mental picture of the cranial structure, the osteopathic mechanic of the human osseous framework will wisely confine his skill to that with which he is familiar. Without this exact knowledge of the cranial articular surfaces, he is almost certain to hesitate in accepting the writer's claims relative to cranial membranous-articular strains.

In my experience, this knowledge can be obtained only through diligent study of the articular *surfaces* as they exist on the separate bones of a *disarticulated* skull. After this knowledge has been acquired in minutest detail, the mechanism of articular mobility in the basilar area can be better understood by placing the sphenoid, occiput and the two temporals in their correct relationships and retaining them in this position with rubber bands and small screws in a manner affording free movement at the articulations.

In most cases of migraine, there is a "side-tip" of the sphenoid, which causes a greater prominence of the greater sphenoidal wing in relation to the side affected. This can be readily diagnosed by any osteopathic physician who has a well-trained tactile sense. This has been tried at several state conventions, and in nearly every instance, members of the profession have been able to satisfy themselves on the point. Thus far the clinical demonstrations at the conventions have been confined to members of the profession and their families. The following letter from a Doctor of Osteopathy relates to a case involving articular mobility in the basilar area:

> I thought you might be interested in this information about my wife whom you treated for migraine at the state convention last spring following your lecture. Since that treatment until now, four months later, she has had no real headaches...She has expressed herself this summer as feeling better than in years. She has more "pep" and life, and feels different generally. This is the longest I have known her to go without headaches...Certainly you have something in this idea of yours that is workable and of great interest.

In this case, the prominence of the greater wing of the sphenoid was greater on the right side and was verified by each D.O. who examined it, with the exception of two. A demonstration of the technique was made and reduction obtained, following which another tactile test was made by the same group who gave testimony of change made in the comparative prominence of the greater wings.

As is quite common in demonstration at conventions, this diagnosis was necessarily hurried, a procedure that should not be followed in private practice. The case serves, however, to illustrate what occurs in the basilar area in cases of migraine when the tactile sense reveals that one greater wing of the sphenoid is more prominent than the other.

If the careful investigator will place the sphenoid, occiput and temporal bones together as previously described, and then establish by manipulation of the articulations this same difference in the prominence of the greater wings of the sphenoid, he will readily see what occurs in the basilar area. He will recognize the "side-tip" of the sphenoid. This change in the position of the sphenoid also involves a change in the temporal bone articulations. This restricts normal mobility in the basilar area and–what is more important–likewise restricts vascular channels through a consequent tension of the related membranous tissues. It was for this reason that I named the condition "cranial membranous-articular" strain.

Part II

1933.

A penned notation on the original manuscript states: "Edited by Dr. C.B. Rowlingson, editor of The Western Osteopath, *who was 'called home' before publication." A copy was sent later to Dr. J.B. McKee Arthur, editor of* The Osteopathic Profession, *for exchange of thought.*

> Note: Anatomical texts describe the cranial and facial bones in detail, *except for one very important feature*–that of the *articular surfaces.* Hence, the writer will endeavor to confine this chapter to the articular *surfaces,* as he observes them in his study.

In considering cranial articular mobility, convenience is served by making three divisions of the subject: (1) the *mobility of the basilar area*, including the sphenoid, the two temporals and the basilar area of the occiput; (2) the sutural accommodative function of the vault, including the two parietals and the sutural area of the occiput; (3) the mobility of the facial bones.

Mobility of the Basilar Area

The sphenoid bone articulates with eleven others and is of primary importance to the mobility of the basilar area as well as to the vault and facial divisions. Hence, we first consider the sphenoidal articular *surfaces.*

The superior articular surface of the greater wing, where it contacts the frontal bone, represents a small L-shaped area and, although tiny in comparison, is somewhat similar to the larger L-shaped area found in the sacroiliac articular surfaces. There being two greater wings, there are two of these L-shaped areas, and it is probable that they function in the manner of a fulcrum joint affording and limiting mobility at the various other articulations of the sphenoid.

Posterior to these L-shaped areas are the superior surfaces, which change into internal beveled surfaces that have articular contact with similar external beveled surfaces on the frontal and parietal bones. This arrangement affords gliding mobility.

The posterior articular surfaces of the greater wings begin in sharp angles where the superior surfaces end. It is notable that they change at this point from internal to external bevel surfaces. These continue throughout the upper half and then change again to the internal, in a small, angular niche midway, that continues throughout the lower half. These external and internal articular surfaces have alternating internal and external contrast contacts with the anterior articular surfaces of the squamous portions of the temporal bones.

Note well this difference between the greater wings and the squamous portions–the greater wing external on its upper half and the squamous portion internal on its upper half, while the greater wing is internal on its lower half and the squamous portion external on its lower half. The angle niche, situated midway between the upper and lower halves of the posterior surfaces of the greater wings, should be considered in connection with an angle projection on the anterior surface of the temporal squama. This mechanical articular contact between the greater wings of the sphenoid and the squamous portions of the temporal bones in itself, without reference to many other indications of articular mechanics, portrays the design of the master plan for cranial basilar mobility. The shape and form of the anatomical detail in this region, together with all mechanical implications, constitute the specific study required in the necessary formulation of the mental picture that is indispensable in the diagnosis of cranial membranous-articular strains and their treatment.

The anterior articular surfaces of the sphenoid will be left for consideration later in the division pertaining to facial bone mobility. The junction of the body of the sphenoid with the basilar process of the occiput (the sphenobasilar symphysis) is a cartilaginous union early in life. Its movement is best described as flexibility, rather than articular mobility.

The two temporal bones are of next importance in basilar mobility. The study of one provides the mental picture of the articular surfaces of both. The superior articular surface of the squamous portion is continuous with the surface that articulates with the greater wing of the sphenoid and is likewise beveled internally. It contacts with an externally beveled surface on the parietal bone, and the arrangement indicates gliding mobility. As we reach the mastoid portion of the superior articular surface, we find a change to rough corrugations in a surface that faces upward. Its contact with the inferior surface of the mastoid angle of the parietal provides for a rocking movement, necessary for accommodative service to the rotary and undulatory mobility of the petrous portion.

The posterior articular surface of the mastoid portion in contact with the occiput is somewhat similar in design and likewise affords the rocking accommodative service. The inferior articular surface is slightly corrugated where it contacts an upward facing surface on the occiput until we come to a groove just posterior to the jugular notch. This groove runs crossways on the articulation and contacts with a crossway ridge on the occiput. This crossway groove and ridge, when considered in detail with the change to the lateral articular surface of the mastoid portion, indicate our claim of "a combined rockshaft and pivot-bearing articulation in the mastoid articular surface with the occiput and parietal," of which first mention was made in our article, "Cranial Membranous-Articular Strains," in *The Western Osteopath* for December 1931.[1] This mechanism should be studied in all detail,

1. Mechanically speaking, a rockshaft is an oscillating rod used to transmit motion, as in the connection between an engine and a wheel. The end of the shaft rests and turns in a bearing that functions as a pivot–the area around which the rod rotates or oscillates. Dr. Sutherland viewed the occiput as the pivot-bearing part and the temporoparietal mechanism as the rockshaft.

in order to grasp an important mental picture relating to basilar mobility, keeping in mind that the petrous portion runs in a somewhat diagonal direction inwardly from the mastoid portion.

The inferior articular surface of the petrous portion is marked by a longitudinal groove which has an important mobile contact with a longitudinal ridge-like articular surface on the basilar process of the occiput. This provides the keynote that indicates rotary and undulatory mobility in the cranial base.

The anterior articular surface of the squamous portion corresponds in contrast with the posterior surface of the greater wing of the sphenoid as mentioned above.

The further study of the occiput will be made later in connection with the vault and the serrated, dovetail sutures between the occiput and the parietals, since the mechanism of the articular surfaces of the basilar part of the occiput has been interpreted in connection with the study of the petrous and mastoid portions of the temporal bone.

The bones of the cranial base (sphenoid, occiput and two temporals) can now be united as described in our last article. We are now ready to consider a case picture taken from private practice to illustrate the *mental picture* to be formulated in *some* cranial membranous-articular strains.

It might be well to say, in connection with this case, that head complaints are mere indications or symptoms in many respects. These symptoms are often found to be complex in their manifestations and thus make the diagnosis rather indefinite. The family physician, an experienced M.D., previously in charge of this case, therefore is not to be censured for making the guarded diagnosis of meningitis.

The symptoms, as I first observed them, showed a loss of all voluntary facial muscular action, widely dilated pupils, conjunctivitis and a tendency of the eyeballs to roll upward. In conjunction with the head symptoms, the patient was unable to raise his right arm outward from the shoulder, although it was under normal voluntary control otherwise, including a vigorous handgrip. The history revealed a severe attack of tonsillitis with a tonsillar abscess on the right side. This had received efficient care from the physician previously in charge–the head symptoms, or complications, following thereafter. I was likewise cautious in the diagnosis. A history of pushing on a stalled car previous to the tonsillitis led helpfully to procedures for clearing up the arm difficulty. I found a strained clavicle, the proper reduction of which eliminated the arm difficulty from its connection with the head symptoms. Manipulation of cervical tissues was avoided because of the danger of stirring up the tonsillar infection, although they were very tense on the right side in relation to the site of the tonsillar abscess. Upper dorsal treatment was also not attempted. Although it might have proved advantageous, it was later found to be unnecessary.

The case was then examined "skull notionally." In a case of this nature one might expect a tensity of membranous tissue intracranially at the basilar area, with expansion at the cranial and facial articulations. This tensity of membranous tissue would alter the vascular channels. It was likewise among the possibilities to relax the intracranial tissue at the basilar area by cranial treatment and thus release the vascular channels without disturbing the infectious area of the tonsillar abscess. The examination revealed the right greater wing of the sphenoid markedly prominent as compared with that of the left. This greater wing prominence on the right side corresponded with the side of the tonsillar abscess and indicated that articular expansion was greater on that side. I reasoned that there was a "side-tip" of the sphenoid, with the greatest intracranial membranous tensity at the basilar area on the right side. Cranial technique was then applied in the following manner:

> With the patient reclining in the supine position, the right thumb was placed on the mastoid portion of the right temporal bone, just posterior to the external auditory meatus, and the left thumb on the left greater wing of the sphenoid. Gradual strong pressure was then applied on the right mastoid portion and pulled in a backward direction. At the same time, the left thumb pressed upward, backward and inward with the same degree of gradual, strong pressure on the left greater wing of

> the sphenoid. The object was to draw the petrous portion of the temporal bone backward and outward at its basilar area with the right thumb, while rotating or rolling the basilar area of the sphenoid with the left thumb on the left greater wing, thus relieving intracranial membranous tension at the basilar area and freeing the vascular channels.

The result was agreeably surprising to both physician and patient. "Doubting Thomases" will question the statement, yet it is a fact that normal voluntary control of the eyeballs returned immediately, the widely dilated pupils returned to normal size, and there was slight voluntary muscular control of the eyebrows. At the next visit, all the facial muscles were under their normal voluntary control. While a tonsillectomy was indicated and advised, the immediate response of the "head symptom complex" carried an affirmative argument substantiating the contention of Dr. George Reid that: "...there are no true synarthrodial joints in a normal body and that immovable joints are always abnormal."

If the investigator will take the basilar bones and fasten them together in a manner affording movement at their articulations, and then apply the technique used in this case to these bones, he will grasp the *mental* picture of the cranial membranous-articular strain and how the technique proved beneficial in relief. This case undoubtedly was a secondary complication in the tonsillar infection. Yet it can be truly said that the cervical tensity or rigidity disappeared without any cervical manipulation. That fact is something to think about.

The trunk of the mighty oak possesses flexibility to a certain degree until it becomes a sapless log. The tall Norway pine flexes and sways to the wind. A dead Norway pine of the same diameter and height standing nearby is as rigid and inflexible as a telephone pole. A Great Master Mechanic designed the human skull. Like the live oak and pine, it possesses flexibility to a certain degree within its most solid osseous structure and also mobility at its articulations while the life-giving stream remains.

The Sutural Accommodative Function of the Vault

In the study of this division, it is well to keep in mind that "the bones at the base of the skull originate in cartilage while those of the vault originate in membrane." This will assist in the interpretation of the writer's view of mobility in the basilar area and the *necessary compensation thereto* as provided by the expansile and contractile accommodative sutural service of the vault.

The study begins with the lambdoidal sutural *surfaces* of the occiput and the two parietal bones. These two sutures, right and left, curve outward and downward from their superior angle at the lambda in a manner somewhat like the shape of a large wishbone. Beginning at the lambda, the junction with the posterior terminus of the sagittal suture, it is well to note specifically how the articular surfaces of the serrated processes on the occiput are beveled internally as you follow downward to a midway point, where they change to an external bevel in articulation, continuing thus downward to the asterion where the occipitomastoid and parietomastoid sutures meet with it.

Note also and specifically how the internal and external articular surfaces of serrated processes have external and internal contact with the parietal bones. That is, the upper portion of the articular surface on the occiput is internal and articulates with an external articular surface on the parietal, while the lower portion of the articular surface is external and articulates with an internal articular surface on the parietal. This is another mechanical feature of the design of the articular surfaces indicating cranial articular mobility. In some skulls, the lower portion is marked by several small divisions of bones and accompanying sutures. This is the region of the mastoid fontanels of early life which accounts, in part, for the differences in skulls.

The articular surfaces of the sagittal suture, common to both parietals, are marked by wider and fewer serrated processes along the posterior portion as compared with those along the anterior portion. That is, the serrated processes are finer and closer together along the anterior portion. This differentiation indicates a provision for a wider expansile area at the posterior portion in order to cooperate with the expansile service at the junction with the lambdoidal sutures.

The serrated articular surfaces of the coronal suture might be said to alternate externally and internally in their articular contact between the frontal and the parietals. This is another special provision for the expansile and contractile accommodative service of the vault.

The other articular surface contacts were mentioned in connection with the basilar area study and do not require repetition here.

We are now ready to fasten the frontal and the two parietal bones together. They are joined at one point only–at the junction of the sagittal and coronal sutures. This affords free movement of the sutures necessary in the study of the mechanism. After this connection has been made, draw the two parietals outward at their inferior borders and note how the frontal bone moves anteriorly at its lower articulation with the parietals. Study this movement carefully in connection with articular surfaces of the coronal suture. Also note how the sagittal suture expands or widens at its posterior portion.

Now place these three bones in articulation with those of the basilar division and temporarily fasten the two divisions with a band over the crown and below the base. This temporarily holds the two divisions together and allows movement for their study as a whole. Next, take a two-inch bandage, four inches longer than is necessary to pass once around the head, and fasten the ends together. Pass the bandage around the skull, over the brow on the frontal bone and, with the tied ends at the rear, just over the junction of the lambdoidal suture with the sagittal. Next, with a lead pencil, apply a tourniquet pressure at the rear with the bandage. Note how this lifts the frontal bone anteriorly away from its lower articulation with the parietals. Next, note that the occiput is approximated at the upper portion of the lambdoidal sutures while, at the same time, it is drawn backward at the lower portions. While held in this position with the tourniquet bandage pressure, press inward and downward on the zygomatic processes of the temporal bones; you will then grasp the mental picture of the rotary and undulatory mobility that occurs at the petrobasilar articulations, as well as the combined rockshaft and pivot-bearing mechanism of the mastoid portion as it nestles between the parietal and occipital bones. Also note the gliding mobility at the bevel articulations, especially those of the sphenoid with the squamous portions of the temporals which are external and internal in their alternating mechanical feature.

Now, complete the study of basilar mobility and sutural compensation by applying the same tourniquet bandage compression to your own animated skull, in the same manner that you applied it to the specimen. Be sure to have the bandage pass high over the brow of the frontal bone in front and over the junction of the lambdoidal suture with the sagittal at the rear. Apply the tourniquet compression mildly at the side. Then press inward and downward on your zygomatic processes. As a testimony to the effect, note the feeling of mobility in the basilar area and the compensation occurring through the sutures of the vault and, what is more important, the agreeable change in the circulation to the head as well as an added sparkle to the eyes.

Try this technique further upon a fellow practitioner. Purchase a heavy-grade texture of chamois leather and cut a strip two and a half inches wide by about 30 inches long and sew or tie its ends together. The chamois is soft and comfortable and also washable. It makes a workable apparatus. In the division relating to mobility of the facial area, we will cite a severe case of sinus congestion as an illustration of technique.

The Mobility of the Facial Area

We found the sphenoid bone of chief importance in the articular mobility of the basilar area. It is likewise of primary significance in relation to the facial articular mobility.

At the midway point on the superior-anterior articular surface of the sphenoid body, we find the little ethmoid spine, a small flat projection that has articular contact with a corresponding niche on the ethmoid. It suggests a "jigger" movement of the ethmoid. Immediately below this spine lies the ethmoid crest, having flexible articular contact with the perpendicular plate of the ethmoid, indicating lateral flexibility.

Below the crest lies the rostrum, a little beaklike process in the midline of the inferior surface of the body. It has articular contact with a cup-like articular surface on the vomer that suggests a function similar to that afforded by a universal joint. Running laterally outward from the ethmoid spine on the superior-anterior articular surface of the sphenoid, we find the articular surfaces slightly beveled superiorly. These have articular contact with similar inferiorly beveled surfaces on the ethmoid. Study these bevel surfaces carefully on both bones as they will help materially in the interpretation of facial bone mobility. For instance, grasp the *mental* picture of the sphenoid as rocking in suspension on its L-shaped fulcrum joint areas. One may visualize the sphenoid as rocking in the manner of a teeter board. The sella turcica area of the sphenoid represents one end of the teeter board, while the facial bones represent the other end. The sella turcica area undulates downward during expiration and the facial bones upward, the sella turcica area upward during inspiration and the facial bones downward.

The anterior articulation of the greater wings in their orbital contact with the frontal suggest expansile accommodative function only.

The articular surfaces of the pterygoid processes of the sphenoid in contact with the palatine bones indicate a rocking mobility. These articular areas are frequently strained in the process of the extraction of upper molar teeth under novocaine anesthesia in my experience. Three very painful cases of neuralgia of several weeks duration, following molar extraction, give testimony of instant relief with reduction of this type of strain.

In the study of the ethmoid, it is well to remember that the crista galli fits through the notch in the frontal bone and that it provides the attachment for the falx cerebri on the inside of the cranium. This attachment is an important factor in cranial articular mobility. Laterally, on the superior articular surfaces, we note an articular contact with the frontal that suggests either rocking mobility or flexibility. There are likewise two lateral articular surfaces inferiorly on the ethmoid bone that have their contact with the maxillae. They are of similar design, suggesting flexibility.

The inferior turbinates are not easily understood in their articular contact because of their frailty in construction as found on the disarticulated skull, but their construction suggests flexibility or, rather, expansile function.

The vomer was mentioned in connection with the anterior surface of the sphenoid. Its other articular areas suggest expansile service.

In the maxillae we find two articular surfaces which have important contact with the zygomatics. These might be called the "sacroiliacs" of the facial bones and are instrumental in providing oscillatory movement. The maxillary articular contact with the frontal suggests flexibility. Their articular contact with one another, as well as with the palatine bones, indicates expansile function.

The articular contact of the zygomatics with the frontal indicates flexibility, while their semi-oblique contact with the zygomatic processes of the temporals suggests a rocking accommodative function in connection with basilar mobility.

Now, a case picture to illustrate the study of expansive membranous-articular strain occurring in sinus congestion: This case was of a severe type and of long standing. A middle-aged lady had been under the frequent care of an eye and nose specialist and had undergone several surgical operations for relief. At the time of her first visit to the office, she was making weekly visits 90 miles distant for local drainage by the specialist. In spite of the local drainage, all sinuses were practically filled with what seemed to be a putrid type of congestion. She was suffering greatly from pain and inability to breathe through the nasal area at the time she entered the office. It was easy to recognize the extended expansion of the facial articulations that had come about through the congestion.

I applied the soft chamois leather bandage over the brow of the frontal bone and over the lambda and then made *mild* tourniquet compression at the side, also pushing downward and inward on the zygomatic processes. There was immediate relief from pain, and local drainage through the nose came about without local application. The compression also brought about postnasal drainage and then drainage from other areas. There was a marked change in the active circulation to the entire head and face. In other words, in addition to the natural drainage, the nourishing stream of blood that heals had also been freed, a factor which the application of local methods had failed to accomplish.

This is not to be critical of the methods used by the specialist but to picture the possibilities of accomplishment without the use of local methods. This was the chronic type of case. I gave six succeeding treatments to help out the active blood stream. That was ten months ago. During the interval, the patient has not found it necessary to resort to local drainage and is gradually improving. Even the very facial contour has changed.

The mental picture required in the structural diagnosis viewed the basilar area as upward in its undulatory movement, while the facial area was downward with a decided increase in facial bone articular expansion, that is, instead of a side-tip strain of the sphenoid, as described in a case of migraine, *both* greater wings of the sphenoid, as observed in tactile diagnosis, were found *downward* or depressed. It was reasoned that the patient's efforts toward normal breathing had brought about an inspiratory movement at the expense of the expiratory and that this was an inspiratory type of membranous-articular strain in the cranial mechanical structure. In consequence, there was restriction of membranous tissues intracranially that blocked the normal vascular drainage. In such cases it would be impossible to provide active arterial supply without first securing venous and lymphatic drainage–as impossible as trying to refill the crank case of a motor with fresh oil without first draining out the old carbonized oil.

The mental picture in treatment through the application of the chamois bandage tourniquet viewed the frontal bone as lifting and moving anteriorly away from its lower articulation with the parietals, and the occiput moving backward at the lower articular surfaces of the lambdoidal sutures. In connection, we saw the basilar process of the occiput and the sella turcica of the sphenoid undulating downward, the petrous portions of the temporal bones rotating inward and undulating downward with the basilar process, while the greater wings of the sphenoid were gliding upward and the facial bones in the same direction.

This changed the inspiratory strain to that of the normal expiratory position of its mobility, thus freeing intracranial membranous restriction that was obstructing normal drainage and allowing a refilling of active circulation for proper nourishment.

This gross picture lacks many of the important details that would require considerable space to describe. Yet it provides a working knowledge for the practitioner. This technique will be found especially efficient in the treatment of the various types of nasal, postnasal, eye and ear congestive complications so common in respiratory infections.

We have mentioned the inspiratory type of membranous-articular strain. It will be well to include the expiratory type also. In the latter, expiratory efforts act at the expense of the inspiratory, and there is active circulatory congestion, which in some instances might be erroneously called high blood pressure. This is just the opposite of the passive congestive type common to the complications related to influenza and colds. The complications of the expiratory type probably are secondary to concussions, shell shock and similar initiatory factors. In these complications, we expect to find a restriction of the cerebrospinal fluid activity along the longitudinal sinus in addition to the increase in the active circulation of the blood.

As an interpretation of our meaning concerning the expiratory working at the expense of the inspiratory and vice versa, we might compare occupational voluntary muscular exercise of the right arm to the lack of muscular exercise of the left arm–the muscles of the right arm working at the expense of the left. The intracranial membranous tissues possess neither muscular nor elastic fibers, yet they possibly function through alternating tension and relaxation. For instance, the membranous walls of the longitudinal sinus, including those in relation to the subspaces, become tense as the sagittal suture is in accommodative expansion and relax while the sagittal suture is in contraction. Such alternating membranous tension and relaxation probably aid in the regulation of venous blood, lymph and cerebrospinal fluids along the longitudinal sinus channels. Hence, we might expect restriction of cerebrospinal fluid activity during the expiratory type in addition to the excessive arterial activity of the blood.

This channel is but a small tributary in the activity of the cerebrospinal fluid and is mentioned only as a part of the membranous restriction for illustration. Further restriction interpretation must wait until we reach the study of the intracranial membranous tissues in their relation to the activity of the brain.

In this type, the structural picture views the basilar area in the downward undulation and the greater wings of the sphenoid and facial area in an upward position. The accommodative sutural service necessarily moves the frontal bone anteriorly, outward from its lower articulation with the parietals, while the sagittal suture becomes widened or expanded at its posterior portion. This expansile or widening accommodative sutural function increases the tensity of the longitudinal sinus membranous tissue intracranially, which accounts for the restriction of the cerebrospinal fluid activity–one of the symptoms being a dull, heavy or weight-like ache in the top of the head in the area of the pacchionian depressions.

A case in point was one wherein a previous medical diagnosis had indicated encephalitis in an early stage. I was inclined to disagree, believing the condition to be that of excessive arterial activity, as well as a restriction of cerebrospinal fluid flow as a complication to a shock–the complaint having followed an electrical shock from a bolt of lightening which killed a cow nearby. The case was under the care of the family physician of the old school who had been making the customary spinal puncture to relieve cerebrospinal fluid pressure. There had been occasional temporary relief from the punctures. It might be added that the man had lost an arm earlier in life, yet until the electric shock was physically more active than many with two arms. He then began to lose physical strength.

Palpation revealed both greater wings of the sphenoid upward in their position, this being the opposite of that found in the passive or sinus congestion case. The cranial treatment must be applied in a manner somewhat in reverse of that applied to the sinus case. The same chamois leather bandage is applied further down, over the orbital area of the frontal bone in front and immediately *above* the lambda behind–that is, not directly over the junction of the sutures as in the sinus case but immediately in front of the junction and over the sagittal suture only. This compresses the frontal bone inwardly or posteriorly at its lower articulation with the parietals instead of lifting anteriorly when the bandage is placed higher up on the brow. At the same time, the *mild* tourniquet compression draws the sagittal suture closer together into contractile accommodation, thus releasing the intracranial membranous tensity or tension along the longitudinal sinus and restoring normal function to the cerebrospinal fluid. It likewise restores physiologic balance to the expiratory with the inspiratory movement at the basilar area and aids in reducing the excessive activity of arterial circulation. One may press upward on the zygomatic processes of the temporal bones or inward on the mastoid processes as an aid in the technique.

This case was treated in this manner one year ago. I had not seen the patient for six months until recently when he volunteered this remark: "I haven't had a headache since you placed that bandage on my head." The headache was of the dull, heavy or weight-like ache in the crown. The blood had ceased its excessive rushing to the head during the least physical activity, as had been its previous habit, and he is gaining in strength and "pep." What is most satisfactory of all, further spinal punctures were found unnecessary.

These cases cited, taken from private practice, are to be considered only in relation to the head symptoms to illustrate the types of cranial membranous-articular strains and the method of applying the technique. They are not intended as full case reports.

Editor's Note: This article was written in 1933 while experimental techniques were developing along with cranial research. As these evolved, as skill in their use increased and as reasoning was verified in results, the use of all extraneous agencies–bandages, hemostats etcetera–were discarded for all time.

They served a temporary need until replaced solely by manual technique which Dr. Sutherland developed and taught.

Part III

Date unknown.

A penned notation by Dr. Sutherland on this manuscript states: "Chapter Three in hands of Dr. Arthur for exchange of thoughts. Not ready for publication." (Dr. Arthur is Dr. J. B. McKee Arthur of New York, editor of The Osteopathic Profession.*)*

In answer to a question from Dr. John A. MacDonald a few years previous that concerned the falx, Dr. Sutherland said that he could not say anything on his existing knowledge but that he thought that two more years of study should give him the lead that he expected. This article merely deals with the "lead" formulated during that two year period of study, plus two more years in addition. It was a mere hypothesis. It beckoned and led into a period of prolonged study.

The Incitation of Cranial Articular Mobility

The cranial articulations, lacking an intermediary agency of muscular propulsion, prompt the question to arise: Through what intermediate, propellant agency does cranial articular mobility derive its activity?

The study of the incitation of cranial articular mobility commences with the ventricles and convolutions of the brain and includes the pial, arachnoid and dural membranes. The brain is *alive* with incito-motor potentiality and has subsequent activity in its ventricles and convolutions; it moves and has its being within the skull. Therefore we may hypothesize: that inasmuch as the brain incites the intermediary muscular activity propelling all other articular mobility it can, by its own incito-motor potentiality and subsequent activity of the ventricles and convolutions, incite cranial articular mobility by way of the intermediate, propellant tension agency of the pial, arachnoid and dural membranes, the intermediary membranes functioning as propellant tension bands between the convolutions and articulations in place of otherwise necessary intermediate muscular activity.

If we were to make a flexible rubber cast from the ventricles, the formation would somewhat resemble the body and wings of a bird; attaching the convolutions of the two cerebral hemispheres to the wings of the rubber cast would aid in the interpretation of the writer's hypothesis. For instance, the hypothesis views the cerebral "wings" as folding and the walls of the ventricles contracting during inspiration and the cerebral wings as unfolding or expanding–somewhat like the wings of a mother hen squatting to cover a flock of chicks–and the ventricles dilating during expiration. During this ventricular functioning, the convolutions of the hemispheres coil and uncoil as the cerebral wings fold and unfold and thus incite cranial articular mobility by way of the intermediary, propellant tension agency of the pial, arachnoid and dural membranes. *The falx cerebri and tentorium cerebelli, especially, function as intermedial, propellant tension bands between the convolutions and the articulations as well as balance-reciprocants in the equalization of articular mobility.*

In the consideration of this hypothesis, it is well to bear in mind that the walls of the third ventricle are practically formed by the thalami, while the walls of the fourth ventricle are within the boundary of the cerebellum, pons and medulla oblongata. Also, recall that the third ventricle is a narrow, deep, median crevice lying on a plane below the lateral ventricles and has a correlation in the functioning of the upper brain, while the fourth ventricle is *rhomboidal* in shape and has a functional correlation with the lower brain. One might visualize the walls of the fourth ventricle as functioning in the manner of a rubber bulb on a syringe. For instance, imagine the fibers of the cerebellum and pons as squeezing the ventricle and then relaxing the squeeze. One might say that the cerebrospinal fluid is a compression lubricant, functioning much in the manner of the lubricant utilized in a hydraulic lift apparatus.

It is also well to recognize the fact that wherever we have a circulating fluid in the body, there is necessarily activity of the vascular channels to accommodate the flow. The cerebrospinal fluid fills the ventricular system and the subarachnoid space. Pathology informs us that in many instances where there are adhesions or other anomalies of the dural, arachnoid and pial membranes that restrict the flow of cerebrospinal fluid, we find dilation of the ventricles, especially the third ventricle. One might call this a physiological dilation rather than pathological.

In connection with our study, the much discussed pituitary body is visualized as possessing activity in correlation with the intermediate membranous propellant agency. We visualize the pituitary body as "riding in the saddle" of the sphenoid bone–that is, like the riding movement of one's ischial tuberosities as they would ride in a saddle during a gallop on horseback–alternately shifting forward and backward during inspiration and expiration. We are inclined to believe that inactivity of this movement of the pituitary body in the sella turcica through mechanical membranous-articular restriction is the primary cause of pituitary secretory disturbances. In other words, we believe that pituitary secretory disturbances are due to mechanical restriction–that of a cranial membranous-articular strain. In this line of thought, I quote from a recent letter, viz:

> I have been reading a book called *Glands Regulating Personality* by Louis Berman, M.D. of Columbia University. He stresses so much the influence of the pituitary lobes and the influence of the mechanical features on the gland (inability of the gland to accommodate itself to the bony cage, or failure of the cavity to expand to suit the gland); and the variable characteristics developing when one or the other lobes predominate; and yet does not seem to say why the gland might thus shift in its anatomy.... I wonder if you can set up a chain of scientific reasoning between your cranial strains and the pituitary strains. In one place or more I believe Dr. Berman ascribes migraine headaches to this squeezing by the bony saddle.

Thus far I have not been able to secure a copy of the text and the quotation verbatim. However my correspondent's recollection thereof provides the thought of mechanical disturbance.

Adding prestige to the thought is my personal experience through cranial treatment of migraine. In these cases, tactile sense indicated a "side-tip" of the sphenoid bone wherein there was a greater prominence of the greater wing on one side in differentiation from the greater wing of the opposite side, reduction of the side-tip securing results in the majority of cases. As further testimony, a test was made in a case of migraine before a group of osteopathic physicians at a state convention. With the exception of two in the group, there was an agreement in the diagnosis of greater prominence of one greater wing in contrast to the other. The reduction was then made and the same group verified the change to normal position. The side-tip of the sphenoid restricted normal articular mobility, with the subsequent restriction of the "gallop" of the pituitary body through an added tension of the membranous tissues in relation thereto.

8. Correspondence 1933

Dear Doctor,

Your patient called yesterday afternoon. Thank you for the referral.

It is an interesting case of cranial membranous-articular strain. For want of a better term, I call it an expansive external rotation of the petrous portion of the temporal bone that causes membranous restriction of the dural membrane enveloping the trigeminal ganglion. The expansion is quite evident at the squamoparietal contact. One might picture the squamous portion as gliding downward and outward and the parietal as outward and upward. Please understand that as a minute picture enlarged for illustration–the specific “lesion” is in the basilar area, namely, the external rotation of the petrous portion.

The external rotation of the petrous portion increases the tensity of the dural membrane between the apex and the root of the greater wing of the sphenoid. As you know, the trigeminal ganglion lies lodged in the dural membrane on the apex of the petrous portion, which means that this increased tensity results in membranous restriction surrounding the trigeminal ganglion.

Now, the technique: I take a chamois skin bandage of firm but soft texture, some three inches wide and 38 inches long, and pass it around the skull. I fasten the ends together with a hemostat, but they can be tied together as well. The lesion being on the left side, I place the left thenar eminence on the left mastoid angle of the parietal beneath the bandage. Then, with a pencil or small stick, I apply tourniquet pressure with the right hand. [*The technique described here, with the use of the chamois bandage, was temporary and confined to the period when manual techniques were being created.*] This springs the mastoid angle of the parietal inward and away from its articular contact with the temporal bone. This allows the squamous portion to glide upward and inward and, of course, the petrous portion naturally rotates inward at the basilar area, thus relaxing the tensity of the membranous restriction in the dural membrane enveloping the trigeminal ganglion. One may aid in the technique by pulling upward on the zygomatic process of the temporal bone with the free fingers of the left hand while the thenar eminence is springing the mastoid angle of the parietal. This pulling of the zygomatic process upward draws the squamoparietal contact into closer approximation.

There are likely other basilar membranous restrictions in a lesion of this type, but the trigeminal ganglion is enough for you to reason by.

Fraternally yours,
W.G.S.

9. Treatment of "Modified Vertebrae" in Respiratory Influenza

The Osteopathic Profession, *September 1934.*

The basilar bones of the skull, originating in cartilage and resembling "modified vertebrae," have many mechanical indications for the accommodation of normal articular mobility. Provided that normal basilar articular mobility may be proved through research activities, osteopathic technicians may then expect to find abnormal limitation of basilar articular mobility to be of as frequent occurrence as is the abnormal limitation of articular mobility in the spinal vertebrae.

The vault bones of the skull, originating in membrane, have many mechanical serrate indications for the accommodation of normal sutural expansion and contraction.

The trunk of the mighty oak, swaying to the impulses of the wind, proves the feature of flexibility in its structure until it becomes a sapless log. The vault bones have many indications for the accommodation of structural flexibility until the "sap" departs. Provided that the vault structural flexibility may be proved through research activities, osteopathic technicians may then consider vault structural flexibility in connection with normal sutural expansion and contraction.

The professional experience of the writer, in the treatment of various types of cranial membranous-articular strains, suggests the solemn fact that normal basilar articular mobility and normal vault sutural expansion and contraction are as essential to health as is the normal articular mobility at the occipitoatlantal and other vertebral areas. This cranial-technical experience adds prestige to the contention ventured by Dr. George Reid of Worcester, Massachusetts, some 20 years ago, that "there are no true synarthrodial joints in a normal body–immovable joints are always abnormal."

While this cranial-technical experience includes various types of cranial membranous-articular strains, this article will be confined to the limitative expansive type common to respiratory influenza.

In this type, the tiny infective organism *initiates* its destructive ramble *within the skull*. As a dire consequence, the intracranial membranous tissues, so physiologically important to the normal channels of blood and lymph, become increased in tensity and restrict drainage and nourishment to the primary physiological centers. This possibly interprets the phenomena of pathological complications occurring here and there throughout the body. These complications include the various spinal muscular contractions.

The exaggerated tensity of the intracranial membranous tissues also restricts the normal basilar articular mobility and the normal sutural expansion and contraction. The lambdoidal sutures at their lower areas will be found in limitative expansion and in limitative contraction at their upper areas, which condition may be readily diagnosed by tactile sense. The mastoid portions of the temporal bones will also be found expansively outward, and in consequence, the petrous portions are rotated externally at their articular contacts with the basilar process and become limited in their normal functioning of internal and external rotary articular mobility. This is the mere gross picture. We will not go into detail because of lack of space but will describe the cranial technique which has been found effectual in the treatment–a technique that any osteopathic technician with mechanical skill can apply, thus testing the writer's hypothesis.

Reestablishing Normal Mobility

The intent of the treatment is to reestablish normal basilar articular mobility and normal sutural expansion and contraction and thus free vascular channels throughout the intracranial membranous tissues and restore normal drainage and nourishment to the primary physiological centers.

We utilize a chamois skin bandage of soft firm texture, about 30 inches in length and three inches in width. The bandage also has two lateral appendages, about six to eight inches in length and three in width. We also have a concave fulcrate cap remodeled from a wooden chopping bowl. The fulcrate cap is padded in front and behind with a free concave space of about six and one half inches between, to afford leverage applied over the crown without pressure contact to the sagittal suture. The pads rest upon the frontal bone anterior to the coronal suture and upon the occipital bone posterior to the junction of the lambdoidal sutures with the sagittal. The fulcrate cap is nine inches in length and four inches in width at the center.

Editor's Note: This appliance was used temporarily during this early transitional stage when Dr. Sutherland was developing the manual techniques which were his goal and which he later taught to those who sought cranial instruction. No appliances or adjuncts ever substituted for the trained tactile sense upon which he insisted.

With the patient lying supine, we place the chamois skin bandage snugly around the head and fasten the ends together with an arterial forceps over the frontal bone. The fulcrate cap is then placed over the crown with the front pad resting on the frontal bone anterior to the coronal suture and the rear pad resting on the occiput posterior to the lambda. The lateral appendages of the bandage are then drawn upward over the fulcrate cap and the ends fastened together with an arterial forceps. We then roll or turn the forceps in such a manner as to tighten the lateral appendages. This draws the inferior borders of the parietal bones inward and upward while the fulcrate cap holds the frontal and occipital bones downward.

One might say it lifts the vault bones inward and upward away from the basilar bones, a necessary primary procedure in the reduction of all the various types of cranial membranous-articular strains about which we may speak later. The drawing inward and upward of the parietal bones allows the squamous portions of the temporal bones to glide inwardly. As they glide inwardly, the petrous portions of the temporal bones necessarily rotate inwardly from their position of limitative external rotary strain found in respiratory influenza.

The technique is aided in some cases by springing inwardly upon the mastoid portions of the temporal bones with the palms of the hands, but in most cases this is unnecessary. Keep the parietal lift pressure in contact until a change in the active circulation of the head becomes noticeable. This change is often accompanied by an agreeable sensation of warmth intracranially throughout the occipital area. Do not be surprised to observe the majority of patients rubbing their noses as an indication of a decided change in the active circulation of the head; further, do not be surprised to find the cervical muscular contractions relaxing in the wake thereof, nor to find similar muscular relaxation occurring throughout the entire spinal area. In addition, a notable change in respiration and other physiological activities may be noted. These results may remind you that a change in the active circulation to the head usually precedes the crisis of pneumonia as a favorable indication.

Case Histories

Respiratory influenza: male, age 35, occupied as an insurance adjustor; seen at the twelfth hour following the initiation of the ailment. Temperature 102° F., onset sudden with chill, labored pulse and respiration; heavy dull ache intracranially in cerebellar area, cervical and upper dorsal muscles contracted with a toxic feel; other spinal musculature contracted with no apparent osseous lesions of the vertebrae. Complaint of a general "grippy" ache through the whole body. Tonsils slightly congested; nasals clogged; slight laryngitis; bronchial and lung tissues negative.

One mild application of cranio-technique as described above was quickly followed by an agreeable intracranial sensation of warmth in place of the dull ache in the cerebellar area; the forehead became hot, the eyes brightened and the nasals cleared. "It is like waking up," the patient said. Osteopathic tactility detected a warm sensation, moving, running or flowing upward in the cervical area, a sensation that one might encounter with a hand placed upon a pipe leading to a hot water radiator in the case when the pipe has been cold and frosty and is changing to warmth as the water begins to heat down in the furnace.

Immediately following the change from passive to active circulation in the head, there was a change to normal respiration and to normal pulse. The toxic feel oozed from the cervical tissues and muscular contractions relaxed *without any local manipulation whatsoever.* We interpreted this phenomenon as an indication that the "arterial supremacy" was now actively busy and further treatment was unnecessary. It was time to "leave the tissues to their own repair." The fever receded. The patient, though feeling quite well, remained in bed as a safety procedure until the following morning and then returned to office duties. Although previously doubtful of the efficiency of osteopathic methods, he was much impressed with the prompt reversal of his acute distress.

Respiratory influenza with complication: female, age 42, married; seen on the seventh day following the attack. The patient had taken her own temperature at the beginning as 103° F., had remained in bed and used home methods. We found the fever still raging in its endeavor to combat the ailment. Respiration was labored and pulse somewhat accentuated. There was slight bronchitis, but the lung tissues were negative in indication. According to the patient, she had a "swell sore head" and was suffering intensely on account of "inability to blow the nose." Relief from this was what she most desired.

The sinuses were aggravatingly congested. Slight congestion at the left mastoid. Eyes were dull with conjunctiva very red and lacrimal ducts blocked. Tonsils were absent. Cervical and upper dorsal muscular tissues were markedly contracted on the left side with a drawing of the atlas to the left. The first and second ribs were drawn upward, probably secondary to contraction of the scaleni. There was difficulty and pain in endeavors to raise or turn the head as in torticollis. We will not report the story of complications natural in a case presenting a history of previous chronic ailments.

One application of the cranial-technique provided the immediate relief which she specifically desired in the nasal area, through a copious suppurative discharge. This immediately followed the change from the passive to the active circulation of the head. The cervical tissues relaxed and the toxic feel oozed from the region. The atlas spontaneously returned to normal alignment, but the ribs required local attention with consequent upper dorsal muscular relaxation. The patient rested comfortably throughout the night. Feeling well on the way to complete recovery the next day, she made the mistake of sitting up about the house and brought about a relapse. A second application of the technique with instructions to stay in bed cleared up the case without further attention.

The point in the narration of these two case reviews is to emphasize the change from the *passive* to the *active* circulation to the head. It indicates what we are striving for in any osteopathic treatment. It indicates that the arterial supremacy is busy, and it is time to leave the tissue to their own repair.

10. "Modified Vertebrae" in Tic Douloureux

The Osteopathic Profession, *May 1935.*

In an article in the September 1934 issue of *The Osteopathic Profession*, reference was made to the indications–relative to limitative basilar articular mobility and intensified tensity of intracranial membranous tissues restricting the blood and lymph channels to the primary physiological centers–as suggesting the interpretation of the various complications in respiratory influenza. In this article I will try to interpret limitative basilar articular mobility and consequent intensification of the tensity of membranous tissue pertaining to the intracranial ganglia as tic douloureux has provided an example.

In tic douloureux, osteopathic technicians may expect to find a unilateral limitative petrous portion internal rotary strain–just the opposite of external rotary strain as described in respiratory influenza. This type usually occurs secondary to trauma such as pugilistic blows beneath the jaw, falls on the chin, extraction of lower wisdom teeth under novocaine anesthesia or, as the history in one case strongly indicates, during a tonsillectomy under general anesthesia, which will be mentioned later.

A pugilistic blow beneath the jaw or the extraction of a lower wisdom tooth apparently jams the petrous portion inwardly and posteriorly against the basilar process and thus causes a slight separation between the apex of the petrous portion and the root of the greater wing of the sphenoid. This result stretches, or intensifies the tensity of, the dural membrane enveloping the trigeminal ganglion which lies embedded between the folds of dural membrane upon the apex of the petrous portion and upon the root of the greater wing of the sphenoid. This disturbs the functioning of the ganglion and suggests the interpretation of the phenomenon of tic douloureux.

In addition to the limitative articular strain at the petrous portion, the sphenoid is pulled downward and laterally, signifying additional stress to the separation between the root of the greater wing and the apex of the petrous portion. This position of the sphenoid may be readily diagnosed by skilled tactile sense beneath or near the junction of the zygomatic process with the temporal process of the zygomatic bone, the greater wing of the sphenoid being expansively prominent and downward in contrast with the greater wing of the opposite side. This type is usually accompanied by occipitoatlantal lesions, either as primary or secondary thereto, or may be simultaneously sustained. Reduction of the occipitoatlantal lesion apparently does not remove the limitative basilar articular strain, but on the other hand, reduction of the limitative basilar articular strain frequently relaxes suboccipital and submaxillary tissues and releases occipitoatlantal lesions into self-reduction.

In the technique it is necessary to "lift" the vault bones away from the basilar, so we utilize the chamois skin bandage and fulcrate cap appliance as described in the article dealing with respiratory influenza. [See article 9, "Treatment of 'Modified Vertebrae' in Respiratory Influenza."] While the vault bones are held in the "lift," we place a palm or thenar eminence on the mastoid portion immediately posterior to the external meatus and draw inward and backward to release the limitative articular mobility and then press forward while with the thumb of the free hand we push upward upon the greater wing of the sphenoid. Simple and effective.

Editor's Note: The appliance described above was used temporarily during the early stages in the development of the manual techniques, which were Dr. Sutherland's goal and which he later taught. No appliance or adjunct ever substituted for the trained tactile sense upon which he insisted.

Dr. Perrin T. Wilson describes a successful technique in connection with tic douloureux in an editorial case report in the issue of the *Journal of the American Osteopathic Association* for October 1933, wherein the "mandible was drawn downward and forward to free the tissues and soft tissue work done under the angle of the jaw."[1] He also called attention to Dr. Still's statements in *Research and Practice* that in all cases of tic douloureux which he had treated, mandibular lesions had been found and that treatment directed to them had brought relief in nearly every case.[2] Dr. Still frequently referred to the "tail" of the osteopathic "squirrel" as still sticking out from the "hole in the tree."[3] In his mandibular treatment, it is likely he was merely gripping the tail. The body of the squirrel still lies within the tree. My hypothesis of limitative basilar articular mobility barely touches the rear end of the squirrel, that is, it is still holding the tail. Our research activities are still confronted with a "breech presentation" prospective to a complete delivery of the body of the squirrel.

Considering the position of the petrous portion, jammed internally and posteriorly against the basilar process as we see it in limitative basilar internal articular mobility, the glenoid or mandibular fossa is consequently out of its normal alignment, and this accounts for the mandibular lesion and its accompanying clicks and trifacial "tics."

Case History

We cite a case to strengthen our hypothesis: high school girl age 14 with tic douloureux symptoms of seven years duration, dating from or following a tonsillectomy under general anesthesia. In this case

---

1. Perrin T. Wilson, D.O. (American School of Osteopathy, 1918) was president of the American Osteopathic Association (AOA) in 1933, chairman of the Osteopathic Manipulative Technique and Clinical Research Association in 1938-39 and president of the Academy of Applied Osteopathy (AAO) in 1944-46. Along with Thomas L. Northup, D.O., Dr. Wilson helped to create an opportunity for Dr. Sutherland to present his ideas at the scientific seminar of the AOA in July, 1946. The impetus to create the Osteopathic Cranial Association as an affiliate of the AAO came out of this meeting.

2. Still, *Research and Practice*, pp. 268-269 (n. 636). In that text Dr. Still uses the term "lower maxilla," which is an older term for the mandible.

3. Dr. A. T. Still presented osteopathy as a science, a philosophy and an art whose potential was not fully realized, much as a squirrel only partially seen within a hole in a tree would not be fully visualized. He stated that only the tail of the squirrel was currently in view.

there was a markedly expansive position of the greater wing of the sphenoid with consequent disfigurement of the face through the sphenoid's articular contact with the facial bones, a disfigurement that might mar the girl's beauty for life. The mastoid process was expansively more prominent than the process of the opposite side. There were no occipitoatlantal or other cervical lesions, though there may have been, as the patient had "taken chiropractic treatment for cervical lesions."

The case had passed through the usual expert fields of observation with very little encouragement for a scientific diagnosis or suggestion of a proper treatment. It then fell into the chiropractic field, which included the electronic diagnostic machine and its treatment, the machine diagnosis signifying a "sinus affection." One course of chiropractic and machine treatment failed to give relief.

We informed the parents of our doubts about the diagnosis and said that if they wished we would exercise our skill on a trial basis only. We followed the above described technique, feeling our way cautiously. Considerable relief followed the first trial. We kept up these cautious endeavors for a period of three months with weekly intermissions. In the meantime the facial disfigurement gradually receded, which was very gratifying to the girl, and the "tic" gradually subsided, which was still more gratifying to all concerned.

Thus far, in 35 years of osteopathic practice, we have not claimed to have "cured" a single case of any malady, and we certainly do not intend making a claim of cure in this case. However, considering the period of duration and the change that is bound to occur in bony structure during the growth period ahead, we feel that we succeeded where others failed. The endeavor strengthens our contention of normal basilar mobility, of limitative articular mobility as abnormal and that such abnormality may be successfully treated by skilled osteopathic technicians.

11. A New Mechanism in Cranial Technique

The Osteopathic Profession, *August 1935.*

In the September 1934 and May 1935 issues of The Osteopathic Profession, *Dr. Sutherland described how he used a rather revolutionary technique in the treatment of influenza and tic douloureux. The equipment he used at that time was homemade, and the mechanism illustrated below is the outgrowth of further study and experience along the lines of this "cranial technique."*

The accompanying illustration portrays an improvement effected in the mechanism that we now utilize in cranial technique. The mechanism affords the application of lateral compression to the cranium at desired specific areas without anterior-posterior contact and also anterior-posterior compression without lateral contact. It may be applied specifically over the lambdoidal sutures, the mastoid portion, the mastoid processes, the squamosal sutures, the maxillae, the zygomatics, the parts of the sphenoid and other bones according to the necessity of specific compression in relation to the different types of cranial membranous-articular strains.

The mechanism operates somewhat in the manner of the automobile brake-type application of compression. There are two concave wooden clamps that conform to the convexity of the cranium, eight and one-fourth inches long and four inches wide. Four small buckles are attached to one clamp and four small straps are attached to the other clamp. There are also two cranial contact pads, made from rubber sponge material and encased in soft leather of the same length and width as the wooden clamps, the contact pads being about three inches in thickness, affording a soft mild compression and at the same time one that is forceful. Compression is applied as desired by adjustment of the straps.

12. Correspondence 1935

Dated November 11, 1935.

Dear Doctor,

I am pleased to note your enthusiasm in your recent letter. As you "dig on," you will find that the cranial idea does open a field of various possibilities; not only in head conditions but in systemic conditions also. Yes, I have found the technique effective in headaches and in eye complaints including changes in the orbital cavity. I have not become enthusiastic about results in deafness up to now, but there have been enough limited responses to keep me digging into the problems more deeply.

As the hearing mechanism is enclosed in a bony compartment, it requires deep digging. The paragraph from "Skull Notions" that is enclosed gives the cue to my thought thus far about most cases of deafness.[1] The "sand rubbing" sensation which you write of in your mother's case may have some relation to the internal carotid artery. This might be concerned with some intracranial membranous restriction of the artery near the petrous portion of the temporal bone. If so, the lateral compression would be worthy of a trial. My own mother is 86 years of age and has been deaf for quite a number of years. While visiting me last winter, I tried the lateral compression on her and there was improvement in her hearing. This is saying a great deal considering her age.

As background for the technique used in influenza, let me say that the normal basilar articular movement of the sphenoid is a "nosedive" during inspiration and an ascent during expiration. There is also a

---

1. The specific paragraph to which Dr. Sutherland refers is unknown; however, one possibility is that he was referring to the first paragraph of article 5: section 2, "Skull Notions: August 1931."

"side-dip" movement that affords breathing through one nostril at a time–that is, with inspiration through the left nostril the left greater wing side-dips and with expiration it rises. When breathing through the right nostril, the side-dip occurs on that side. In respiratory influenza, you may expect to find a limitation in this area of the sphenoid movement.

The treatment is to adjust the "nasal carburetor" to normal movement. Place the clamps for lateral compression as described in the August issue of *The Osteopathic Profession*. [See article 11, "A New Mechanism in Cranial Technique."] Then close the left nostril with a finger of the left hand. At the same time, place a finger or thumb of the right hand upon the right greater wing of the sphenoid and press downward, instructing the patient to inspire three or four times through the right nostril. Release the pressure on the greater wing during the expiration period. Then reverse the procedure to the opposite side. The treatment not only secures normal basilar articular mobility but also intracranial and postnasal drainage. It also frees up the area of the sphenopalatine ganglion and thus furthers nutrition to the nasal and postnasal tissues. The technique is effective in the treatment of sinus complaints also.

Fraternally,
W.G.S.

13. Spinal Technique

The Osteopathic Profession, *December 1935.*

Dr. Virgil Halladay's animated skeleton[1] suggests spontaneous ligamentous reduction of the abnormal articular fixations that are commonly found by osteopathic technicians in spinal movement, provided the articulations are properly guided by the thinking-feeling-seeing osteopathic fingers. Were it not for the presence of spinal muscular activity in the living body, this skeletal suggestion would prove of practical value in technique, and not only in technique but in diagnosis.

With this skeletal suggestion in mind, the writer devised a method of substituting rubber tissue for muscular tissue. In this substitution, a Firestone 7-50-18, high-speed, heavy-duty inner tube is utilized. The tube is first cut in two, crossways, then cut through the outer edge from one end to the other, securing a serviceable piece of rubber some 60 inches in length and 17 inches in width. One end of this rubber piece is then cut downward through the center some 22 inches, providing two strips for passing over the shoulders.

With the patient in a standing posture, the two strips are passed over the shoulders, the lower end extending down along the spine and over the sacrum where it is passed between the legs and then drawn upward over the abdomen and fastened to the shoulder strips with arterial forceps. By this adaptation, we have apparently dissected the patient of his erector spinae muscles and others in relation. The

---

1. Virgil Halladay, D.O. (American School of Osteopathy, 1916). Author of *Applied Anatomy of the Spine*, Dr. Halladay was a professor of anatomy at the American School of Osteopathy in Kirksville, Missouri. He developed a chemical process by which the natural flexibility of the ligaments in cadaveric specimens could be preserved. He prepared such specimens of the spine, rib cage and pelvis that were often called the "animated skeleton."

patient now lacks spinal muscular activity, which has been replaced by rubber tissue activity. One might say that the patient has become a Halladay animated skeleton.

It is now easy to reach beneath the inner tube and palpate for the detection of any abnormal articular fixation while one flexes, extends, sidebends and rotates the patient's spinal column throughout the normal range of movement. This may be accomplished with the patient sitting or standing. After the proper diagnosis has been made, it is just as easy to guide the articulation during the desired degree of flexion, extension, sidebending or rotation while the ligamentous tissue spontaneously accomplishes the reduction. One may feel the articulation gliding and occasionally jumping into normal position.

The stubborn upper dorsal and upper rib fixations respond readily to the adaptation as well as fixations at other areas of the spine. The low back and sacroiliac strains are especially responsive.

Many low back and sacroiliac strains are sustained, or occur, while standing, and consequently, we have found the standing posture advantageous while making the reduction. However, the adaptation proves practical in the sitting posture and other table positions. The pajama type of patient apparel is worn by women patients.

14. Cranial Respiratory Mechanism

The Osteopathic Profession, *November 1936.*

Many members of the profession are apt to view this line of thought as hypothetical. It is, rather, an interpretation of various phenomena occurring in my research activities with the anatomical structure that "lives, moves and has its being."[1] Case records, including members of the profession, provide the testimony. The anatomical laboratory provides additional testimony in many ways, provided the skull articulations are studied in all their mechanical detail.

There is one articulation at the basilar area that is easily recognized: that of the normal articulation of the sphenoid with the basilar process of the occiput. In testimony, I refer to the skull specimen with which I demonstrated in Detroit at the American Osteopathic Association convention as well as at the Minnesota, Iowa and South Dakota state meetings. This specimen shows a normal articulation between the sphenoid and the basilar process of the occiput that indicates the presence of an intervertebral cartilage adapted for and affording undulatory and rotary mobility. I have another specimen possessing the same characteristics. These two specimens are not sawed in two as is common with most disarticulated skulls.

In connection with these two convincing specimens, Dr. Charlotte Weaver provided additional testimony in the presentation of several specimens, prenatal and postnatal, which show the normal articulation. One of the latter shows an "intervertebral disc" still intact. See her article on page 333 in the March 1936 issue of the *Journal of the American Osteopathic Association.*[2]

---

1. "For in him we live, and move, and have our being...." Acts 17:28, King James Version.

2. Dr. Weaver lectured and wrote on the subject of "cranial vertebrae." Her published articles on the subject appeared in the *JAOA* between 1936-1938.

Quoting Dr. John A. MacDonald: "The awakening of the respiratory center seems to be on the knees of the gods, but the operation of the diaphragmatic mechanism one might dare to say is somewhat in our hands."[3] While the "awakening of the respiratory center" still remains "on the knees of the gods," the cranial articular and intracranial membranous respiratory mechanism, within which the respiratory center is a habitant, is also adaptable to regulation of its mobility by osteopathic hands.

The ethmoid breathes and moves in articular activity with 13 other bones, swinging the falx cerebri and the tentorium cerebelli forward and backward. The sphenoid moves in articular activity with eleven bones and, piloted by the pituitary body in its sella turcica, undulates and rotates upon a normal articulation at its junction with the basilar process of the occiput and assists in the swinging of the falx-tentorium. Activity of the falx-tentorium creates membranous movement to the intracranial membranous sinus walls without which there would be a stasis in intracranial circulation.

Respiratory ailments initiate through the nasal realm and affect abnormal fixations in the normal range of ethmoidal, sphenoidal and falx-tentorium activity, thus limiting the flow of the venous and cerebrospinal fluid circulation.

Specific compression, applied intelligently by the thumbs or thenar eminences over the maxillae immediately below the orbits and between the zygomatic bones and the nose, reestablishes the normal range of activity. A downward pressure toward the teeth influences the movement occurring during inspiration, and an upward pressure influences the movement toward the orbits occurring during expiration. In the sinus complications, the area of compression will be found sensitive....

All animate tissues are in constant rhythmic motion. The brain is not a quiet lifeless mass of nerve tissues. Its convolutions coil and

---

3. Dr. MacDonald was president of the American Osteopathic Association in 1929 and had an early interest in Dr. Sutherland's ideas.

uncoil, and the ventricles dilate and contract in rhythmic unison with the alternating cranial articular-membranous activity in relation to respiration. Hence, abnormal fixations occurring in the normal range of cranial articular-membranous activity also limit brain and ventricle movement.

The pituitary body is not the seat of intelligence. It is a mere little "body" that rides in the saddle of the sphenoid that is governed by the seat of intelligence. It has a mechanical movement, and limitation of its movement is more important than its function relating to secretion.

In influenza, the tension at the junction of the tentorium with the falx becomes intensified. This restricts normal activity in the realms of the diencephalon, mesencephalon and metencephalon, thus restricting normal dilation of the aqueduct and the third and fourth ventricles and accounting for the dull intracranial aches occurring in this area, common in influenza. Specific compression over the lambdoidal sutures at the location where the lateral sinuses cross over from the occiput to the parietal bones is effective in releasing the falx-tentorium tension.

In the treatment of abnormal cranial fixations due to respiratory ailments, it is well to consider possible fixations due to traumatic causes, as fixations of the latter nature are as common in the cranial articulations as in those of the vertebral column. Diagnosis should be considered accordingly before applying cranial technique.

15. Dental Traumatic Cranial Lesions

The Osteopathic Profession, *April 1937.*

One of the common traumatic types of cranial membranous-articular strains is that occurring during dental surgery. This type included a membranous-articular strain, or fixation, in relation to the temporal, sphenoid and superior and inferior maxillae. [The "superior maxilla" is more commonly known as the "maxilla" and the "inferior maxilla" as the "mandible."] The temporal bone on the lesion side is inward with its petrous portion in internal rotation; the pterygoid process of the sphenoid upward and lateral; the superior maxillary downward; and the mandible in malalignment at its temporomandibular articulation.

The lesion occurs in the following manner: The patient's occiput rests on a V-shaped headrest on the dental chair in such manner as to compress the mastoid portion of the temporal bone immediately anterior to the lambdoidal suture.[1] The dental surgeon chisels around a lower molar or wisdom tooth and applies a specially adapted forceps that extracts the tooth with an inward side-leverage movement, that is, not a straight upward lift or pull. This inward side-leverage upon the tooth tends to increase the compression on the temporal bone by way of the temporomandibular joint. At the same time, this side-leverage twists or throws the mandible on the opposite side downward quite forcibly, thereby causing a severe tension on the sphenomandibular ligament. This pulls the sphenoid downward and lateral and swings the pterygoid process on the lesion side upward and lateral.

During the extraction of an upper molar, the same side-leverage is utilized, which twists the superior maxilla laterally and downward. In

---

1. The V-shaped headrest is no longer encountered in the modern dental office.

some cases, the pterygoid process will be so far laterally as to crowd the coronoid process of the mandible. This crowding of the coronoid process, together with the malalignment at the temporomandibular articulation due to the inward position of the temporal bone, causes overbiting.

This type especially affects the normal functioning of the trigeminal and sphenopalatine ganglia, facial neuralgia usually following. The internal rotation of the petrous portion of the temporal bone affects or twists the cartilaginous portion of the eustachian tube, and in some cases ear complications arise. There is also tension of the intracranial membranes, especially on the lesion side.

The lateral position of the sphenoid bone widens the sphenomaxillary fissure within the orbital cavity, and in cases of long duration, eye pathology occurs. A study of the orbital cavity and the eye mechanism indicates a design for mobility in the various osseous articulations and a mechanical function of the sphenomaxillary fissure other than its service as a passageway for nerves and vessels. The sphenomaxillary fissure provides a widening and narrowing service to the orbital cavity to accommodate a forward and receding movement of the eyeball. The orbital cavity is not one solid osseous cavity like the acetabulum but is formed by parts of the frontal, sphenoid, maxillary, zygomatic, ethmoid, palatine and lacrimal bones which articulate with each other at many joints. Any fixation of the sphenoid is bound to disturb normal functioning or movement of the orbital cavity, and eye pathology follows. Furthermore, a fixation of the sphenoid affects the normal position of the ethmoid with its turbinates, the vomer, and the palatine bones, and this may account for many of the irregularities in the nasal region.

This type is not difficult to diagnose. In some cases, the removal of an upper plate for observation tells the story, the impression on its surface reflecting the irregularities of the roof of the mouth and the downward position. Direct observation of the roof of the mouth shows the degree of this effect. In some cases, the downward position of the maxilla is to the extent of a three-ply cardboard and in others, to the extent of a sheet of paper. The writer has one upper plate that shows the three-ply cardboard extent of the downward position. Following reduction in this case, it became necessary for the patient to secure a new plate in order to have a proper fit to the maxilla.

The upward and lateral position of the pterygoid process is diagnosed by inserting an index finger between the upper lip and the gums, traveling backward to the posterior area of the maxillary, then turning up under the zygomatic and then further posteriorly until contact is made with the pterygoid process. The pterygoid process on the lesion side will be found upward and lateral in contrast to the pterygoid process of the opposite side. In most cases it will be found crowding the coronoid process of the mandible on the lesion side. Palpation of the mastoid portions of the temporal bones will reveal the lesion side as inward in contrast to that of the opposite side.

Reduction is made by inserting the index finger gently on the pterygoid process of the lesion side in the same manner as in the examination. The finger holds the pterygoid process firmly while the patient is instructed to close the jaw gradually upon the finger. This movement exaggerates the lesion. When the finger senses the proper tension, the patient is again instructed to open the jaw gradually. Usually the pterygoid process releases and springs back into normal position, being guided by the finger.

In most cases, reduction of the pterygoid process also reduces the maxillary and the temporal fixations. In cases to the contrary, a gentle pull downward on the maxilla and then allowing it to spring backward accomplishes the reduction; increasing the inward position by compression on the temporal and then releasing secures return to the normal. Cases of short duration, within the period of a year, usually respond in one treatment. Those of longer duration require several treatments before reduction is accomplished.

> Note: The dental traumatic type of cranial membranous-articular strains occurs frequently. This type in itself, without reference to the various other types such as traumatic and viscerosomatic, opens a vast field of new possibilities to osteopathic practice. It likewise

invites cooperation by the dental profession. The writer is indebted to a leading Saint Paul dental surgeon for authentic information regarding the technique employed in surgical extraction. When I thanked him for the conference, he volunteered cooperation and said that he had gained more from the interview than I had.

16. Standing Posture Technique

The Osteopathic Profession, *October 1939.*

Many low back, mid-back and high back strains or lesions occur during standing or stooping postures. The reduction of such lesions indicates the application of standing posture technique, wherein it becomes possible to gain the effective maximum with a minimum of energy. According to an editorial statement in *The Osteopathic Profession*, "The wise physician pays great attention to developing a technique which will be maximally effective with a minimum of energy."

Low back lesions sustained during standing or stooping postures are not true sacroiliac or spinal types as a rule, although they may have diverse indications posturally. This type of patient usually hobbles into the office with the aid of a cane, assuming an exaggerated stooped and sidebending-rotation posture, especially manifested in the low back region and indicating sacroiliac and lumbar trouble.

These indications may be secondary to a primary femoral-acetabular lesion or twist initiated through muscular traction on the psoas major and iliacus muscles. In these types, reduction of the sacroiliac and lumbar lesions seldom secures the return to normal posture, and the patient is apt to hobble out in the same manner in which he made entrance because the femoral-acetabular twist continues its traction on the psoas major and iliacus muscles and causes rotation of the lumbar vertebrae.

The femoral-acetabular lesion, having been sustained during a standing or stooping posture, responds easily if the technique is applied in the same posture. The writer usually places a chair on the operating table, and the patient may rest his arms on this while in the standing posture. The patient should face the table while the technician sits in a chair at the lesion side.

The fingers of one hand fixate back of the trochanter, and the fingers of the other hand grasp the common tendon of the psoas major and iliacus near its insertion. The patient is then instructed to turn the opposite side of the pelvis forward and backward. The method is like the turning of a nut on a bolt rather than the turning of the bolt into the nut, or the turning of the acetabulum on the head of the femur rather than the laborious task of turning the head of the femur within the acetabulum. Old-timers at the American School of Osteopathy[1] will remember the method of turning the head of the femur within the acetabulum, wherein the patient reclined on the table while the leg was fixed on the abdomen and rotated externally and then held in external rotation with the operator's chin on the knee during extension of the leg.

The technician will find it an easier task to turn the acetabulum on the head of the femur in the standing posture wherein the patient furnishes the effective maximum and the physician the minimum by fixing the bone and tendon and guiding with trained, tactile skill.

The sacroiliac lesion is reduced in the standing posture while the technician sits at the lesion side, by fixating the ilium with one hand and the sacrum with the other and then holding and guiding as the patient turns or sidebends the opposite side of the pelvis.

In sacrolumbar lesions the technician is seated. One hand is placed on the sacrum near the fifth lumbar and the other passed around in front of the pelvis to the crest of the ilium. The patient is then instructed to keep the feet firmly on the floor and the arms upon the chair and to push the pelvis backward and rotate it from side to side while the technician guides the lesion.

Mid-back and high back lesions may be reduced advantageously during the standing posture also, as the posture provides normal relaxative movement throughout all the articulations of the vertebral column. The same method of fixation of the lesion site by the

---

1. The American School of Osteopathy was established in Kirksville, Missouri in 1892 by Dr. A. T. Still and was the first osteopathic school. Dr. Sutherland was a member of the graduating class of 1900.

technician's fingers is applied while the patient is instructed to flex, extend or sidebend in accordance with the movement necessary to reduction.

Certain types of upper rib lesions often typified by difficulty in reduction are sustained usually during a standing posture through overreaching efforts: the reaching effort commonly occurring in an upward and backward direction and causing traction on the serratus magnus muscle, which traction would be responsible for initiation of the rib lesion. In these types, the serratus magnus muscle may need attention before correction of the rib is begun.

There is apt to be a "charley horse" beneath the scapula tending to hold the rib in malposition. The technique is used during the standing posture. The technician places the fingers of one hand carefully and gently beneath the scapula from its anterior border below the glenoid fossa; the fingers travel as far backward and as near to the posterior border as possible and fixate the rib. The fingers of the opposite hand are placed over the acromioclavicular articulation. The patient is then instructed to lean toward the technician and to turn the opposite shoulder forward and then backward while the technician guides with trained tactile skill, which should include a mental picture of what is occurring at the vertebral facets.

The charley horse in the fibers of the serratus magnus is usually encountered by the fingers as they travel backward beneath the scapula. This condition should be overcome before making the rib reduction. It is accomplished by springing the scapula outward.

Lower rib lesions may be handled nicely in the standing posture technique.

Prolapsed organs of the abdominal region may be raised through the cooperation of the patient during the standing posture. The technician places his hands or fingers beneath the organ, and the patient is instructed to stand on tiptoe and push the pelvis backward and then forward, finally lowering the heels back to the floor, the technician guiding the organ meanwhile.

17. The Core-link Between the Cranial Bowl and the Pelvic Bowl

Bulletin Number Forty-Five, International Society of Sacro-Iliac Technicians.

This lecture was given at the meeting of the International Society of Sacro-Iliac Technicians during the annual convention of the American Osteopathic Association in St. Louis, Missouri in June, 1940. The Society functioned as "A Post-graduate Section of Special Research in Osteopathy." It is no longer active as an organized group.

Osteopathic technicians are familiar with the sympathetic, efferent and afferent nerve impulses functioning in relation to the head and pelvis. They understand as well the established osteopathic facts relative to pathological consequences resulting from ligamentous-articular fixations or lesions occurring at the sacroiliac joint. Hence it is unnecessary to review that section of the subject. The intraspinal membranes that surround the spinal cord act as a reciprocal tension tissue that links and regulates the cranial articular mechanism with the pelvic articular mechanism during the periods of respiration, according to indications from practical experience. I will endeavor to crawl into the cranial and vertebral core and consider the view from within rather than a view from without.

In my book, *The Cranial Bowl*, attention was called to a reciprocal tension membrane that regulates the articular mobility of the cranial bones, the membrane including the falx cerebri and the tentorium cerebelli. This reciprocal tension membrane has an anterior superior pole of attachment on the crista galli of the ethmoid, an anterior inferior pole on the clinoid processes of the sphenoid, lateral poles on the petrous portions of the temporal bones and a posterior pole on the occiput. During respiration, the reciprocal tension membrane, at the inhalation period, allows the ethmoid to drop downward while drawing the sphenoid and the petrous portions upward and the occiput forward. At the exhalation period, it allows the sphenoid and petrous portions to drop downward and the occiput backward while drawing the ethmoid upward.

The brain and spinal cord function in *unison* during the respiratory periods, the spinal cord drawing upward during inhalation and dropping downward during exhalation. There is a *unity* of the cranial articular mechanism with the spinal articular mechanism, *the latter including the sacrum of the pelvic bowl.* The intraspinal membranes surround the spinal cord and are the *main threads* upon which our subject *hangs*.

The intraspinal membranes are continuations of the intracranial membranes. It is well to take note of the anatomical facts that the dural membrane is lacking in attachment to the periosteum of the vertebrae as it is within the cranium. It has only two attachments below the occiput: one in the upper cervical region and the other at the sacrum.[1] I wish to point out to you that the intraspinal membranes *hang*, or are *suspended, through* the vertebral column until they reach their attachment on the sacrum. I wish to reason toward a purpose that may be served by the design in this special arrangement. The arrangement indicates a specific reciprocal tension tissue to regulate articular mobility at its two points of attachment: at the cranial articular mechanism and at the pelvic articular mechanism. So, in addition to the reciprocal tension membrane functioning between articular poles within the cranium, we have a reciprocal tension membrane likewise functioning between

---

1. Subsequent anatomic studies have demonstrated that the dura mater is attached to the vertebral canal in the lumbar region. The anterior attachments are short and strong while the posterior attachments are weaker and longer. The anterior and anterolateral connective tissue bands attach to the posterior longitudinal ligament. The bands are strongest at the L5-S1 level and less strong in the upper lumbar region. The dural nerve root sheaths are also attached to the posterior longitudinal ligament anteriorly and to the periosteum of the inferior pedicle laterally. Cf. Parkin and Harrison, "The Topographical Anatomy of the Lumbar Epidural Space," *Journal of Anatomy* 141 (1985):211-217, and Spencer, Irwin and Miller, "Anatomy and Significance of Fixation of the Lumbosacral Nerve Roots in Sciatica," *Spine* 8, no. 6 (1983): 672-679.

the cranial articular mechanism and the pelvic articular mechanism, the two reciprocal tension membranes functioning in unison during the respiratory periods. During exhalation the sphenobasilar area of the cranial mechanism extends in its mobility while the sacrum drops forward on its sacroiliac articulations, and during inhalation the sphenobasilar area flexes while the sacrum draws backward on is sacroiliac articulations.

Another function of the reciprocal intraspinal membrane is that of fluctuating the cerebrospinal fluid within the vertebral column. As the sphenobasilar area extends and the sacrum drops forward, the membrane fluctuates the fluid, and as the sphenobasilar area flexes and the sacrum draws backward, the membrane again fluctuates the fluid within the vertebral column.

Articular fixations at the sacroiliac limit this functioning, and as time runs along, articular fixations become established secondarily within the cranial articulations. Chronic articular fixations of the cranial mechanism limit the activity of the cerebral convolutions, and nerve impulses are disturbed that lead to pathologies in the pelvis.

Attention to the reduction of cranial articular fixations as well as to the sacroiliac articular fixations is important. Attention thus given to the cranial mechanism has many surprises to offer in overcoming pelvic pathologies. While not criticizing our ambulant surgical practitioners, I prefer trying osteopathic methods that get back to fundamental etiologic factors rather than the application of local treatment. My endeavors in this direction have borne fruit.

Tests of this core-link movement aid in the diagnosis of sacroiliac articular fixations and even in the differential diagnosis of one sacroiliac from the other.

18. Standing Posture Technique in Relation to the Sacroiliac

Bulletin Number Sixty-five, International Society of Sacro-Iliac Technicians.[1]

In St. Louis your attention was directed to the relationship of cranial articular mobility to the sacroiliac. Mention of these facts was made: that there are no muscular agencies of propulsion concerned in cranial articular mobility and that there are no muscular attachments between the sacrum and the ilia. It was stated that muscular agencies are unnecessary in cranial mobility as its activity is *involuntary*, occurring as the periods of respiration, and that the sacroiliac articulations are also *involuntary* in their activity, likewise occurring as respiratory periods. We also stated that the intracranial and intraspinal membranes function as the agencies of this *involuntary* activity. Recognition of this viewpoint interprets some of the various ideas of others concerning lesions at the sacroiliac, as well as my own.

Today your attention is called to a *postural* mobility at this articulation as well as to the *involuntary*. In the involuntary, the sacrum rotates between the ilia, and in the postural, the ilia rotate on the sacrum. The involuntary operates through the accommodation of the intraspinal membranes during respiratory periods and *the postural through the accommodation of the sacroiliac and sacrosciatic ligaments, brought about by gravity and indirect leverage.* [The sacrosciatic ligaments are the sacrotuberous (greater sacrosciatic) and sacrospinous (lesser sacrosciatic) ligaments collectively.] Although there are muscular attachments from the sacrum and ilia to the trochanters, as well as from the pubic arch to the femur, these muscles have very little to do, if anything, in the

1. The International Society of Sacro-Iliac Technicians was an informal organization of osteopathic physicians who met annually to explore new viewpoints and concepts in the field of osteopathy.

accomplishment of articular activity at the sacroiliac. Dr. Virgil Halladay presents a similar thought in his *Applied Anatomy of the Spine* [p. 138]. The sacroiliac ligament as well as the greater and lesser sacrosciatic, in their special arrangement of transverse and oblique portions, act as *check agencies* in accommodation of postural mobility. The intraspinal membranes act as *check agencies* in accommodation of the involuntary.

Many, possibly the great majority, of sacroiliac lesions occur during the standing or stooping posture. These usually happen through indirect leverage when the femurs are in abduction. For example, a patient spreads the legs wide apart while pushing a stalled car out of a snowbank. While pushing he is inclined to inhale deeply and hold the breath. Consequently, there is extreme tension placed on the intraspinal membranes as well as upon the sacroiliac ligaments, and the bones move beyond their normal range of mobility. The same forces operate during a stooping posture and even in a sitting position, for example, a farmer sitting on a milking stool with femurs in abduction. There is one case on record in my files where a farmer sat on the ground with his femurs in abduction around a hill of corn during the light task of weeding. He found it necessary to call for help and later came into the office by the aid of a crutch.

While experimenting with Dr. Halladay's animated pelvic specimen[2], first on exhibition in Chicago at the American Osteopathic Association convention in 1919, I discovered that abduction of the femurs causes the ilia to rotate posteriorly, or inward on the sacrum, and that the sacrum drops forward, thus narrowing the lateral diameter of the pelvis and that abduction of the femurs rotates the ilia forward and widens the lateral pelvic diameter. This experimentation

---

2. Virgil Halladay, D.O. (American School of Osteopathy, 1916). Author of *Applied Anatomy of the Spine*, Dr. Halladay was a professor of anatomy at the American School of Osteopathy in Kirksville, Missouri. He developed a chemical process by which the natural flexibility of the ligaments in cadaveric specimens could be preserved. He prepared such specimens of the spine, rib cage and pelvis that were often called the "animated skeleton."

changed my previous ideas regarding diagnosis and technique at the sacroiliac.

Diagnosis: The diagnosis is advantageously made with the patient in the standing position while testing for immobility at the articulation. A chair is placed flat on the table to increase the height as well as to act as a support for the patient's arms or hands. The patient faces the side of the table with arms or hands resting on the chair while the physician sits comfortably in a chair immediately back of the patient. The test for immobility is first made with the patient's legs close together. He is instructed to push the hips backward and forward as well as laterally while the physician's fingers contact the ligaments to note their tensity as well as the mobility of the articulation. The patient then abducts the legs, and the same procedure follows in the test. He then crosses the legs followed by similar procedure. This concerns the postural test for immobility. The patient stands in a normal posture and is instructed to inhale deeply and to inhale with the brain rather than the diaphragm. In case of a fixation or immobility, the ilium or ilia will move upward along with the sacrum.

Technique: In all spinal technique, it is my custom to have the patient exercise his own natural forces rather than the application of mine. There are no thrusts, no jerks nor the application of another or distal end of the anatomy as a lever. The principle is that used and taught by Dr. Still, namely, exaggeration of the lesion to the degree of release and then allowing the ligaments to draw the articulations back into normal relationship. This same method is applied in sacroiliac technique.

The patient faces the side of the table in the standing posture with hands or arms resting on the chair, as in diagnosis. The physician sits in a chair at the patient's back. In case of a fixation on the right side, indicated as anterior or forward rotation of the ilium, the patient abducts the legs as far as possible, and the physician places the left palm on the sacrum at its lower area and the right hand on the crest of the right ilium. The patient is then instructed to push forward with the right hip and backward with the left, to exaggerate the lesion to its degree of release, at which degree he is instructed to push backward on the right hip and forward on the left, the physician's hand, in the meantime, guiding in the direction of the desired movement.

Another method is to have the patient bend the knees while the femurs are in abduction. In this position the ilia merely hang in suspension upon the sacrum, one might say, suspended like a skeleton, and manipulation thereof is as easy as it might be applied to the skeletal specimen. In some cases one may allow the patient to drop the pelvis down on the physician's knees, the knee functioning in the manner of the Old Doctor's sacroiliac chair.[3] The pubic arches are shifted from side to side or forward and backward as desired in accommodation to reduction of the lesion. As easy in accomplishment as trotting a baby on one's knee. The technique is applicable with the femurs in adduction, if so indicated, in which case the patient crosses one leg over the other.

Note: In many cases of low back lesions occurring in the standing or stooping posture, a twist or rotation of the head of the femur within the acetabulum is often the primary one at fault. This lesion limits either external or internal rotation of the leg and causes leverage through the acetabulum affecting the sacroiliac articulation, as well as tension on the psoas major and iliacus muscles, with consequent rotation throughout the lumbar area. This lesion should have primary attention.

---

3. In his later years, Dr. A. T. Still was respectfully referred to as the Old Doctor.

19. Pelvic Technique

Mankato, Minnesota, June 13, 1941.

Written for the sections of technique and manipulative therapy given at Atlantic City, June 1941.

Fraternal Greetings:

To the intelligent and experienced group of osteopathic physicians of forty years and more, the group who went forth into a field of experience in guiding bodily tissues into normal relationship without other equipment than "ten little fingers" trained in the skillful art of thinking, feeling and seeing, and the group who through that wonderful experience not only proved for themselves but also demonstrated to the world that Dr. Andrew Taylor Still's scientific therapeutic principle is superior to all others.

As one of these "forty yearlings" I have been requested to include "some brief description of a bit of osteopathic technique that can be applied to some specific condition and be depended upon for results. Something that I know from experience *works*."

As an indication that my experience concerns the pelvic bowl as well as the cranial bowl, my "bit" relates to the muscular floor of the pelvis. During that early day experience I found it necessary to compete with the needle. So, when modern ambulant proctology methods entered our fold, my fingers began thinking, feeling and seeking out another pathway in competition, this competitive venture being in the nature of force of habit and the pleasure of personal accomplishment, rather than criticism of the modern method. The venture was quite satisfactory, and it *works* for others, judging from a recent letter from a 1922 graduate to whom it has been my pleasure to pass along the technique. He writes: "It has been astonishing a time or two when I raised the pelvic organs or other organs that have migrated to the pelvis by your method. How it changed the patient's symptomatology."

In this method, the patient stands facing the table with hands resting thereon. The physician sits comfortably in a chair behind the patient. Two fingers, the first and second, are gently inserted between the external wall of the rectum and the internal area of the ischium. The patient then sits gently downward upon the fingers which are gently crawling upward into the pelvic bowl. When they have reached a desired field, detected only by trained tactile sense, they hold gently and firmly while the patient takes a slow deep inspiration. As the patient slowly exhales, the organs that have migrated down into the pelvis "jump" upward away from the fingers.

In answer to the question regarding experience in pneumonia: *Yes*, I would not only or solely be willing, I would insist upon *competent* manipulative treatment and good nursing in my own case as well as in a case in my family.

20. Correspondence Undated

Excerpts from a letter.

...you have that scientific mind, searching for scientific interpretation of cranial mobility. Yet it seems from your questions that you have the "cart before the horse," and quite different from my hypothesis. Our first endeavor, scientific, is to prove the fact of cranial articular mobility. Until we can furnish such proof, I would much prefer that nothing appear.... When we have the proof, Dr. Hulburt is ready to accept scientific articles from scientific members of the profession like yourself.[1] So please do not prepare anything at present. As soon as we have something definite I will gladly acquaint you with the facts as we find them.... Now, I will endeavor to answer the questions, although it is difficult between busy hours of interruption:

One–Primarily, it is the restriction of the normal fluctuation of the cerebrospinal fluid that causes the changes in the pH and CO_2 findings. Remember that *all* the physiological centers, including the physiological center of respiration, are located in the medulla oblongata or the floor of the fourth ventricle. Their operation is secondary to the operation of the primary respiratory mechanism, as I have stated elsewhere. While the pH and CO_2 changes do affect the physiological centers, the same cranial lesion can and frequently does cause "kinks" in the cerebral aqueduct. The cerebrospinal fluid (mechanically, in its fluctuation) acts somewhat like an hydraulic brake system and locks the movement of the brain, a part of the power mechanism of primary respiration. The "Breath of Life" is the spark, primarily, and not the breath of *air.* The breath of air is merely one of the material elements that the Breath of Life utilizes in man's walkabout here on

---

1. Ray G. Hulburt, D.O. (1884-1947: American School of Osteopathy, 1920) was the editor of the *Journal of the American Osteopathic Association.*

earth.[2] In fact, the brain, the cerebrospinal fluid, the intracranial membranes, the physiological centers and so forth are merely secondary elements in the walkabout on earth.

Two–Keep in mind that primarily it is the normal fluctuation of the cerebrospinal fluid that is back of all the changes in the ingredients. The changes affect the nuclei secondarily.

Three–Yes, according to a recent text the cerebrospinal fluid receives products from the pituitary body. However, *motion* of the pituitary is more important than the function of its secretion. Without the motion that occurs as the sphenoid moves upward and downward during respiratory periods, there would be no resultant secretion by the pituitary. The interchange occurring between the cerebrospinal fluid and the blood at the areas of the choroid plexuses is more important. Here is where the chemical interchange occurs.

Four–Possibly.

Five–...the dural membrane is tense, acting as a "check ligament" as well as an agency of propulsion between the articular poles of attachment, as I have stated elsewhere.

Six–...

Seven–The temporal bone is like a wobbling wheel in its mobility. Take a disarticulated temporal bone. Hold the bone with a thumb and forefinger, finger on tip of petrous portion and thumb back of the external meatus. With a finger of the opposite hand, move the zygomatic process upward and downward. Note that as the petrous portion rotates externally, the mastoid portion is prominent externally and the mastoid process is depressed inwardly. As the petrous portion rotates internally, the mastoid portion is depressed internally and the mastoid process becomes prominent externally. As the basilar area of the occiput moves forward during inhalation, or flexion,

---

2. For a fuller discussion of Dr. Sutherland's use of the Breath of Life see article 23, "Untitled Talk 1944." Cf. "And the Lord God formed man of the dust of the ground, and breathed into his nostrils the breath of life; and man became a living soul." Gen. 2:7, King James Version.

the mastoid portion will move backward, and as the basilar area of the occiput moves backward during exhalation, or extension, the mastoid portion will move forward.

Fraternally,
W.G.S.

21. Correspondence November 1943

Excerpts related to the "Lippincott Notes," A Manual of Cranial Technique.[1]

There is *much* that might be included in the "Lippincott Notes" were the *much* not so "fanatical" to the customary reasoning of mice and men. The *much* concerns information gained through personal experiences as the "guinea pig" during my earlier days of cranial progress. Those early personal experiences are the source of my endeavor to answer your question as to "both voluntary and involuntary activity within the cranium not connected with skeletal activity."

One can voluntarily control the involuntary activity, independently of all skeletal activity–that is, one can voluntarily activate the cerebral hemispheres into the same normal involuntary activity that occurs during the periods of respiration and also voluntarily activate the cerebellum into the same involuntary activity that occurs during the periods of respiration. During the voluntary activity, one can *feel* the cerebrospinal fluid being drawn from beneath the arachnoid membrane into the fourth ventricle and fluctuated up into the third and lateral ventricles during the period of inhalation.[2] Likewise, one can *feel* the cerebrospinal fluid being drawn from the lateral and third ventricles into the fourth and then fluctuated out into the area beneath the arachnoid membrane during the period of exhalation. In fact, I found that one may "compress the bulb," that is the fourth ventricle, through voluntary activity of the cerebellum independently

---

1. Howard A. and Rebecca C. Lippincott, *A Manual of Cranial Technique.* This manuscript was often referred to as the "Lippincott Notes" and was prepared from material supplied by Dr. Sutherland. It was later incorporated into Harold I. Magoun's *Osteopathy in the Cranial Field,* 1st ed.

2. This report stems from the series of experiments on his own skull with bandages, etc. See article 28, "Obtaining Knowledge Versus Information" for a greater discussion of these experiments.

of the skeletal factor. This early experimentation led to my hypothesis concerning the fluctuation of the cerebrospinal fluid and also to the compression of the bulb technique as now given in cranial instruction.[3]

That personal knowledge is something that one must feel inside his own skull in order to understand the action. The problem lies in how to teach it to others, for one can only lead up to it in the instruction through primary avenues like the study of the mobility of the cranial bones. Thus far, the instruction is none too easy.

In the appendix to the "Lippincott Notes," attention is called to the importance of teaching the patient to breathe with the brain instead of with the secondary respiratory mechanisms. It is another step in the progressive study aimed to grasp the body of Dr. Still's "osteopathic squirrel" still within the "hole in the tree."[4]

I certainly agree with you concerning the importance of thorough study of what you term the "opposing structures, such as the cervical muscles, fascias and muscles of the face and pharynx. Also that the structures about the jugular foramen play a part in the whole picture." As you outline it, "The respiratory effort" *is* divided "into abdominal, thoracic and cervical areas," but they occur secondarily to the *primary* cranial respiratory effort which may act independently of the secondary. Aside from the structures around the jugular foramen, have you thought about the nine muscles subadjacent to the mandible? Multiplied by two, there are 18 of these muscles. Tack on to these the levator and tensor palati, the soft palate and the tongue. Any sphenobasilar or temporal bone lesion is bound to disturb the normal activity of these muscles and should always be included in the anatomical-physiological mental picture in diagnosis and technique.

---

3. The technique "compression of the bulb" was later renamed "compression of the fourth ventricle."

4. Dr. A. T. Still presented osteopathy as a science, a philosophy and an art whose potential was not fully realized, much as a squirrel only partially seen within a hole in a tree would not be fully visualized. He stated that only the tail of the squirrel was currently in view.

22. Correspondence 1943

Excerpt from a letter dated November 30, 1943.

Inasmuch as the cranial thought is yet a mere "breech presentation" of Dr. Still's "osteopathic squirrel" in the "hole of the tree"[1], the "amplification of the basic consideration of cranial technique" needs scientific minds like yours. It is gratifying to note your interest, and I shall be pleased to hear from you regarding the subject at any time. I will endeavor to answer as adequately as possible. I might predict that there will be many diverse opinions relative to that basic consideration in the years ahead. There may be as many theories as now exist relative to the method of formation of the cerebrospinal fluid and the concept of a dialyzing equilibrium with the blood plasma. There is a reason for the continuation of theorizing about the processes concerned with the subject. It is because that *hidden* "Breath of Life" is left out. I have frequently called attention to the fact that I do not refer to the "breath of air," which I consider to be one of the *material* elements utilized by the Breath of Life in man's walkabout on earth.[2]

It was recognition of the supreme potency of the Breath of Life as the *initiative spark* to involuntary activity that interpreted my hypothesis relative to the primary respiratory mechanism. When you, in personal experiment, use your own cranium as a "guinea pig," as I have done in the years past, you may perhaps understand the involuntary

---

1. Dr. A. T. Still presented osteopathy as a science, a philosophy and an art whose potential was not fully realized, much as a squirrel only partially seen within a hole in a tree would not be fully visualized. He stated that only the tail of the squirrel was currently in view.

2. For a fuller discussion of Dr. Sutherland's use of the Breath of Life see article 23, "Untitled Talk 1944." Cf. "And the Lord God formed man of the dust of the ground, and breathed into his nostrils the breath of life; and man became a living soul." Gen. 2:7, King James Version.

activity as initiated by the Breath of Life. Call it what you may, it is the "something" that starts the movement of "some form of energy dissipation which has to be derived from somewhere." (Your quotation).

...one might say that there are *both* maximal and minimal degrees in the movement of the brain. The maximal occurs during deep inhalation and exhalation, and the minimal during the "idling of the motor" that occurs following compression of the fourth ventricle. Compression of the fourth ventricle is followed by the situation wherein the periods of respiration manifest changes of rhythm in the shorter or minimal degree.

Should you care to experiment, the following method may aid in the understanding of the degrees of motion. Lie supine on a table. Clasp the hands over the sagittal suture at the lambda and compress firmly over the mastoid angels of the parietals and the lambdoidal sutures. Hold continually while you exhale step by step to the lowest degree of exhalation, and then inhale step by step to the highest degree of inhalation. Repeat the respiratory steps several times and then release the compression. Following this, note carefully the outward movement of the mastoid angles of the parietals and *feel* the expansion of the hemispheres of the brain. Try the same procedure on a patient.

The construction of a mental picture might help you in the recognition of the *feel* of the movement of the hemispheres. A way of doing this is to crawl inside the cranium mentally and assume a reserved seat on the foramen magnum and thus have a position for *visualizing* the activity as well as *feeling* it. One of the fundamental keys to diagnosis and technique is the ability to get within the cranium mentally and visualize all the activities going on. In answer to your question about the changes elsewhere in the brain, the following picture contains the highlights. As the hemispheres expand upward and outward during inhalation, the third ventricle dilates in a V-shaped manner. This draws the floor of the ventricle upward and thus lifts the pituitary body upward. The pituitary body, being firmly strapped down to the sella turcica by a strong dural membrane, naturally lifts the posterior end of the sphenoid upward and tips the anterior end into its "nosedive." Then, during exhalation, the third ventricle contracts, and the floor of the ventricle recedes downward and drops the pituitary body and posterior end of the sphenoid downward with consequent upward movement of the anterior end. The falx cerebri and tentorium cerebelli, being tense at all periods, participate in the movement in a reciprocating manner and act as check ligaments. They, together with the arachnoid membrane, fluctuate the large body of cerebrospinal fluid that surrounds the brain. I would not say that the expansion of the hemispheres against the membranes does the "pushing."

23. Untitled Talk 1944

This talk was given without notes during a course of instruction at the Des Moines Still College of Osteopathy and Surgery in 1944. The talk was transcribed from either shorthand notes or a recording. A mounted disarticulated skull, separate cranial bones and many anatomical charts were on display, as was customary in Dr. Sutherland's courses of instruction in cranial osteopathy. These and the actual demonstration of techniques are frequently referred to in the talk.

At the time of my talks before the Academy of Applied Osteopathy meeting in Chicago, a member of the profession put two questions to me: "Is the cranial concept a religious one?" and "Where did you find the bug to think out this stuff?"

While meditating on a promise to write an autobiography–that it seems there will never be time to fulfill–I have wondered if I might devote the opening chapter to a consideration of these two questions. My answers at the time were as follows.

If the recognition by Dr. Andrew Taylor Still of God as creator of the human body is religious, then the science of osteopathy, in concept, is religious. If the science of osteopathy is religious, then the cranial concept *in* osteopathy is religious. The science of osteopathy is a specialty and those who practice that specialty are specialists. The cranial concept itself is not a specialty. It is osteopathy, and the credit belongs to Dr Still.

The concept of the science of osteopathy came during a sad period in Dr. Still's life when he had lost members of his immediate family. The experience was related to his loss of faith in orthodox medical methods. The new concept came at an hour when a sincere prayer went up to his Maker for guidance.[1] Dr. Still studied the living human body

---

1. In the spring of 1864, spinal meningitis killed three of Dr. Still's children despite

in great detail and developed a knowledge of its anatomical-physiological mechanisms that became the keynote of his phenomenal skill in diagnosis and technique. In all of his lectures and talks, he never neglected to refer to his Maker, the Maker of the human body.

Where did I find "the bug" to think out this "cranial stuff?" Some 46 years ago, while a student at the American School of Osteopathy in Kirksville, Missouri, my attention was drawn to the bones of a disarticulated skull that Dr. Still had on display among other anatomical specimens. The thought came, like a bolt from the blue: "*Beveled like the gills of a fish; indicating articular mobility for a respiratory mechanism.*" Because of my doubt of the possibility of such mobility, that guiding thought became a compelling whip, stimulating me to dig and find out. It became "the bug" in my system.

In my study of the intricate articular surfaces on the cranial bones, I found that every detail on those articular surfaces indicated mobility for a respiratory mechanism. In the continued study, I eventually began experiments on my own skull–even to the point of creating cranial lesions for the study of their effects. Some of these effects were quite serious, but they helped to show the way.

Someone has said, "To the dreamer who can work and to the worker who can dream, life surrenders all things." That might be modified to read, "To the dreamer who will dig and to the digger who can dream, the science of osteopathy provides possibilities superior to all other therapeutic methods."

You already know from Dr. Kimberly's lectures covering the anatomy of this region[2] that you are going to have many dreams and

---

the best efforts of both preacher and physician. It was a time of great spiritual crisis for Dr. Still, the resolution of which resulted in the birth of the science of osteopathy ten years later. See Still, *Autobiography*, pp. 87-88, 303-304.

2. Paul E. Kimberly, D.O. (Des Moines Still College of Osteopathy, 1940) was a professor of anatomy at the Des Moines Still College of Osteopathy. Beginning in 1944, he arranged for Dr. Sutherland to use the college facilities to conduct classes in "Osteopathy in the Cranial Field." At these courses Dr. Kimberly would extensively review the anatomy of the human head.

that there is reason for meeting with others in monthly study groups to dig into this subject further. Remember that Dr. Still said in reference to osteopathy, "We merely have a grip on the tail of the squirrel in the hole of the tree." Much of the osteopathic squirrel is still within "the hole of the tree." The cranial concept is but a portion of the whole. There are undreamed of possibilities in the science of osteopathy as conceived by Dr. Still. Each dream may initiate the working out of an hypothesis. It is necessary to have a beginning.

We learn of the creation of man that, "the Breath of Life," not the breath of air, "was breathed into the nasals of a form of clay and man became a living soul."[3] I consider the breath of air as one of the material elements utilized by man in his walkabout here on earth. The human brain is a motor; the Breath of Life is a spark of ignition to the motor, something that is not material, that we cannot see.

In my hypothesis, I have described what we call the primary respiratory mechanism. This mechanism includes the brain, the cerebrospinal fluid, the intracranial membranes and the articular mobility of the cranial bones; also the spinal cord, the intraspinal membranes, the same cerebrospinal fluid and the involuntary mobility of the sacrum between the ilia. Critics have pointed out to me that there are no muscles attached to the sacrum and the ilia to provide for articular mobility between them. Yet mobility between them has been demonstrated. It has also been pointed out that there are no muscles attached from bone to bone in the cranial structure to provide articular motion between them. It is therefore apparent that the mobility of the sacrum between the ilia and the mobility between the cranial bones is not provided by muscular agencies. It is not the voluntary articular mobility that is motivated by muscular action. The mobility of the cranial mechanism and also the mobility of the sacrum between the ilia is an involuntary movement, and the whole functions

---

3. "And the Lord God formed man of the dust of the ground, and breathed into his nostrils the breath of life; and man became a living soul." Gen. 2:7, King James Version.

as a unit during the periods of respiration. The mechanical interpretation of the design of the articular surfaces of the cranial bones, such as the beveled articular surfaces, indicates mobility related to a respiratory mechanism. This does not refer to the respiratory mechanism concerned with the breath of air. As all the physiologic centers of the human body, including the respiratory center, are located in the floor of the fourth ventricle, a primary respiratory mechanism that includes all the elements already named would be primary to thoracic respiration through the center of respiration.

As a beginning in the study of the primary respiratory mechanism, consider a cast of the ventricles of the brain and spinal cord. Notice its bird-like form. Here we have the body of the "bird," and the cerebral aqueduct with the fourth ventricle and the central canal of the spinal cord resembling the tail of the bird. Notice where these lateral ventricles are attached. They are located as one would find the wings of a bird attached at the superior anterior border of the third ventricle. Thus we can use the lateral ventricles as an illustration of the wings of the bird that flies. We will take this cerebral hemisphere and put it around that lateral ventricle in its normal position. This develops the wings of the bird. Now put the Breath of Life in there with the spark that ignites the motor, and visualize the convolutions of the hemisphere expanding. What does the bird do when it flies? The wings move outward posteriorly during the inhalation period of respiration. Now watch the third ventricle. See the third ventricle dilating in a V-shape manner. Note that the floor of the ventricle moves upward and that the roof stretches out.

What is attached on the floor of the third ventricle? The infundibulum which runs down to the little pituitary body riding in the sella turcica, or the saddle. The body is not riding freely in the saddle but is strapped down into the sella turcica by dural membrane. The infundibulum draws that little body upward at the posterior area of the sphenoid during inspiration. Consequently, the anterior end of the sphenoid goes downward. The brain does not require muscular agencies for the movement of its structure within the cranium. It lifts the little pituitary body upward and tips the sphenoid into a "nosedive" during the period of inhalation. What happens during the exhalation period? Birds fly, light on trees and fold their wings down. The upper area of the third ventricle where the wings are attached moves inward, the roof of the third ventricle crowds together, the floor drops down and the little pituitary body drops downward while the anterior end of the sphenoid elevates.

Hilton stated in *Rest and Pain* [p. 24], "...the central parts of the base of the brain...rest upon this collection of cerebrospinal fluid which forms for it a most beautiful, efficient and perfectly adapted water bed." To this I add, not only rests, but rocks its cranial articular cradle. There are two "water beds," the cisterna interpeduncularis and the cisterna magna.

In the study of the spinal column, you learned that the ligaments hold the vertebrae together and allow a range of mobility. You might call them "check ligaments" or "reciprocal tension ligaments." Direct your attention to the reciprocal tension membrane here in the cranium, the falx cerebri and the tentorium cerebelli. I have told you that the membrane continues down the spinal column, hanging like a hollow tube, with firm attachment only at its upper area around the foramen magnum and one or two of the upper cervical vertebrae, and at its lower area to the sacrum.[4] Here, in the falx cerebri and the tentorium cerebelli, we have the reciprocal tension membrane between poles of articular attachment in the cranial mechanism. As the sphenoid is lifted during inhalation, the reciprocal tension membrane lifts

---

4. Subsequent anatomic studies have demonstrated that the dura mater is attached to the vertebral canal in the lumbar region. The anterior attachments are short and strong while the posterior attachments are weaker and longer. The anterior and anterolateral connective tissue bands attach to the posterior longitudinal ligament. The bands are strongest at the L5-S1 level and less strong in the upper lumbar region. The dural nerve root sheaths are also attached to the posterior longitudinal ligament anteriorly and to the periosteum of the inferior pedicle laterally. Cf. Parkin and Harrison, "The Topographical Anatomy of the Lumbar Epidural Space," *Journal of Anatomy* 141 (1985):211-217, and Spencer, Irwin and Miller, "Anatomy and Significance of Fixation of the Lumbosacral Nerve Roots in Sciatica," *Spine* 8, no. 6 (1983): 672-679.

the petrous portions of the temporal bones into external rotation from the median line. At the same time, we see the foramen magnum move forward, lifting the intraspinal membranes and drawing the sacrum posteriorly between the ilia. During exhalation, the reciprocal tension membrane moves the opposite way: The posterior part of the sphenoid drops down, the petrous portions rotate internally and the intraspinal membrane drops the sacrum anteriorly between the ilia.

Beneath the dural membrane we have the arachnoid membrane, beneath which the cerebrospinal fluid fluctuates within the brain, around the brain, around the spinal cord–like an hydraulic brake mechanism in an automobile. It has an intracranial force. The emergency brake system in an automobile can really stop the car. The cerebrospinal fluid is not only an hydraulic mechanism but also has chemicals within it similar to those found in arterial blood plus something else–elements of which more may be known in the future. The arterial stream may be supreme but the cerebrospinal fluid is in command.[5]

Out on the battlefields today, terrific explosions are creating heavy vibrations. In many instances these affect the membranes of people in the environment, locking them down over the little cerebral lakes of cerebrospinal fluid. We will be meeting this effect in our practices of the future.

These cases will have the same problem as one I will cite that arose from a combination of toxic and physical causes. The instance occurred on the shore of Lake Erie where there is a long stretch of shallow water. The man had been imbibing moonshine liquor of poor quality, for it was in the days of prohibition. He had waded out into the water and was suddenly taken with a meningeal shock where the depth was hardly above his knees. His companion carried him back to shore where they worked over him with methods of respiratory resuscitation even though there was no water in his lungs.

I was a guest in a nearby cottage, and we hastened to the scene

---

5. Reference is being made to Dr. Still's principle that the rule of the artery is supreme and Dr. Sutherland's addition that the cerebrospinal fluid is in command.

upon hearing the commotion. The man was blue and stiff as a cadaver with no sign of respiration. He appeared to be dead. I grasped his temporal bones and threw them into external rotation. A warm sensation appeared and respiration began. I released my grasp and respiration ceased. Bystanders called out, "Why doesn't someone send for a doctor?" I repeated the technique, and the same warm sensation resulted as respiration returned. The man turned his head and spoke to his sister. The Breath of Life, not the breath of air, was still present. It was the spark that ignited the motor. I merely "cranked the starter mechanism" of material respiration.[6]

The ventricles are expanding during inhalation. Visualize that body of cerebrospinal fluid fluctuating through the fourth ventricle during inhalation as well as through the third and the two lateral ventricles. The ventricles dilate during this period. During exhalation, the ventricles contract and the fluid fluctuates in the opposite direction, fluctuating also around the brain and the spinal cord. It is an hydraulic mechanism which we utilize with respiration in the reduction of cranial lesions.

We have an articular mobility in the cranial base which is formed by bones that ossified in cartilage. This is the cranial bowl, and mobility would be impossible here without some compensation in the vault whose bones are formed and ossify in membrane. This compensation is achieved by two features. One is the provision for sutural movement indicated in the serrated design of the articulations between the bones that form the cranial vault. The other is the flexibility throughout the structural portions of these bones that form in membrane. The diploe has two walls. The inner wall is smooth and the outer is rough. There is fluid between the two walls. Thus, to repeat, the bones that are formed in membrane provide compensation to articular mobility between the bones of the cranial base that are formed in cartilage.

---

6. This story is also told in Sutherland, *Cranial Bowl*, p. 54.

Here we have a schematic sketch designed to clarify the movement of the sphenoid and occiput. The sphenoid, including the sella turcica, is shown as a wheel with spokes. As the sphenoid circumrotates, or revolves, the various locations on the wheel move as suggested by the spokes. The movement of the sphenoid is not a backward nor a forward movement. The occiput, too, turns like a wheel. The two wheels turn at the same time. During inhalation, the sphenoid wheel turns anteriorly and the occiput posteriorly; thus you see the sella turcica and the anterior end of the basilar process of the occiput both moving upward. During exhalation, just the opposite occurs: The sphenoid bone turns posteriorly and the occiput anteriorly. Thus the sella turcica drops downward, the basilar process drops downward and the jugular foramen and the foramen magnum turn with the wheel, as represented by the spokes.[7]

The junction of the sphenoid and the basilar process of the occiput is an arch. It is somewhat like one of those bridges on the Chicago river that opens up and closes down, both sides together. Although it moves downward, it remains an arch as it lowers. This is an important point in visualization when it comes to cranial technique. This junction has been likened to a symphysis. It is most important as an area in the cranial mechanism, an area which you cannot feel directly but which you must visualize. It is like the area of the vertebral bodies in that you cannot palpate the body of a vertebra, but you have the mental picture. Your sense of touch observes the transverse processes and that observation tells you of the position of the body. You can learn to tell the position at the junction between the body of the sphenoid and the basilar process of the occiput by the sense of touch. This is not difficult, although it may seem so to you right now.

Now we come to the study of the two temporal bones as they join in the movement of the cranial base. First we consider their form and location between the sphenoid and occiput, and then we note

---

7. Illustrations of this general concept may be found in Sutherland, *Teachings*, pp. 26, 29.

what the study of their articular surfaces tells us about the mechanics of their motion, as the sphenoid and occiput circumrotate into flexion and extension at the sphenobasilar "symphysis." This mental picture will give us the understanding of the normal motion going on all the time in the cranial bowl. From this mechanical understanding of the normal we will be able to observe and interpret the variations and abnormalities to be understood when we meet them in our patients. For we must have a working diagnosis before we come to consider lesions of this area and techniques for correcting them. Two basic motions that occur in the cranial base, other than flexion and extension, are sidebending and torsion. The temporal bones enter into these significantly. In fact, I sometimes think of them as mischief makers.

The temporal bone moves like a wobbling wheel. If you hold one in your hand with one finger on the tip of the petrous portion and another at the base of the mastoid process, and then contact the zygomatic process with the other hand, you will observe that when you pull down on the zygomatic process, the petrous portion rotates externally, that is, away from the medial line. As I lift up on the zygomatic process, you see that the petrous portion rotates internally toward the medial line. Now you note that the petrous portions are located on a diagonal that points forward into the head. Place them into the cranial base between the occiput and the sphenoid, and fit the grooves on them to the tongues on the sides of the basilar process of the occiput, and you have the picture for motion. When the sphenoid and occiput move into flexion during the inhalation period, the petrous portions rotate externally. When the sphenoid and occiput turn into extension, the petrous portions rotate internally.

When the petrous portion of a temporal bone rotates externally, this mastoid portion moves outward and this mastoid process moves inward–that is, in external rotation of the petrous portion we find the mastoid portion more prominent on the outside of the skull, and the mastoid process less prominent. When the petrous portion rotates internally, it is the other way around. Then the process moves outward and the portion inward. Thus we have evidence on the outside of the skull of the comparative rotations of the petrous portions on the inside of the skull. This evidence can be palpated and used in the construction of a mental picture of the positions in the sphenobasilar area. Because of the tongue and groove articulations between the basilar process of the occiput and the petrous portions of the temporal bones, the relation between them is direct, and from the evidence on the outside as to the rotation of the petrous portions, we can interpret the position of the basilar process of the occiput. The mechanism of the movement between the occiput and the temporal bones is quite intricate and needs detailed study. In some degree, the temporal bones move with the occiput because they are carried by it on the jugular processes. The strange part lies in realizing that when the basilar process, as a spoke on the occipital wheel, turns, the petrous portion of the temporal turns along with it. Yet, at the same time, there is a motion between the two bones that resembles the motion between a fruit jar and its cap.

The circumrotation of the occiput not only turns the basilar process but also the foramen magnum and the jugular processes. We view the jugular process as a combined pivot and fulcrum process, an arrangement on which the petrous portion is fixed. Thus, if the basilar process moves then the pivot moves along with it, yet that pivot also allows the tip of the petrous portion to move forward and the lower area of the mastoid portion to turn backward. This occurs in inhalation, or flexion, at the sphenobasilar symphysis. As the basilar process turns backward during exhalation, the pivot moves along with it and the tip of the petrous portion moves backward as the lower area of the mastoid portion turns forward. As with the fruit jar and its cap, when you turn the jar in one direction and the cap in the other, while the pivot and the petrous portion move forward, the basilar process moves in one direction and the petrous portion in the opposite. You can now see why we have that concavity right back of the jugular processes and the pivot, and why the lower area of the mastoid portion is convex.

During inhalation, the anterior end of the sphenoid makes a "nosedive," that is, moves down as the area of the sella turcica moves up. What happens at the sphenosquamous articulation? We find that the upper half of the greater wing is beveled externally and the upper half of the squamous portion of the temporal bone is beveled internally, and then at a niche–at about the infratemporal line–the beveling changes so that the lower half of the greater wing is beveled internally and the lower half of the temporal is beveled externally. In the early days of my explorations, I was able to disarticulate the temporal bone from a skull that I owned, by prying it apart with a small blade of a penknife. Because of my mental picture of this mechanism, I knew how to take it apart. If you will place the fingers of one hand beneath the mastoid process and spring in on the greater wing of the sphenoid with the other hand, or better, with another finger of the same hand, you will feel the action that this sphenosquamous design permits. It is not difficult.

To feel the intricate movement between the occiput and the temporal bones, first feel along the occipitomastoid suture and locate each bone. In getting acquainted with the area, use light palpation and locate the groove on the undersurface medial to the mastoid process; then feel the pulse of the occipital artery. The articulation is medial to this. Draw your fingers along it at the same degree of palpation. You can detect the movement like the fruit jar and its cap of which I spoke. The movement is somewhat like a crease in a piece of cardboard. It moves outward and inward. Do not press in and obstruct the movement. This is an intricate mechanism, and your touch must be very light in order to sense the movements and interpret them in making your diagnosis. You do not do this to fix a suture. You feel it.

When you have the feeling, it is necessary to visualize the mechanism and how it works in order to understand what you feel and learn to know the difference between the normal and abnormal from experience. You have the pivot going forward and the petrous going along with it during inhalation, and yet the petrous is turning in the opposite direction at the same time. You have the pivot and fulcrum moving backward in exhalation, and yet the temporal bone is turning in the opposite direction. As you study this mechanism, you will find that this is a lateral and inferior area. But when you examine this pivot, it is more of a superior articular surface, a little turning point that means a lot in that mechanism. The pivot moves forward and the temporal bone turns on the lateral surface. That picture must be in mind when you come to a lesion. You are twisting it in the concave and convex surface.

What is a cranial lesion? Suppose we use flexion as an example. If the sphenobasilar symphysis had moved a little beyond its normal range of movement in the direction of flexion and become fixed in that position, there would be lack of mobility that would prevent the movement in the direction of extension. For diagnosis, you would have all the appearances that go with the flexion position, and when you tested for motion, you would find that the area could move in the direction of flexion but not in the direction of extension. So you would call it a "flexion lesion." The opposite would be the case with an "extension lesion." We will also discuss sidebending and torsion lesions of the sphenobasilar area. Thus, for diagnosis and technique, we will have these four sphenobasilar patterns to work with. There are these factors to think about: the mechanics of movement that the anatomical design of the articular surfaces permits; what each of the four patterns looks like and feels like on the outside of the head; how to test for motion in making a working diagnosis; and how to use that diagnosis in applying a technique that will correct the lesion in the easiest and most successful way.

What happens in flexion of the cranial base?

We have seen that when the occiput turns as a wheel, the basilar process is turned forward and the jugular process and foramen magnum are also turned forward. The petrous portions of the temporal bones rotate externally, and we have the mastoid portions more prominent on the outside of the skull and the mastoid processes inward. The upper area of the temporal bones is turned forward, and the area at the parietomastoid articulation is outward.

The sphenoid wheel also turns at the same time, and as the anterior end goes into its nosedive, the greater wings move forward. This movement carries the eyeballs forward, the angles of the frontal bones outward, and there is thus a receding at the metopic suture where the two frontal bones join. We find that the ethmoid notch in the orbital plate of the frontal is widened posteriorly, and the ethmoid bone is moved backward. The lateral parts of the ethmoid contain a collection of air chambers and the fragile turbinates curl and uncurl during inhalation and exhalation like the leaves of a tree. In the midline, you have the perpendicular plate of the ethmoid articulating with the ethmoidal crest on the front of the sphenoid body and with the vomer, which in turn articulates with the body of the sphenoid at the rostrum. The vomer runs out over the palatines and maxillae like a plowshare, and with the perpendicular plate of the ethmoid makes up the bony part of the nasal septum.

As the sphenoid circumrotates, there is movement between the ethmoid and the vomer, a little gliding movement. The pterygoid processes hang down below the body of the sphenoid, and as we follow their movement as spokes of the wheel, we find that they go downward and backward. They turn, as you know, in grooves or tracks on the back of the little palatines. The palatines fit into the maxillae, so that the pterygoid processes turn the maxillae through them outward and posteriorly, the same as the angles of the frontal bones are turned. You will find that the teeth, the upper incisors, will have a receding movement the same as the frontal bones. As the greater and lesser wings of the sphenoid form part of the orbital cavities, and as four of the extrinsic muscles of each eyeball have their origin around the optic foramen between the roots of the lesser wing, the forward movement of the greater wings makes for a forward position of the eyeballs in flexion.

The greater wing of the sphenoid articulates with the zygomatic bone in the lateral wall of the orbit. As the wing comes forward in flexion of the cranial base, it tips the zygomatic bone outward. As the zygomatic process of the temporal bone is moved in external rotation of the petrous portion, it also aids in external rotation of the zygomatic. The sphenoid does not, as a rule, articulate with the maxilla, and neither does the temporal bone, but they do articulate with the zygomatic, which in turn articulates with the maxilla. In the orbital cavity, there is the sphenomaxillary fissure, which we see can provide for a widening and narrowing of the cavity.

In the flexion type lesion at the sphenobasilar area, we have what we call a wide type of skull, with the wide orbital cavity and the forward eyeball. This gives you an observation cue for diagnosis. You palpate for motion to confirm your diagnosis through observation. In the extension type lesion, we have the case where the physiologic motion in the direction of extension has gone beyond the normal range at the sphenobasilar symphysis. You may find it in cases of bronchitis and asthma. The petrous portions have rotated internally, and so you find the mastoid portions and the mastoid angles of the parietals to be medial, and the mastoid processes prominent. The effect is a narrow shape of the skull. The sphenoid is backward, the frontal inward and the ethmoid notch is narrowed posteriorly. The maxilla is up and drawn inward, and the zygomatic bone has turned inward, thus narrowing and deepening the orbital cavity. The eyeball is receded into the deepened space. Here you have a factor to consider when thinking about the shape of the eyeballs as related to near and distant vision.

You see that patient coming in with a narrow skull and receding eyeballs. Observation indicates the sphenobasilar extension type. Palpation tells the story. Why? because you have the anatomical-physiological understanding and the ability to apply the keynote of Dr. Still's technique, namely, thinking-feeling-seeing-knowing fingers. Osteopathy still has undreamed of possibilities to yield. It is not a specialty in the sense of applying to just one region of the body, but it does provide the opportunity, should you wish, to specialize osteopathically in the treatment of eyes, ears, nose and throat.

Now to consider the sidebending type of sphenobasilar lesion. In a sidebending-rotation of the sphenobasilar junction with the convexity to the left, the greater wings of the sphenoid would be tipped so that the right wing would be higher than the left, while the sphenobasilar junction would rotate down on the left. At the same time, the occiput tips upward on the right and downward on the left side. The basilar process is included in this so that it is tipped upward on its right side and downward on its left side–on the side, not the end. Whenever the basilar process tips up on one side and down on the other side in this way, the effect on the position of the petrous portions of the temporal bones is direct. The petrous portion on the high side is carried into the position of internal rotation, and the petrous portion on the low side is carried into the position of external rotation. So, again, the evidence as to the position of the petrous portion of the temporal bones tells you about the position of the basilar process of the occiput. On the face, there will be a wider orbit and a forward eyeball on the side of the higher great wing and a narrower orbit with a receding eyeball on the side of the lower great wing. Thus, with sidebending to the left, the great wing being high on the right, the wider orbit and the forward eyeball will be on the right. Sidebending-rotation at the sphenobasilar to the right would be just the opposite.

Here we have what we call a torsion lesion, meaning here a twist at the sphenobasilar junction. In this case, the greater wing is high on the right and the basilar process is high on the left. You see that the basilar process is tipped in the opposite direction to the tip of the sphenoid. Now, whenever the basilar process is tipped up on its side, you will always find the petrous portion in internal rotation on that side. In this case, the left petrous portion is in internal rotation. With the greater wing high on the right, we have the wider orbit and the forward eyeball on the right and the externally rotated temporal on the right. On the patient's left side, we have the narrower orbit with the receding eyeball and the internally rotated temporal.

Now look at these differences as they can be seen in the general effect they make on the contours of the head as a whole. In the sidebending type, you will see that the side of the head, from front to back on the side where the sphenoid and occiput are high, is flatter, even concave in some instances, and on the other side it is longer and fuller, even convex to a marked degree in some instances. This can be verified by palpation. With this picture in mind, you then make your real working diagnosis by the feel for mobility.

Now you can't get your feel down to the area of the sphenobasilar junction itself, but you can grasp the sphenoid in front and the occiput in back and turn each of them gently, carefully, so as to get the range of mobility or possible motion. If you find that the range of mobility is more in extension, then it is the extension type of lesion. If you find that the greater wing moves up farther on the right and the occiput farther on the left, then it is the torsion type with the greater wing high on the right. If you find that the greater wing moves up farther on the right and the occiput also moves up farther on the right, then you have the sidebending type with the convexity to the left. With the necessary anatomical-physiological knowledge, your fingers can determine the type you are dealing with.

In technique we endeavor to follow Dr. Still's methods–that is, getting the point of release with no jerking and then allowing the natural agencies to return the bones to their normal relations and positions. What are the natural agencies? The ligaments, not the muscles, are the natural agencies for this purpose of correcting the relations and positions at joints. Dr. Still's application of the technique is the gentle exaggeration of the lesion that allows the natural agencies to draw the bones into place. Dr. Still has taken my hand in his and allowed me to feel the lesion as it was being exaggerated and then as the natural agencies pulled the bones back into place. There is reason for applying that technique in the cranial mechanism. The difference between spinal technique and cranial technique is like the difference between an automobile mechanic and a watchmaker. We do not force anything into place in the reduction of the lesion. We have something more potent than our own forces working always in the patient towards the direction of the normal.

What are the normal agencies in the cranium? They are: (1) the brain–the motor of respiration; (2) the cerebrospinal fluid; (3) the reciprocal tension membrane.

When we exaggerate the cranial lesion to the point of articular release, we have the patient cooperate through respiration–that is, exhaling as deeply as possible and then holding the breath as long as possible. When unable to hold it longer, there is a sudden inhalation over which the patient has no power. It moves in the normal direction, and we find that the motor causes the cerebrospinal fluid to fluctuate in the membranes. Have you seen a force pump? Often that is the change that occurs in a motor. It is always operating in a direction toward the normal. That is intracranial force.

At this time Dr. Sutherland was demonstrating the methods he was speaking of and the members of the class were located two to a table about the room as they practiced what he was teaching.

In application, the flexor profundus digitorum muscles are used for leverage. The origin of these muscles is in the forearm and the action is in the finger. I liken these muscular agencies to the handles of a pair of pliers. The fingers are interlaced and I pull or draw with the digits. The force is guided along the index finger, then along the little finger, then the middle fingers. One finger does one thing, another does another, while lifting the parietal bones upward. In this lift, you lift these angles of the parietals outward and upward. At the same time, you can lift the mastoid angle and pull it forward by exercising the index finger.

In this test, you place one palm over the occiput with the fingers extended. Be certain that you are on the occiput and not on the temporal bone. The other hand grasps the greater wing of the sphenoid. Rotate the greater wing anteriorly and the occiput posteriorly, gently and carefully, to see how much movement there is in the upward movement at the sphenobasilar junction. Do not tilt the head. You are moving the sphenoid and occiput only. Some of you place your hand beneath the sacrum to see if you can detect evidence of the motion at the sphenobasilar symphysis. Now throw the sphenobasilar junction downward, just the opposite of what you did to produce flexion, and repeat the movement into flexion. Notice the temporal bone when it rotates externally, moving along at the same time that the bottom part turns backward and the squamous part forward, the mastoid process going inward. Place the index finger over the parietomastoid suture. Have the patient inhale deeply. Note the action that takes place. Visualize mentally the picture of the cerebellum moving with the foramen magnum and the body of cerebrospinal fluid in the cisterna magna. See the cerebellum expanding–the fourth ventricle expanding. The cerebrospinal fluid is in command. The tentorium cerebelli is above the roof of the fourth ventricle. Here you have the temporal bones, the petrous portion in external rotation. During inhalation, see the membranous connection with the cerebellum and the tentorium.

Throw the sphenobasilar into extension and note the petrous portion rotate internally. The pivot on the occiput goes backward and so does the foramen magnum. The intraspinal membranes drop down and the base of the sacrum falls anteriorly. As the occiput turns in this direction, it carries the petrous portion backward. The mastoid portion is inward and the lower area goes forward as the squamous portion moves posteriorly. In exhalation, the mastoid process will be outward. In inhalation, the mastoid process is inward, the parietomastoid suture is prominent, and the mastoid portion is outward by comparison with the process.

Try to bring the left greater wing up as you also bring the occiput up on the right. This tests the sphenobasilar position of the sphenoid up on the left and the basilar process up on the right. Detect the mobility at the sphenobasilar junction. Now try the sphenoid up on the right and basilar process up on the left. Next try the sidebending-rotation. Move the sphenoid up on one side and the sphenobasilar junction rotates to the other. Test the sidebending-rotation to the right. Turn the sphenoid and occiput up on the left. This rotates the sphenobasilar junction to the right.

Now that you have the picture of the rotation of the temporal bones, you can learn to fluctuate the cerebrospinal fluid by alternate rotation of the temporals. In this method, the tentorium cerebelli fluctuates the cerebrospinal fluid not only in the cranium but also in the entire spinal column. You can use the method for testing the mobility of the temporal bones. You can throw the petrous portion into external rotation, and by changing the pull, you can throw them into internal rotation. Thus you tell the mobility of the temporal bones. Do not compress. With the same sense of touch, drop onto the lambdoidal suture. You will sense a movement somewhat like a crease in a cardboard.... Use those thinking-feeling-seeing-knowing fingers!

Now, have your patient hold his breath out. Visualize the compression of the fourth ventricle. The patient is doing more compressing than you are. Then there comes a sudden involuntary inhalation. Then a sensation of warmth is felt through the area of the third and fourth ventricles. The movement of the diaphragm changes. When that point is reached, all the fluids of the human body change, including those of the eyeballs, toes, fingers, heart, etcetera. You start the motor that runs this. A branch of the arterial inflow runs up through the body of the cerebrospinal fluid, up on the roof of the third ventricle, out onto the walls of the lateral ventricles and another on the roof of the fourth. These go to make up the choroid plexuses. They lie on the outside of the neural tube and within the arachnoid membrane. The choroid plexus on the roof of the third ventricle stretches out during inhalation.

In thinking about the choroid plexus, realize that Dr. Still was a thousand years ahead of us in his mental picture. What does he mean when he says that the brain is God's drugstore, having in it opiates, acids and every other drug thought necessary for human happiness and health?[8] If you become a mechanic of the cranial mechanism by correcting a cranial lesion, you then become the pharmacist. There is no end to this thought. It is not a new thought. Swedenborg, 200

---

8. Still, *Autobiography*, p. 182. Note that in the 1908 revised ed., Dr. Still changed the word "brain" to "body;" cf. the original 1897 ed., p. 219.

years ago, said there is movement of the brain.[9] Have we anything totally new? No.

The juices of the body are most important, especially the cerebrospinal fluid. I call attention to the fact that the little pituitary body is surrounded by a wall of blood on every side. Speransky would have recognized a movement of the brain and cranium as a respiratory mechanism, if he had gone further in his experiments.[10]

In my experiments, I had to use my own skull. Why? Because it was I who had to possess the personal knowledge. I found that not only did the cranial articulations have mobility, but that there is also movement of the intracranial and intraspinal membranes and, best of all, a fluctuation of the cerebrospinal fluid. I also found that I could feel that fluid in the cranium of my patient. Take a can of water and give it a shake and set it down. Place your hand on the can and you will feel the water within it fluctuate. You can feel such a movement in the cranium. You know what you are feeling for. When I used a parietal lift on my head, the effect was as though someone were milking my fingers, toes, etcetera.

---

9. Emanual Swedenborg (1688-1772) was a Swedish scientist and mystic who studied anatomy in order to find the soul. His ideas blended spirituality with science and were incorporated into the Spiritualist movement in 19th century America, and are said to have influenced Dr. Still in his thinking. See Trowbridge, *Andrew Taylor Still.*

10. A.D. Speransky was a Russian scientist who conducted a wide variety of experiments, including those on the nature of the cerebrospinal fluid. See Speransky, *A Basis for the Theory of Medicine.*

24. The Cranial Bowl

Journal of the American Osteopathic Association, *April 1944.*

This paper was delivered before the annual meeting of the Eastern Osteopathic Association, New York City, April 3, 1943. In the journal article, introductory comments were made by the editor, Ray G. Hulburt, D.O. [American School of Osteopathy, 1920].

Eight years ago this spring, Dr. Russell C. McCaughan [American School of Osteopathy, 1914] and the editor published a series of papers entitled, "Osteopathic Research Imperative." In the third of these papers, in March 1936, we quoted Dr. Della B. Caldwell as urging the investigation and evaluation of various discoveries made, and methods used, by osteopathic physicians, including the diagnosis and treatment of cranial conditions as taught by Dr. W. G. Sutherland.

For many years previous to that, Dr. Sutherland had been studying skulls–in fact, since his early days in osteopathic college. He examined them dead and dry, on the dissection table, and in his patients, young and old. More recently, he has been appearing with greater frequency on convention programs, where the bare outlines of his methods were brought to the attention of increasing numbers of osteopathic physicians, since no convention sessions are long enough to cover the ground. And he has been giving individual instruction to those greatly interested, so that cranial technique is now being practiced by more and more doctors, from coast to coast.

Like any other specialty in osteopathy, cranial technique is not to be learned from casual observation, or even from study of an article or two in a magazine. Therefore, there has been hesitation about putting anything about it in print. The presentation which Dr. Sutherland made at the Eastern Osteopathic Association meeting last spring was such as he has made at various other places. It calls for many drawings and for the examination of the skull and the various bones which make it up, most of which do not lend themselves well to representation on a flat surface. The illustrations reproduced herewith are not intended to clarify the text adequately, but they do exemplify the drawings used freely by Dr. Sutherland in his presentations. It is hoped that the text will excite interest in many who are not familiar with the principles underlying this aspect of osteopathic diagnosis and treatment and that to some who already are somewhat familiar with it, it will serve as a review.

It is by no means to be understood that this is the first appearance in print of material relating to the effects, the diagnosis or the treatment of cranial lesions. Dr. Sutherland brought out a book in 1939, *The Cranial Bowl*, which is no longer in print. In that book, there were references not only to the earlier editorial mention of his work in the *Journal* but also to his articles in *The Northwest Bulletin* and *The Western Osteopath.*

Dr. Charlotte Weaver has for years lectured and written on the cranial vertebrae. She had articles on the subject in the *Journal* for March, April, May and June 1936. This series was followed by a symposium by Drs. Charles L. Naylor, Earle E. Sanborn, Edward T. White, N. A. Ulrich and Charlotte Weaver, running in the *Journal* from November 1937 to March 1938. In the *Journal* for June 1942, Dr. Perrin T. Wilson had an article in which he referred to Dr. Sutherland's work and told of his own application of a modification of it.[1]

–Editor (Ray G. Hulburt, D. O.)

Our subject is "The Cranial Bowl," but that is not a detached unit, any more than is any other part of our complicated body machine. In my interpretation, we take into consideration a mechanism which includes the brain, the intracranial membranes, the cerebrospinal fluid and the articular mobility of the cranial bones, and also the spinal cord, the intraspinal membranes, again the cerebrospinal fluid, and the articular mobility of the sacrum between the ilia.

The cranial thought belongs to Dr. Andrew Taylor Still, founder of osteopathy. The Old Doctor frequently referred to the osteopathic "squirrel in a hole in a tree." He had a grip on the squirrel's tail, and

---

1. Perrin T. Wilson, D.O.: see article 10, "'Modified Vertebrae' in Tic Douloureux," note 1.

we had to go on and pull it out. The cranial thought is simply a part of the process of getting the body of the squirrel out. The thought provides an avenue for "digging on" through scientific research.[2]

We remember Dr. Still's dictum: "An osteopath reasons from his knowledge of anatomy. He compares the work of the abnormal body with that of the normal body." In this avenue of scientific research, one must primarily possess a *knowledge* of the cranial structure, within and without. It is true here, as in any part of the body, that, as Dr. Still said again: "We must *know* the position and purpose of each bone and be thoroughly acquainted with each of its articulations. We must have a perfect image of the normal *articulations* that we wish to adjust."[3]

His anatomical-physiological knowledge was the keynote of his diagnosis and his corrective adjustments. The cranium is an *intricate mechanism* and requires especial study of its complicated articular surfaces. For the perfection of skill required in cranial diagnosis and technique, it is necessary, primarily, to possess a perfect anatomical-physiological mental picture.

As a preliminary to further study, attention is called to these illustrations. [*Two pictures of the sphenoid and one of the sphenoid and occiput joined at the sphenobasilar junction were shown.*] Observe the L-shape of the superior articular surface of the greater wing of the sphenoid bone. The two of these, one for each greater wing, articulate with L-shaped articular surfaces beneath the frontal bone. At birth there are two frontal bones, and in some adults, the sagittal suture continues down

---

2. Dr. A. T. Still (respectfully referred to as the Old Doctor) presented osteopathy as a science, a philosophy and an art whose potential was not fully realized, much as a squirrel only partially seen within a hole in a tree would not be fully visualized. He stated that only the tail of the squirrel was currently in view.

The phrase "digging on" represents Dr. Sutherland's own approach to his study and the approach he encouraged others to follow. For his telling of the boyhood story that inspired this, see article 26, "Philosophy of Osteopathy and Its Application," note 1.

3. Still, *Research and Practice*, p. 8 (n. 10) and p. 30 (n. 66); emphasis added.

to the ethmoidal notch. Inasmuch as there are two ossification centers, we may reason on the basis of two frontal bones: the sphenoid being suspended from the two as the sacrum is suspended, by the L-shaped articular surfaces, between, or beneath, the ilia. Both bones, the sacrum and the sphenoid, have anterior and posterior rotation articular mobility as well as sidebending movement.

Now observe the little flat process upon the middle of the anterior superior area of the body of the sphenoid. This fits into a small groove upon the middle of the posterior superior area of the ethmoid. It provides the mechanical arrangement for movement of the ethmoid when the sphenoid moves downward. Immediately lateral to this process, on the superior articular surface of the lesser wings of the sphenoid, are two lateral beveled articular surfaces, articulating beneath the two frontal bones, lateral to the ethmoid notch. These provide a mechanical arrangement for the accommodation of articular mobility between the lesser wings of the sphenoid and the frontal bones.

One need not look farther than these two indications, found upon the articular surfaces of the sphenoid, for a truth signifying that a Master Mechanic designed the bones of the cranium for articular mobility. There are many other indications throughout the cranial bones signifying that truth, which also may be found in the anatomical laboratories of our osteopathic colleges as proof to our anatomists, providing they "dig" for it. The proof of the assertion of cranial articular mobility is right there on the articular surfaces, and it does not require even a mechanical mind to recognize the mechanical principle.

Here at the lower middle anterior area of the sphenoid is a beak-like process, called the rostrum. Doubtless the term was given by some anatomist because of its resemblance to the beak of a bird, which corresponds to the bird-like form of the sphenoid with its greater and lesser wings.

Next we consider the vomer. It has a cup-like articular surface, a provision designed to fit over the beak, or rostrum. It provides a movement like that afforded by a universal joint.[4] From the articulation, the vomer extends forward over the roof of the maxillae and palatine bones, which also have mobility.

Down here at this inferior area, we have rockers which are known as the internal and external pterygoid processes. They are convex in shape and hang beneath the bird-like, or boat-like, form from the bottom of the sphenoid. When the sphenoid rocks forward, these rockers rotate downward and backward. They articulate with the concave articular surfaces of the little palatine bones.

Let us study this concave articular surface on the palatine bone in all its details and the articular surface connecting the maxillae with the palatine bones. It almost calls for a magnifying glass to study the orbital surface that sticks up within the orbital cavity.

Dr. Still said: "It is the little things that are the big ones in the science of osteopathy." That tiny orbital surface has a big task to perform in the cranial mechanism. The little palatine bone provides an opportunity for osteopathic specialization in the field of eye, ear, nose and throat.

The sphenopalatine ganglion lies between the palatine bone and the body of the sphenoid. Articular fixations commonly occur which crowd the palatine bone backward onto the ganglion, thus disturbing its functioning. The ganglion sends nerve fibers to the lacrimal gland, the turbinates, the nasal and postnasal areas and the mouth of the eustachian tube.

The sphenoid does not articulate with the maxillae but does with the palatine bones. The palatine bones fit in between the sphenoid and maxillae and function as "speed-reducers" to retard the movement between the sphenoid and maxillae. The sphenoid also articulates with another equalizer in connection with the movement of the sphenoid and maxillae. This is the zygomatic bone, which articulates

---

4. A universal joint is a coupling that permits a swing of limited angle in any direction, especially one used to transmit rotary motion from one shaft to another not in line with it, as in the drive shaft of an automobile.

with the greater wing of the sphenoid *within the orbital cavity*. As the sphenoid rocks forward, the greater wing swings the zygomatic outward and widens the orbital cavity. As the anterior end of the sphenoid ascends, the greater wing draws the zygomatic inward and narrows the orbital cavity. The zygomatic also articulates with the maxillary bone. Hence the movement of the sphenoid, through its equalizer the zygomatic bone, moves the maxillary. The functioning widens and narrows the sphenomaxillary fissure within the orbital cavity. This fact is taken into consideration in the diagnosis of sphenobasilar lesions through observation at a glance. Wide or narrow orbital cavities provide clues which later may be verified by the skilled art of osteopathic palpation.

The orbital surface of the palatine bone is located immediately back of the maxillary, at the beginning of the sphenomaxillary fissure. The infraorbital nerve passes over that tiny orbital surface, just before it enters a groove in the maxillary to find its way to the infraorbital foramen. Were it not for that especially designed little orbital surface, the maxillary bone might saw or wear the infraorbital nerve in two. The orbital surface of the palatine bone is an equalizer that removes the tension from the nerve.

The orbital cavity is not like the solid osseous acetabulum of the ilium, but is formed by the articulation of the frontal bone, the orbital surface of the ethmoid, the lacrimal, the maxillary, the orbital surface of the palatine, the zygomatic and the greater and lesser wings of the sphenoid. It is a cavity designed by a Master Mechanic for mobility.

In addition, the Wise Mechanic placed the origin of the extrinsic muscles of the eyeball around the optic foramen, on the lesser wing of the sphenoid, with the exception of one, the inferior oblique, which He placed a little farther forward, arising from the maxilla. As the sphenoid comes forward, the eyeball comes forward also; as the sphenoid moves backward, the eyeball moves backward. In addition to the infraorbital fissure, we observe another, the supraorbital fissure, which is formed by the greater and lesser wings of the sphenoid. The cavernous sinus leads from this fissure, carrying its volume of venous blood that flows to the exit at the jugular foramen. The ophthalmic veins lead into this cavernous sinus.

In the case of glaucoma, one may reason that the accumulation of fluid points to a condition somewhere back along the intracranial membranous wall of the cavernous sinus, or in the walls of the petrosal sinus, to a membranous restriction affecting the venous return, and back of that, the possibility of a cranial lesion as an etiological factor.

The maxillary bones hang by their nasal processes from the frontal bones, lateral to the ethmoid notch. There is a gap between the nasal processes that is capped by the nasal bones. Now we may imagine the sagittal suture as continuing down to the ethmoidal notch or ending between the nasal processes of the maxillary bones. The ethmoid lies beneath the nasal processes. It has processes known as the superior and middle turbinates. A lesion fixation of the nasal processes of the maxillae would crowd the turbinate bones. These fixations are quite common. Here again is an opportunity for one who would become an osteopathic specialist in eye, ear, nose and throat. Let one who doubts the opportunity stand before a mirror, place a finger in contact with the roof of the mouth, at the junction of the palatine bones with the maxillae, inhale and exhale deeply, and watch the incisor teeth separate and come together alternately. One's own skilled osteopathic fingers will guide him to this opportunity, providing there is no fixation in the maxillae.

Now let us drop back to the posterior articular surface of the greater wing of the sphenoid. The upper half of its articular surface is beveled externally, and it articulates with an internal articular surface upon the upper anterior half of the squamous portion of the temporal bone. At the halfway point lies a tiny niche, which articulates with a tiny projection upon the squamous portion. As we observe the lower half, we note that its articular surface has changed to an internal bevel and that it articulates with an externally beveled articular surface upon the lower half of the squamous portion. These surfaces are designed especially for articular mobility.

Posterior to the squamous portion of the temporal bone, we find serrations running across the articular surface. These articulate with similar serrations that run across the articular surface of the posterior inferior angle of the parietal bone. These provide for a lateral movement between these bones, the temporal and parietal, inward and outward.

At the inferior articular surface, which might be called a lateral articular surface, we find the surface convex. It articulates with a concave articular surface within the condylar area of the occipital bone in such a way that while the convex surface of the temporal bones moves in one direction, the concave surface of the condylar area moves in the other.

Just a little farther forward on the condylar portion of the occiput is a small fulcrum, which articulates with a groove beneath the petrous portion of the temporal. This fulcrum is immediately posterior to the jugular foramen.

The basilar portion, anterior to the jugular foramen, has a lateral ridge on its articular surface. This ridge articulates within a longitudinal groove on the petrous portion of the temporal. Now it is important to observe the peculiar shape of the temporal bone, that of a disk wheel, such a condition as sometimes occurs in the wheels of automobiles and causes them to wobble.[5]

The temporal bone was especially designed to wobble in order to accommodate the internal and external rotation of the petrous portions which, in my opinion, takes place with respiratory movements. When the mastoid portion is outward, the mastoid process will be inward; while the mastoid portion is inward, the mastoid process will be outward. This feature of the wobbling of the temporal bone provides the means of diagnosing, by palpation, a sphenobasilar lesion, the mastoid portion being prominent in one type and depressed in another.

The cartilaginous portion of the eustachian tube is attached to the

---

5. It was popular to have disk, as opposed to spoke, wheels on one's automobile at the time. If the disk warped, however, then the wheel would wobble.

petrous portion. It is my belief that the petrous portion rotates externally during the period of inhalation, that the cartilaginous portion rotates externally also and the mouth of the eustachian tube opens. Likewise, I believe that in exhalation, the petrous portion rotates internally also and that this causes the mouth of the eustachian tube to close. In case of a lesion fixation in the movement of the petrous portion, the movement of the cartilaginous portion would be in the same fixation and the mouth of the eustachian tube would be either wide-open or closed. Here is another opportunity to specialize osteopathically in eye, ear, nose and throat conditions.

The temporal bone, like the sphenoid, does not articulate with the maxilla. It articulates with one of the same equalizers, the zygoma, and the zygoma with the maxilla. This articulation is by way of the zygomatic process of the temporal. The articular surface is semioblique and overlaps the zygoma providing an up and down movement as the petrous portion rotates internally and externally. One may take a disarticulated temporal bone and demonstrate the wobbling wheel motion by moving the zygomatic process upward and downward.

The bones at the base of the skull have their origin in *cartilage*, while the bones of the vault have their origin in membrane. Articular mobility occurs at the basilar area, in the bones having their origin in cartilage. The cranial structure is a *cranial bowl*, and we could not have articular mobility at the basilar area without compensation by the bones of the vault, which are formed in membrane. Here we have another mechanical design by a Master Mechanic who understood His handiwork.

Now it is advisable to take a different view as to the structural consistency of the bones of the vault. We may reason that having been formed in *membrane*, they remain as *membranous tissue* as long as the sap remains, or until life departs, like the soft-shelled egg, flexible throughout their structural portions, as well as at their sutural serrations. The intracranial dural membrane has two walls, or sheets. The inner wall is smooth while the outer wall is rough. On the other hand, the diploe of the vault bones has two walls, an outer and an inner. Like the intracranial dura mater, the inner wall is smooth while the outer wall is rough. Why not continue to call this diploe *membrane*? We have mother dura in the dura mater; why not have a father dura as a dura pater? Father dura is flexible throughout its structural portions as well as having special serrations along the sutural connections that provide sufficient compensation for the articular mobility of the bones at the basilar area of the skull. One may pick up any inanimate skull from an anatomical laboratory and easily flex the structural portions of the vault bones. In the skull of the human being with life still present, how much more easily are we able to flex the vault tissues.

Our Master Mechanic made further provision in the outer wall serrations for compensation to articular mobility at the base of the skull. The serrations at the lower area of the occipital bone are externally beveled while those of the parietal are internally beveled. In other words, the serrations of the parietal lap over those of the occiput at this area. At the upper area of the occiput, these serrations change to an internal bevel while the serrations of the parietal change to the external. This signifies that the occiput laps over the parietal at the upper area–a special arrangement for compensation to articular mobility at the base of the skull. The serrations along the sagittal suture are wider apart posteriorly than they are anteriorly. This provides compensation for a widening and narrowing at the posterior area of the sagittal suture as bones move, upward and outward and downward and inward. The frontal bones fit in between the parietals at their inferior angles at the coronal suture.

Obviously, so large a subject can be covered only sketchily in the space available now. We pass lightly over such dilation and contraction as may take place in the ventricles of the brain with movements of the sphenoid, the effects upon the cerebrospinal fluid, which Hilton in *Rest and Pain* [p. 24] refers to as "water beds" upon which the brain rests. We can but glance at the membranous walls with their content of venous blood, at the pituitary, the sella turcica, the infundibulum. We see the internal carotid artery with its branch which becomes the choroid plexus where, it is stated, an important interchange occurs between the cerebrospinal fluid and the arterial blood, and note that movement, slight though it be, is essential to the freedom of that interchange.

As we look ahead of the cavernous sinuses, we see the supraorbital fissure of the sphenoid bone, the movements of which tense and relax the membranous walls of the sinuses by way of which the venous blood passes. We observe also the ophthalmic veins entering the cavernous sinuses through the sphenoidal fissure. We likewise observe the oculomotor, trochlear and abducens nerves, as well as the ophthalmic division of the trigeminal, passing through the same sinuses. Immediately anterior to the sella turcica, we note the optic chiasm and the optic nerves passing out through the optic foramina in the lesser wings of the sphenoid bone. We remember that the extrinsic muscles of the eyeballs have their origin around the optic foramina, with the exception of one having its origin on the maxillary bone, and note the effect upon these muscles of normal mobility–or its lack–in the articulations of the sphenoid.

Posterior to the sella turcica, we notice the junction of the sphenoid bone with the basilar process of the occiput and remember that, up to the average age of 25 or 30 years, there is a modified intervertebral cartilage present and from then, for a further period, mobility at the sphenobasilar junction is still present. Lateral to this junction, we note the foramina laceratum and see the internal carotid arteries passing into the cranium through individual canals in the petrous portions of the temporal bones. We take cognizance of the fact that these petrous portions extend diagonally forward and inward to their junctions with the basilar process of the occiput. We then remember that the cartilaginous portions of the eustachian tubes have their attachment to these portions, as already pointed out. Upon the apices of the petrous portions, we find the trigeminal ganglia embedded in dural membrane, having attachment upon both the petrous portions and the sphenoid. Then we see the ganglia sending out the branches of the fifth nerves; further along, we view the sphenopalatine ganglia in the pterygopalatine fossae. Is it not obvious that disturbances affecting their functions result from tension of the membranes surrounding these ganglia, caused by lesions of the sphenoid and temporal bones?

Again we must hasten over a part of the picture, at this time giving less attention than should be paid to the fourth ventricle, the floor of which is occupied by various physiological centers, including that of respiration. We pass too rapidly over the dural and arachnoid membranes, the former carrying venous blood over the superior longitudinal sinus into which empty the smaller veins from the brain and the lateral sinuses.

However, in connection with my belief, which I have mentioned, that normally there is movement in many cranial articulations coincident with inspiration and expiration, I believe the venous blood is carried along by membranous activity to the exits at the jugular foramina. We keep in mind the fact that the main venous channels have walls decidedly different within the cranium from those without and that they find their way out of the cranium through exits formed by the articulation of two bones–the jugular foramina as examples. On the other hand, the arterial walls are the same within and without the cranium and have the same nerve system. In addition, the arterial walls are protected on their way into the cranium by passing through individual canals in individual bones. Thus we may reason that membranous restriction disturbs the venous flow and the fluctuation of the cerebrospinal fluid. While cranial lesions may be primary, the intracranial membranes, including the dural and arachnoid, are the real disturbing causative factors leading to disease or disturbed function of the brain.

The intraspinal membranes are included in the picture. They continue with those of the intracranial, being attached to only two or three of the upper cervical vertebrae and the foramen magnum, and without other firm attachment until they reach the sacrum.

Various types of cranial lesions are found in professional practice. Four of these are known as the sphenobasilar types: the sidebending-rotation, the torsion, the flexion and extension lesions. These occur at the junction of the sphenoid with the basilar process of the occiput and are quite common.

The sidebending-rotation lesion is shown in the illustration of the sphenoid and occiput joined. The sidebending is convex to the left. The petrous portions of the temporal bones are included in the lesion, the right in internal rotation, the left in external. The basilar process is tipped upward on the right and downward on the left, while the greater wing of the sphenoid is upward on the right and downward on the left. The cranium, from front to back, is shorter on the right and longer on the left. If one were to observe this type of lesion from the front, he would see the right orbital cavity wider while the left would be narrower. The right zygomatic bone would be turned outward and the left inward. The right eyeball would be forward, while the left would be backward. Such observations would indicate the type of lesion at a glance, and it would be easily verified by palpation.

The torsion types of sphenobasilar lesion are another common pattern. The sphenoid is twisted in one direction at the sphenobasilar junction, while the basilar process is twisted to the opposite. The basilar process is tipped downward on the right and upward on the left, and the greater wing of the sphenoid is upward on the right, and the opposite greater wing is downward on the left. The petrous portion of the temporal bone is in external rotation on the right, while the opposite petrous portion is in internal rotation on the left. From the front view, the observation indication is the same as in the sidebending-rotation lesion, with a wide orbital cavity on the right and a narrow on the left. The zygomatic bone is turned outward on the right and the opposite bone inward on the left. The eyeball is forward on the right, while the opposite eyeball is backward. However, the uniform front to back contours of the cranium differentiate the torsion type of lesion from the sidebending type. The presence and type of lesion may be easily verified by palpation.

The flexion type of sphenobasilar lesion is an exaggeration of the normal flexion position at the sphenobasilar junction. In this type, the front view shows both orbital cavities wider and both eyeballs forward. The zygomatic bones will be turned outward. The greater wings of the sphenoid will be forward, and the petrous portions of both temporal bones will be in external rotation. The lesion may be easily verified by palpation.

The extension type of sphenobasilar lesion is an exaggeration of a normal position at the sphenobasilar junction. From the front view, the orbital cavities will be narrow with backward eyeballs. The zygomatic bones will be turned inward, the greater wings of the sphenoid will be backward, while the petrous portions of the temporal bones will be in internal rotation. The lesion may be easily verified by palpation.

Other cranial lesions come under the heading of traumatic types and in these days of automobile accidents, are frequent. They are described according to the area of traumatic contact.

In the frontoparietal type, the frontal bones have been compressed in between the parietal bones by trauma at the middle area. The inferior angles of the frontal bones will be found inward, thus locking the normal movement of the greater wings of the sphenoid. The lesion may be unilateral when the trauma occurs either to the right or left of the middle, and in such cases, only one inferior angle will be compressed inward at the parietal junction.

In the parietofrontal type, the parietal bones have been compressed downward by trauma at the junction of the sagittal and coronal sutures. There is a consequent lateral position of the anteroinferior angles of the parietals. There is a subsequent malposition of the condyles of the occipital bone which have been forced posteriorly within the facets of the atlas bone. The lesion may be either bilateral or unilateral, according to the area of traumatic contact.

In the parietosquamous type, the parietal bones have been compressed downward between the squamous portions of the temporal bones by trauma occurring at a midway point directly over the sagittal suture. It may be unilateral when the trauma occurs either to the right or left of the sagittal suture. The squamous portions of the temporal bones are forced outward, with consequent external rotation of the petrous portions at the basilar area and a subsequent flexion of the sphenobasilar junction.

In the parieto-occipital type, the parietal bones have been compressed downward by trauma at the junction of the sagittal with the lambdoidal sutures. The trauma tends to force the condyles of the occipital bone deeply into the facets of the atlas, thus tipping the basilar process upward at its sphenobasilar junction and frequently driving the basilar process into the sphenoid. There is a consequent malposition of the petrous portions of the temporal bones in external rotation. The lesion may be either bilateral or unilateral according to the area of contact. These malpositions at the basilar area indicate a rather serious condition in relation to the intracranial membranes that act as channels for the venous flow and which, in my opinion, incite activity of the cerebrospinal fluid.

In the occipitomastoid type, the lateral basilar area of the occipital bone has been forced upward between the lateral articular areas of the mastoid portions of the temporal bones by trauma at the lower region of the occiput. The basilar process of the occiput has been forced into its junction with the sphenoid and the petrous portions of the temporal bones into internal rotation. The lesion may be either bilateral or unilateral according to the area of contact. It is another type indicating serious consequence to the intracranial membranes that act as walls to the venous flow and the fluctuation of the cerebrospinal fluid.

The dental traumatic type of lesion opens a field of new possibilities to members of the osteopathic profession. It should interest the dentist as well. Dentists possess special anatomical knowledge and constructive surgical skill in relation to the facial bones, and this type of lesion invites cooperation by the two professions.

It includes a membranous articular strain in relation to the temporal, the sphenoid, the maxillae and the mandible. The temporal bone on the lesion side is found laterally inward with its petrous portion in internal rotation; the pterygoid process of the sphenoid upward and lateral and the maxilla downward; the mandible in malalignment at its temporomandibular articulation.

According to indications, the lesion occurs thus: The patient's occiput rests upon a V-form headrest on the dental chair in such a manner as to cause compression upon the mastoid portion of the temporal bone immediately anterior to the lambdoidal suture.[6] The dental surgeon chisels around a lower molar and applies a specially adapted forceps that extracts the tooth with an inward lift or pull. This inward side leverage upon the tooth tends to increase the compression upon the temporal bone by way of the temporomandibular articulation. At the same time, the side leverage twists or throws the mandible downward on the opposite side quite forcibly, thereby causing tension upon the sphenomandibular ligament and swinging the pterygoid process on the lesion side up and lateralward. During the extraction of an upper molar, the same side leverage is utilized, which twists the maxilla laterally downward. In some cases, the pterygoid process will be so far lateral as to crowd the coronoid process of the mandible. The crowding of the coronoid process together with the malalignment of the temporomandibular articulation, due to the inward position of the temporal bone, causes overbiting.

This type apparently affects the functioning of the trigeminal and sphenopalatine ganglia, sometimes leading to symptoms of facial neuralgia or tic douloureux. The internal rotation of the petrous portion of the temporal bone affects or twists the cartilaginous portion of the eustachian tube, which explains some of the ear complications that arise. There is tension of the intracranial membranes also, especially upon the lesion side.

The lateral position of the sphenoid bone, as well as the downward position of the maxilla, narrows the sphenomaxillary fissure within the orbital cavity, thus disturbing venous drainage by way of the ophthalmic vein that leads through the sphenoidal fissure into the cavernous sinus, with consequent eye pathology in some cases. The fixation of the sphenoid bone is apt to disturb the normal functioning, or movement, of

---

6. The V-shaped headrest is no longer encountered in the modern dental office.

the orbital cavity and also affect the normal position of the ethmoid with its turbinates, the vomer and palatine bones, and account for many of the irregularities found in the nasal region. The malalignment of the maxillae crowds the turbinates and the palatine bones also. The crowding of the palatine bones affects the sphenopalatine ganglia.

This type of lesion is not difficult to diagnose. In some cases, the removal of an upper dental plate tells the story, the plate being quite irregular in shape and the impression showing the downward position of the superior maxillary. This position may be verified by observation within the mouth.

The upward and lateral position of the pterygoid process of the sphenoid is diagnosed by inserting an index finger between the upper lip and gums, traveling backward to the posterior area of the superior maxillary, then turning up under the zygomatic to move further posteriorly until contact is made with the pterygoid process. The pterygoid process on the lesion side will be found upward and lateral in contrast to that of the opposite side. In most cases, it will be found crowding the mandible on the lesion side. Palpation of the mastoid portions of the temporal bones will reveal the lesion side as inward in contrast to that of the opposite.

The majority of lesions involving facial bones are found in relation with sphenoidal lesions and usually respond to sphenoidal reduction. However, there are many local injuries occurring to the facial bones that require local attention.

The zygomatic bone is found in malalignment frequently. The lesion is recognized readily by observation, comparing the zygomatic on one side with that of the opposite. Its outer and inner borders are found in an outward position, with consequent widening of the rim of the orbital cavity and disfigurement of the face. Its semioblique articulation with the zygomatic process of the temporal bone will be out of alignment. The zygomatic bone forms part of the articular mechanism relating to the eye.

Malalignments of the maxillae occur frequently through local injuries as well as by dental traumatic initiation and should be given consideration as causative factors in nasal, postnasal and pharyngeal affections. In these cases, the nasal processes will be found crowding the turbinates of the ethmoid bone. The malposition affects the width of the sphenomaxillary fissure within the orbital cavity. In extreme types, the lesion crowds the palatine bone backward to the extent of disturbance to the sphenopalatine ganglion.

Malalignments of the palatine bones are usually secondary to those of the maxillae and sphenoid. They are readily diagnosed by observation through the mouth.

While the ethmoid bone belongs to the cranial base, its turbinate processes must be considered with the facial bones. In sinus complaints, the turbinates are found in expansion. The frontoethmoidal articulation might be said to be in expansion also, which causes fixation instead of the normal movement of the ethmoid.

There are various types of birth injury cases common to subnormal types in children, but space limits prevent going into that aspect of the subject now.

25. Lectures on Cranial Osteopathy: Des Moines

The following are five lectures given at the College of Osteopathic Medicine and Surgery in Des Moines, Iowa, in April 1948. The first was an informal lecture presented during an introductory course in Cranial Osteopathy. The lectures that follow were given either during the introductory course or the advanced course and were the only ones taken down in shorthand at that time. Translations were made with considerable difficulty because of what proved to be inexpert shorthand.

1. Introductory Talk

April 5, 1948.

You came here to matriculate for a course in Cranial Osteopathy. In reality, you came to continue your study of the science of osteopathy as envisioned by Dr. Andrew Taylor Still, who in his vision was a thousand years ahead of us.

You see before you a dreamer–one who had to get away from the texts, as did Dr. Still, and follow something he could not explain. Something that kept him digging into his dreams. Which reminds me of the early boyhood days when my father assigned to my brother and me the task of digging potatoes in the garden patch. We dug the potatoes. But the following morning father came around and said, "Boys, go dig again." This was repeated three times or more, and on each occasion we found a generous supply of potatoes.

You know of Dr. Asa Willard of Missoula, Montana, and his broad-brimmed Stetson. Under that hat, he has something that he got from Dr. Andrew Taylor Still. In *The Cranial Bowl* text published in 1939, there is this interpolation by Dr. Asa Willard: "Along in 1874 after years of *independent thinking* there *came* to Dr. Still the concept of osteopathy."[1] I like the thought: "there *came* to Dr. Still." It came during one of the saddest periods of the Old Doctor's life, with the loss of members of his family. A period when a devout prayer went out to his Maker for guidance. The science of osteopathy goes deeper than material interpretation.[2]

On the wall to the right, you will see a quotation from another old-timer who was in close contact with Dr. Still, the late Dr. Harry L. Chiles [American School of Osteopathy, 1901]. It reads: "If one can think osteopathy he will practice osteopathy." It does not say "think osteopathically." If one will "think osteopathy" as Dr. Still thought osteopathy, he will get something that Dr. Still had. Something which we all need in order to practice osteopathy as Dr. Still envisioned it. If you can get that vision in the lines of his *Research and Practice* and his *Philosophy of Osteopathy*, you will practice osteopathy.

Dr. Still was dealing with a practical world. He had to lead step by step, and with the use of material interpretation. As you read the *Philosophy of Osteopathy* and get in between the lines, you begin to see the magnitude of the science of osteopathy. You will think osteopathy... not osteopathically.

Back in my student days in Kirksville, I was endeavoring to think osteopathy. In North Hall there was a collection of specimens belonging to the Old Doctor. Among them were disarticulated bones of the skull. As I viewed them, endeavoring to think osteopathy as Dr. Still thought osteopathy, there came this thought: Beveled, like the gills of a fish indicating a primary respiratory mechanism for mobility. That

---

1. Asa Willard, D.O. (American School of Osteopathy, 1900) was president of the American Osteopathic Association in 1925. Hailing from Missoula, Montana and widely recognized by his Stetson hat, he was a charismatic speaker and very active in osteopathic politics.

2. In the spring of 1864, spinal meningitis killed three of Dr. Still's children despite the best efforts of both preacher and physician. It was a time of great spiritual crisis for Dr. Still, the resolution of which resulted in the birth of the science of osteopathy ten years later. See Still, *Autobiography*, pp. 87-88, 303-304. In his later years Dr. Still was respectfully referred to as the Old Doctor.

is how the cranial concept came. It is not mine. It never has been. Like many of you, I was skeptical, and my first endeavor was to prove that there could be no mobility of the skull. The more I endeavored to prove it, the more my endeavor resembled my boyhood potato digging experience. It went on and on.

Here is a prenatal skull. Are there any bony contacts in that prenatal skull? It is so arranged that it can fold up for its passage through the birth canal. Can any one doubt that there is mobility in that skull in its prenatal existence? See this one at birth...and these...and on up to the fourth and fifth years, and so on...separate, without bony contact. Think of it! The parietal bones folded over the frontal bones. The parietal bones folding over the squama of the occipital bone so it can pass through the pelvis. We can't doubt that! But later we find these bones that form in membrane in the vault, and those that form in cartilage at the base of the skull, forming into a mechanism that has mobility. I did not try to disprove that argument, but I did try to disprove that there was mobility of that [*pointing to an adult skull*]. And the more I tried, well....

In the early days, Dr. Still pointed out the necessity of a knowledge of the articular surfaces between the vertebrae of the spine, and the ribs, and so forth–the articular surfaces that provide a range of motion in that spinal column. Without that mechanical picture, you could not scientifically adjust the spinal mechanism.

I searched through all the anatomical texts, which differ considerably today from that earlier day. We could find a lot about the external and internal surfaces of the bones, but nothing concerning the articular surfaces, the important articular surfaces between bone and bone. I want to specify some of the mechanical features which I found, on which beveling, both internal and external, with opposite articular contacts signified gliding mobility.

From the back of the room can you see this illustration? The sphenoid and the occiput, with the sphenoid up in front? I want to point out to you the beveled articular surface, like the gills of a fish. This [*pointing*] is the posterior articular surface of the greater wing of the sphenoid. At the upper half there is an external articular surface, changing down here to an internal bevel. A little groove between the upper and lower halves articulates with a little projection at the halfway point on the articular surface of this squamous portion of the temporal bone. Above this, the temporal bone is beveled internally and below it externally. Beveling, both internal and external, with opposite articular contacts signifying gliding mobility. Back of that squamous portion of the temporal bone, you will find corrugations that fit into corrugations running across the posteroinferior angle of the parietal bone. Corrugations, not a beveled articular surface, but a corrugated articular surface. We find these corrugations running transversely, diagonally, and so forth, picturing worm-gears, friction-gears, screw-gears. Gears found on the articular surfaces to which no anatomical texts refer.

I had to get away and do some independent thinking. I found the proof by digging into that hill of potatoes, the articular surfaces. Here are a few more: ball and socket, ball bearing, pulley, counter-shaft, and even a cradle. And why were they there but for mobility of those bones? It had to be! I am telling you that the Old Doctor's Ram of Reason hit me a terrific blow.[3] I had to *dig*. Here are still more: equalizers, force-pumps, governors, and even a fulcrum.

Now when you go into the adjoining room, you will begin to make a few tests for mobility. I had to test and prove these things on my own skull, using various contraptions of this and that. The more I tried to disprove, the more I found in the hill of potatoes.[4]

It is not going to be necessary for you to go through what I did. We are endeavoring to make this presentation as simple as possible so that you may see and feel the movement of the skull bones. In that endeavor you will be cautioned to *tone down* your sense of touch. You

---

3. Ram of Reason: Still, *Autobiography*, pp. 355-356, 362-363.

4. For the telling of his boyhood story of digging potatoes see article 26, "Philosophy of Osteopathy and Its Application," note 1.

have been used to dealing with the gross anatomy of the spinal column. In the cranial mechanism, we might say in comparison that you are dealing with the mechanism of a lady's wristwatch. Do not try to force anything within that cranial mechanism. There is something within it that is potent, and intelligent. An intelligent force within that *guides* the mechanism. All you need to do is to give it a little start and allow that "something" to carry it on into the position of flexion at the sphenobasilar junction. We will take you step by step. Your first test will be for recognition of the movement between the basilar part of the occipital bone and the sphenoid bone that occurs during inhalation, and the movement that also occurs in the opposite direction during exhalation. We want to get this into your thinking at this time. We will have more to say regarding "fundamentals" later on.

There is something within the skull that moves the osseous shell mechanism. An osseous shell mechanism with gears for accommodation of that "something" of which we will have more to say, intracranially, as we go along step by step.

I want to leave this thought with you. You know something of the cerebrospinal fluid, and there are textbooks and scientific experiments from the laboratories relative to it. But my knowledge of that body of cerebrospinal fluid differs from the present accepted authorities on the cerebrospinal fluid. Why? Because my knowledge came from experimentation on this specimen [*indicating his own head*]. For experiments, I had to perform upon my own skull, that is, upon a live specimen. I could not take a doctor and use him for a guinea pig. He would have all the knowledge and I would have none. I had to be my own guinea pig. By so doing, I learned something about the cerebrospinal fluid that differs from the texts. And I read between the lines of Dr. Still's writings. Here are quotations from his *Philosophy of Osteopathy*. I want you to endeavor to get between the lines with me in his thought:

> Another period of observation appears to the philosopher.... His mind will explore the bone, the ligament, the muscle, the fascia, the channels through which the blood travels from heart

> to local destiny with lymphatics and their contents.... It does obtain blood abundantly to and from the heart, but the results obtained are not satisfactory, and another leaf is opened of why no good results are obtained, and where is the mystery. [pp. 38-39]

We hear him say that the arterial stream is supreme, but here we get another thought as we think between the lines:

> A thought strikes him that the cerebrospinal fluid is the highest known element in the human body, and unless the brain furnishes this fluid in abundance a disabled condition of the body will remain. [p. 39]

He is speaking of the cerebrospinal fluid, not the arterial stream. You will hear me say from time to time that the arterial stream is supreme but the cerebrospinal fluid and its fluctuation is in command. Then Dr. Still goes on to say:

> He who is able to reason will see that this great river of life must be tapped, and the withering fields irrigated at once or the harvest of health will be forever lost. [p. 39]

Thus, in this cranial concept, we have been thinking with Dr. Still in our endeavor to tap this great river of life, the cerebrospinal fluid, and we hope you may understand how the cranial concept became a contribution of thought, directing attention to a hitherto unexplored area, or channel, in the science of osteopathy. A thought that is in no way apart from the science of osteopathy. Get that! Nothing apart. Not a specialty by itself...not even a therapy. We are dealing with a science! In that thought, we humbly recognize with Dr. Still that the cerebrospinal fluid is the highest known element in the human body.

That is all I will leave with you this morning because you will hear more about that later as we go along step by step. We take you to where you will have that intracranial vision that includes the fluctuation of the cerebrospinal fluid with its highest known element, and the membranes that carry venous return from the brain. Membranous channels that differ from the venous channels without the cranium. Venous channels that require something to move them along.

If this osseous shell did not accommodate that movement, we would have a stasis of venous blood leading from the brain, leading later to pathology of the brain.

Now to the tables, and tests for mobility. Thank you.

2. Cerebrospinal Fluid Fluctuation and Central Nervous System Motility

April 9, 1948.

It is my task to think independently in the presentation of the cranial concept relative to the formation of the cerebrospinal fluid and its function. I realize that I am bucking up against authorities, so-called, who one year from now may differ in their viewpoint. In other words, in their summary, they wind up, "in conclusion there is no conclusion." One of their conclusions refers to an interchange between the cerebrospinal fluid and the arterial circulation of the choroid plexus, and there is a long string of theories as to what takes place.

On the board to my left, there is a drawing taken from an anatomical text with which you are familiar. It was made from the dead specimen in which the walls of the third ventricle are vertical and close together. Dr. Kimberly called your attention to the third ventricle and what happens at death.[5] The roof of that third ventricle is a so-called choroid plexus. It has a curtain between it and the third ventricle. When death came, there was a shortening process, a bunching up of the choroid plexus, as you see it here on the chart. The same thing occurs in the choroid plexus which is in the walls of the lateral ventricles–not in the ventricle–but in the walls. When death occurred, the motility of the cerebral hemispheres contracted. There again you

---

5. Paul E. Kimberly, D.O. (Des Moines Still College of Osteopathy, 1940) was a professor of anatomy at the Des Moines Still College of Osteopathy. Beginning in 1944, he arranged for Dr. Sutherland to use the college facilities to conduct classes in "Osteopathy in the Cranial Field." At these courses Dr. Kimberly would extensively review the anatomy of the human head.

have the shortening or bunched appearance that you see in the anatomical illustration, in the walls of the lateral ventricles. It is the same way in the walls of the fourth ventricle–contraction of the brain stem, and the shortened, or bunched appearance of the choroid plexus, the arterial circulation of the pia mater with the artery running up to it. If I had time, I would take you on a minnow swim through the cerebrospinal fluid, but there is no time this morning.[6] I would show you the artery passing through the cisterna interpeduncularis on its way to the choroid plexus. I would show you a little stream of cerebrospinal fluid flowing along with that artery to the roof of the third ventricle, out on the walls of the lateral ventricles, and out to the walls of the cerebellum for the fourth ventricle. In envisioning this, you are on the outside of the brain, not inside the ventricles. There is a curtain hanging down into the ventricle, but the interchange that occurs between the cerebrospinal fluid and the blood is not within the ventricles. It is on the walls, on the outside of the ventricles. The specimen you are looking at [chart] is in exhalation. Now let us take a look at the live specimen and see what occurs during inhalation.

The third ventricle goes into a V-shape formation, and the roof of the third ventricle stretches out. The bunched up formation of the choroid plexus spreads out on this V-form, a mechanical arrangement for rhythmic balanced interchange between the cerebrospinal fluid and the blood during inhalation and exhalation: stretching out during inhalation, bunching up during exhalation, the fluctuation of the cerebrospinal fluid and that little stream of fluid that follows along with the artery, clear out into the walls of the lateral ventricles. See how in inhalation the motility of the hemispheres expands and the bunched up choroid plexus lengthens. The same thing occurs back in the walls of the fourth ventricle. The hemispheres expand–the cerebellar hemispheres–during inhalation and contract during exhalation. In the cranial concept, that illustrates the mechanism that provides that important rhythmic

---

6. See article 34, "The Tour of the Minnow."

balance interchange between the cerebrospinal fluid and the blood.

There are chemicals in the cerebrospinal fluid, and there are chemicals in the arterial stream. You find that in your texts. They tell you what you will find in the cerebrospinal fluid, yet the same text tells you there is something there they cannot find, something invisible in the cerebrospinal fluid. We call your attention to the Breath of Life.[7] Intelligence. Authorities have various ideas as to how the cerebrospinal fluid originates. They know about as much about it as I do, and that is close to zero. I am satisfied to know that it does originate and that it is replenished from time to time. It has to be, like the water in the battery of your car. As you read between the lines of Dr. Still's writings, you wonder what he means when he says: "The brain is God's drugstore, having within all drugs, lubricating oil, opiates, acids, and every quality of drug that the wisdom of God thought necessary for human health and happiness."[8] He keeps referring to his Maker. He refers to the waters of the brain–the highest known element–then he tells you that the lymphatics drink more of the waters of the brain than all the internal viscera combined.[9]

We have been talking of testing for motion. Of what? The sphenobasilar "symphysis." Now we are going to say something about the motility of the brain. Motility, not mobility, of the cerebral hemispheres

---

7. For a fuller discussion of Dr. Sutherland's use of the Breath of Life see article 23, "Untitled Talk 1944." Cf. "And the Lord God formed man of the dust of the ground, and breathed into his nostrils the breath of life; and man became a living soul." Gen. 2:7, King James Version.

8. Still, *Autobiography*, p. 182. Note that in the 1908 revised ed., Dr. Still had changed the word "brain" to "body;" cf. the original 1897 ed., p. 219.

9. "A thought strikes him that the cerebrospinal fluid is the highest known element that is contained in the human body, and unless the brain furnishes this fluid in abundance a disabled condition of the body will remain." (p. 39); "The lymphatics consume more of the finer fluids of the brain than the whole viscera combined." (p. 104); "The lymphatics are closely and universally connected with the spinal cord and all other nerves, long or short, universal or separate, and all drink from the waters of the brain." (p. 105). From Still, *Philosophy*.

swinging out, expanding during inhalation, the lateral ventricles dilating. As you look at this drawing of the cast of the ventricles, here, we will say, are the wings of a bird. Put a cerebral hemisphere on this wing, and another one on the other. Now visualize that in its motility–expanding–the wings, like the wings of a bird, go back. But where are those wings attached? Up here [*pointing to chart*] at the superior anterior area of the third ventricle. As they go out, visualize that roof stretching out from the third ventricle, taking this form, this V-shape form. There is a floor to that third ventricle, and from that floor you have a stalk which has a hollow tube that extends down, and here we find the little pituitary body, an anterior lobe and a posterior lobe. Some of these authorities tell you that, from the hypothalamus area in the floor, there are about 40,000 nerve fibers running down that infundibulum to the pituitary body. As that floor lifts up, the infundibulum goes along with it.

What happens to the pituitary body which is strapped down to the sella turcica of the sphenoid bone by a firm band of dural membrane? It has either to be torn apart, as in dissection, or it is going to lift that sella turcica of the sphenoid bone and tip the sphenoid into a "nose dive." That is what occurs when the sphenoid circumrotates into flexion during inhalation. So, you have that little pituitary body possessing motility in itself, and also a ridable mobility. Riding in the saddle, riding in the sella turcica–motion and motility–essential for secretion. The little pituitary body, the leader of the flock of the endocrine system. And, if it is going to lead the flock, it cannot be idle. It must be active, up and doing, with motility, and mobility. Riding in the saddle, and at the same time having motility-like pulsation, expansion and contraction. Then, what occurs during the exhalation period? The bunched up appearance here [*roof of the third ventricle*] and the floor of the third ventricle drops down and the infundibulum drops downward. Now then, if you have a restriction in the movement of that sphenoid bone and its saddle, what would happen? A disturbance would occur in the normal secretion of the pituitary body, a restriction in the mechanical mechanism at the roof–a disturbance to that important rhythmical balance interchange between the cerebrospinal fluid and the blood. So, when you become a cranial technician, you become a pharmacist in restoring the mobility of that sphenoid bone, and restoring the activity of the leader of the flock of the endocrine system. You mix the drugs in God's drugstore. You fill the prescription. Remember that you have the cerebrospinal fluid in the lateral ventricles, within the third ventricle, in the aqueducts cerebri, or the Sylvian aqueduct, and back in the fourth ventricle. A constant body of fluid from the fourth ventricle through the doorways leading to the large body of cerebrospinal fluid surrounding the brain, surrounding the spinal cord–oh, that important fluctuation of the cerebrospinal fluid! Something that carries nourishment, something invisible that it gives to the nerve cells in the hypothalamus for instance, with the transmutation following along those fibers down to the little pituitary body. Think of it! The cranial concept goes further and deeper than the mere knowledge of this lifeless bone, of specimens you find in the laboratory.

Dr. Kimberly spoke of the membranes, the falx cerebri and the tentorium cerebelli. They form the main venous channels, do they not, carrying venous blood from the brain. And so in my early writings, especially an article appearing in *The Western Osteopath*, the title was "Membranous-Articular Strains." Notice–not "Articular-Membranous Strains" but "Membranous-Articular Strains." Why? Because it is the restriction in the mobility or movement of that main membranous wall carrying venous blood from the brain. A membranous wall that must have some sort of an osseous shell that allows the blood to move along during the inhalation and exhalation periods–the sagittal suture. You will find in the concave internal area of the mastoid portion of the temporal bone that there is no suture to move the blood along. But you follow the lateral sinus and find it passes over the posterior inferior angle of the parietal bone–that area where you were told that there are corrugations on its inferior articular surface that allow it to move outward during inhalation and inward during exhalation. So we have right there, in the movement of that posterior inferior angle of the parietal bone, something that moves the venous blood along. You know that the petrous portion of the temporal bone rotates internally and externally. You have another venous channel, the superior petrosal and inferior petrosal sinuses. Unless the membranous channels have some movement, you would find a restriction in the venous channels and a backing into the cavernous sinus. And, where is the cavernous sinus? It runs along lateral to the body of the sphenoid bone, lateral to the little pituitary body with a body of cerebrospinal fluid above it. And the infundibulum passing down through that body of cerebrospinal fluid. Membranous walls of the cavernous sinus. If it were not for the motion of the sphenoid bone during inhalation and exhalation, you would have a stasis of venous blood leading to the superior and the inferior petrosal sinuses. Notice that the internal carotid artery passes through that sinus [*cavernous*] in the opposite direction, protected, and having the same arterial wall that is without. The main venous channels are membranous. You do have small cerebral veins with the same venous wall found outside the skull, emptying into this main venous channel. But when you look at the dead specimen, these empty in the opposite direction. During inhalation the mouths turn and empty into the main venous channels, like a plumber's "T." Membranous articular strains–it is the membranous restriction in the main venous channels that leads to the pathology in the brain.

I told you about starting the fluctuation of the cerebrospinal fluid by throwing the petrous portions into external rotation, and in that instance, it is the tentorium that fluctuates the cerebrospinal fluid. Restriction in the movement of that membrane means restriction in the normal fluctuation of the cerebrospinal fluid. Hence we not only have venous channels to consider in restriction leading to pathology in the brain but also a limitation of the normal nourishment from the cerebrospinal fluid to the nerve cells and its transmutation along the nerve path to its terminal.

That is the picture that becomes deeper as you dig into it. I am skipping over the surface. I could talk all day long on this subject. But

I am going to give you just enough so you can get a bite on the hook. Then you will be joining a study group, digging deeper and deeper. Sometime today you are going to be hearing something about compression of the bulb. Now do not think for a moment that you are going to compress a bulb. That is something that came into the terminology because of using a little compressible rubber bulb for illustration of movement of the fourth ventricle during inhalation and exhalation. It contracts during exhalation and expands during inhalation. And why do we apply it to the fourth ventricle? Because all the physiological centers, including that of respiration, are located in the floor of the fourth ventricle. In other words, in "compressing the bulb" we mean compressing the operation of the fourth ventricle, which is done manually, by compressing the outer edges of the squama [*of the occiput*] at its lower area. That is the only place that you can compress the squama of the occipital bone. It is beneath the attachment of the tentorium cerebelli which is above the cerebellum. It is a method of learning how to bring the fluctuation of the cerebrospinal fluid down to a brief idling in its fluctuation.

If I were to take a glass of water and shake this table, the water would spill out of the glass. But if I place my hand gently on the table and transmit a vibration, not a shake, the water will vibrate to the center.[10] That is what we are trying to do when we say "compress the bulb." That is, to bring the fluctuation of the cerebrospinal fluid down to the idling point–a brief idling point period. The cerebrospinal fluid is like that glass of water. When you reach that idling period, you will detect an immediate change, a going down under your fingers like water under thin ice. Not only in the hands, the extremities, but all through the viscera, the connective tissue and the fascia. An interchange that occurs between all the fluids of the body. And I mean *all* the fluids of the body.

Now think back to what I said earlier: All the physiological centers are located in the floor of the fourth ventricle. The endocrine system

10. This is the description of transmitting a vibration to a glass of water to which Dr. Sutherland often refers.

is regulated to the immediate needs of the body, and to interchange between the "leader of the flock" and the endocrine system. The cerebrospinal fluid is in command of metabolism and much of the involuntary operation, and the autoprotective mechanism of the system.

You heard Dr. Howard Lippincott call attention to the fact that secondary osteopathic lesions become less perceptible under the influence of bulb compression.[11] So it is valuable in determining primary spinal lesions. Do you know anything about the penetrating oil that a mechanic uses on a rusty belt? He doesn't tear that bolt off. He puts on some penetrating oil. All through that spinal area, you have a change in the tissues of that osseous spinal column. You have that same cerebrospinal fluid carrying nutrition to the various cells leading out from the spinal column. I am reminded of a guest speaker who had studied with me, who appeared on the Minnesota State Program at the annual convention. What did he do? He called a few of the doctors up front and had them examine a case, the cervical tissue, the spinal tissue, etcetera. Then he told them, "I am going to compress the bulb." He did so, and then called the same men. They could hardly believe their sense of touch. They found relaxation all the way down that spinal column, the cervical tissue, and so forth.

The cranial concept includes what? Dr. Kimberly started in with the brain this morning. Now I am going to reverse that and consider fundamentally the cerebrospinal fluid and its fluctuation, the motility of the cerebral hemispheres and the cerebellar hemispheres, and the motility of the third ventricle and the cerebral aqueduct. Remember that the aqueduct of Sylvius widens during inhalation and contracts during exhalation, that the corticospinal tracts form the walls of the aqueduct of Sylvius, that the third ventricle dilates, and so forth. So we speak of the motility of the brain–the entire brain, including

---

11. Howard A. Lippincott, D.O. (1893-1963: American School of Osteopathy, 1916) was a member of Dr. Sutherland's teaching staff. He became president of the Sutherland Cranial Teaching Foundation following Dr. Sutherland, wrote several publications regarding osteopathy in the cranial field, and conducted an active study group with his wife, Rebecca, in his home in Moorestown, New Jersey.

the stem–and of the spinal cord, the fluctuation of the cerebrospinal fluid all around it and within it. This tide, as we call it, this constant body of fluid. Then we have the intracranial membranes, which we call the reciprocal tension membranes. If we put up a couple of poles and attach a wire to them, we would call that wire a reciprocal tension wire between the two poles. We pull one pole one direction and the other pole comes with it, and vice versa. That is a reciprocal tension wire. So we have the falx cerebri and the tentorium cerebelli which we call a reciprocal tension membrane between articular poles of attachment. As the sphenoid moves in one direction and the occiput moves in another, as the petrous portions rotate externally and internally–that is a tense reciprocal tension membrane. Dr. Kimberly told you how it has attachment at the upper cervicals–not all the upper cervicals–and that the dural membrane then hangs, as described by some anatomical authorities, like a hollow tube, that is, hanging without any other osseous contact until it reaches the sacrum.[12] So we include in that consideration a reciprocal tension membrane continuing on down from the cranial mechanism to the sacral mechanism. And we say that this mechanism includes the articular mobility–not the articular motility–but the articular mobility of the bones of the skull and also the articular mobility of the sacrum between the ilia. Mark that! Between the ilia–not the mobility of the ilia upon the sacrum, that is a postural mobility.

There are no muscles of attachment from the sacrum to the ilium as

---

12. Subsequent anatomic studies have demonstrated that the dura mater is attached to the vertebral canal in the lumbar region. The anterior attachments are short and strong while the posterior attachments are weaker and longer. The anterior and anterolateral connective tissue bands attach to the posterior longitudinal ligament. The bands are strongest at the L5-S1 level and less strong in the upper lumbar region. The dural nerve root sheaths are also attached to the posterior longitudinal ligament anteriorly and to the periosteum of the inferior pedicle laterally.
Cf. Parkin and Harrison, "The Topographical Anatomy of the Lumbar Epidural Space," *Journal of Anatomy* 141 (1985):211-217, and Spencer, Irwin and Miller, "Anatomy and Significance of Fixation of the Lumbosacral Nerve Roots in Sciatica," *Spine* 8, no. 6 (1983): 672-679.

an agency of propulsion of articular mobility. Ever stop to think of that? No muscles of attachment from the sacrum to the ilium. We have ligamentous tissue. We have muscles of attachment leading from the sacrum to the femur. But none from the sacrum to the ilium as an agency of articular mobility. The movement of the sacrum between the ilia is an involuntary mobility that moves in conjunction with the mobility of the cranial mechanism. There are no muscular agencies for the propulsion of the cranial articular mechanism either. It is an involuntary mobility. Gears that formed in adult life to accommodate the intracranial mechanism. That is all it is. So we have these gears, as the sacrum between the ilia, that work in conjunction with gears in the osseous shell of the cranium. Getting tired? Enough for now.

3. Techniques for Incitation and Repression of Cerebrospinal Fluid Fluctuation

April 10, 1948.

In the application of cranial technique, both in diagnosis and in treatment, we have adapted Dr. Andrew Taylor Still's wrist technique, wherein we utilize only the flexor digitorum profundus and flexor pollicis longus muscles: the flexors–you know where they are located. We use no force from the shoulder! Instead we utilize these muscles. That enables you to tone down your technique from the gross spinal technique to that of the delicate mechanism of the cranial structure. At the same time, utilize these feeling-seeing-thinking-knowing digits in both diagnosis and technique.

Previously, I have called your attention to the man rescued on the shore of Lake Erie, where I threw the petrous portion of the temporal bones into external rotation, and pictured to you the movement of the tentorium as fluctuating the cerebrospinal fluid.[13] That was done

---

13. See the story associated with note 7 in article 23, "Untitled Talk 1944;" and Sutherland, *Cranial Bowl*, p. 54.

with a contact on the temporal bones, using the flexor digitorum profundus muscles as the motive power to throw that petrous portion into external rotation. In other words, we "cranked the car" and started the fluctuation of the cerebrospinal fluid.

Today, we want to call your attention to what we call incitation of the cerebrospinal fluid fluctuation. That is what we did to the man on the shore, with a bilateral movement of the petrous portions of the temporals in the same direction. In this technique today, we are going to alternate the movement–"throw" one petrous portion into external rotation and, at the same time, throw the other into internal rotation, and vice versa. First one side, and then the other, as a unit wherein the entire mechanism moves as a unit, and that same tentorium fluctuates the cerebrospinal fluid.

On the board, you will notice the term "incitive application," that is, to activate or incite cerebrospinal fluid fluctuation. Now visualize the tentorium fluctuating the cerebrospinal fluid, and the mechanism operating as a unit. The sphenoid bone, first on one side–see the torsion activity there? The physiological torsion activity that we have been demonstrating. An incitive application to activate the cerebrospinal fluid. Now then, with this same contact on the temporal bones–it is a contact only, more like a pulse beat of the middle fingers–now barely turn, one in one direction, and the other in the opposite direction. Your contact on the temporal bones is like a gentle pulse beat in its movement of the petrous portions of the temporal bones, one in the direction of internal rotation, the other in the direction of external rotation, and vice versa. As you use your motive power here, it is a very short, barely perceptible movement, and what do we call it? "Palliative application to initiate repression of the cerebrospinal fluid fluctuation."

Yesterday, you were given the application of compression of the fourth ventricle, or "compression of the bulb" so-called.[14] What did

---

14. The technique called "compression of the fourth ventricle" was originally termed "compression of the bulb."

you do? You brought the fluctuation of the cerebrospinal fluid down to the same point we get here in the palliative application for repression. We are bringing the fluctuation down to that desired point, that brief rhythmic period of fluctuation of that body of cerebrospinal fluid inside the cranium, all around the brain, within the brain, all around the spinal cord, within the spinal cord. Again I want you to visualize the movement of that body of cerebrospinal fluid in its fluctuation, as I compared it to a glass of water with a transmitted vibration by which the water all came up to a central point. Quite different from a shake of the table by which the water spilled over. It is what we want to get in "compression of the bulb." And it is what we want to get in the palliative application type of technique, which I likened to the pulsebeat, where you bring the fluctuation to a central point in vibration, the motor is idling, and that interchange between all the fluids of the body occurs.[15]

I am going to take Dr. Kimberly to task for one expression he used this morning, when he spoke of "the outflow" along the nerve fibers. It is not the outflow so much as a change or transmutation in that fluid–something that goes out from that quiver–an invisible something, which you might call the nerve force, and it follows along out to the area where its terminals dwell with the lymphatics. A change in its constituents or elements, through a transmutation. This is quite different from transmission, or an outflow. A transmutation, a change in the fluid, that changes infection that has accumulated in the lymph nodes, as we call them, and that same transmutation changes that infection before it empties into the cisterna chyli, before it is emptied into the venous channels. There is "something" in the cerebrospinal fluid–many so-called authorities refer to it–but they do not know what it is. Dr. Still in his vision referred to it as "the highest known element in the human body." Now I want you to see this highest known element in the human body going out in that transmutation

---

15. Cf. "Lectures on Cranial Osteopathy: Des Moines," lecture 2, "Cerebrospinal Fluid Fluctuation and Central Nervous System Motility."

from the nerve cell along the fibers to the terminal–a transmutation–something that is changed, carrying this highest known element. Then you will understand more clearly, perhaps, what Dr. Still meant when he tells you that the lymphatics consume more of the "waters of the brain" than the entire viscera.[16] Now we are thinking between the lines of Dr. Still's philosophy as he expressed it in material terms. In reading *Philosophy of Osteopathy* and *Research and Practice*, think with his thoughts in order to get his viewpoint and vision.

He mentions there that *all* the nerves "drink from the waters of the brain." Visualize that transmutation of the highest known element, rather than an outflow of the cerebrospinal fluid, clear to the venous channels. A transmutation, and a change in the cerebrospinal fluid in that transmutation.

We are going to pause now and let that thought sink in. I am going to make a special endeavor to stress the fluctuation of the cerebrospinal fluid as the fundamental principle in the cranial concept. The "sap of the tree"–something that contains the Breath of Life–not the breath of air.[17] Something invisible, referred to by Dr. Still as the highest known element–replenished from time to time. Do you think we will ever know from whence it cometh? Probably not. But it is there. That is all we need to know.

Next week we will tell you how to control that tide of cerebrospinal fluid in another direction. How to utilize it in diagnosis and in technique. We want you to understand the fundamental principle. We want to simplify your technique. To get away from the use of any external force. But enough for now. Thank you.

---

16. See note 9 in this article for the full quotations. Still, *Philosophy*, pp. 39,104,105.

17. For a fuller discussion of Dr. Sutherland's use of the Breath of Life see article 23, "Untitled Talk 1944." Cf. "And the Lord God formed man of the dust of the ground, and breathed into his nostrils the breath of life; and man became a living soul." Gen. 2:7, King James Version.

4. Diagnosis and Treatment Using the Tide

April 12, 1948.

The same old subject! Fluctuation of the cerebrospinal fluid. You have been learning how to control that fluctuation in the "compression of the bulb,"[18] and also in the incitant and repressive techniques which some of you have heard me allude to as the "pussyfoot" and the "cat's paw" technique, to convey gentleness.[19] This morning we are going to endeavor to illustrate how you can use that directing of the tide, or potency of the fluctuation of the cerebrospinal fluid, in diagnosis.

We have among us here one who has a fractured squama of the occipital bone on the left side. If you were to make with your fingers a slight pressure on the *left* side of the frontal bone so as to direct the fluid over to the *right* lambdoidal suture, you would find in this case a very free movement in the right occipitomastoid articulation. But by changing your direction from the *right* frontal bone to the *left* occipitomastoid area, you would find some restriction back here in the area of the left occipitomastoid articulation, on the side, that is, of the fracture in the squama of the occipital bone. That is a diagnostic feature. It points out to you the limitation of the movement in the occipitomastoid articulation and shows you a limitation in the movement of the temporal bone. It would not be necessary for you to test that through any physiological motion to see if there was a fixation in that temporal bone. Your direction of the tide from the right frontal bone diagonally across would show you that there was not the separation at that articulation which you do get by pressing from the left diagonally over to the right, where you had the free movement. On

---

18. The technique "compression of the bulb" was later renamed "compression of the fourth ventricle."

19. Dr. Sutherland also used these terms to "make the point of different degrees of excursion and different rates in turning the petrous portions of the temporal bones for controlling the [cerebrospinal fluid] fluctuations." See Sutherland, *Teachings*, p. 174.

the other hand, you can test the movement of the greater wing of the sphenoid bone and the frontal bone by directing your tide diagonally from this area forward to the left frontal area, and test whether that tide moved over and whether you had a movement of the left greater wing of the sphenoid, or the movement of the frontal bone that occurs during exhalation and inhalation. If you found a restriction, you would know you had a fixation of some kind beneath it, in the left greater wing of the sphenoid, or, the left frontal bone. Take for example a frontosphenoidal lesion: a traumatic lesion wherein the frontal bone on that side has been driven posteriorly on the greater wing of the sphenoid or vice versa, anteriorly by a blow up here [indicating vertex], forcing it anteriorly on the greater wing of the sphenoid. So a restriction when directing that tide in the movement of that bone over here would be positive indication–you would not have to test it for motion. That in itself is a test for motion.

I again call your attention to the glass of water and the shaking of the table that would cause the water to spill, whereas the transmission of the vibration from the shoulder would cause the water to vibrate to the center.[20] Now we are going to put a cap on the top of that glass of water, and instead of seeing that quiver to the line on the top of the glass, I want you to see the whole tide coming to what we call the "balance," as balance between two scales. That is the point where the mechanism is idling, neither ebbing out or flowing in, but right on the neutral point. That is why we say, "rhythmic balance interchange." The period where all the fluids of the body have an interchange.

Now then, back to that glass of water. This time let us look at it as in a plastic glass, something flexible. I put my finger on that flexible glass, or plastic arrangement, and I see that water being fluctuated to the opposite side. I am directing the tide in that glass of water. I can put pressure down here at the bottom of the flexible container and direct it to the upper area. Or, from the top I direct it to the lower

---

20. For a description of this transmitted vibration see note 10 in this article.

area. That is an uninvolved illustration of what we mean by directing the potency of the cerebrospinal fluid. In so doing we are directing not only a potency, but a potency that has intelligence within it–a body of fluid that has the Breath of Life, that has "something" invisible, not only of potency but an Intelligence spelled with a capital "I." In that potency of the fluctuation, you have an unerring intracranial and intraspinal force, with the tendency toward the normal as the motive power for the reduction of the lesions. Now in this squama fracture of which I spoke, we have made a diagnosis. In the correction, we can use that same directive force from the right frontal area diagonally over to that point, and if you did nothing else, that tide would in time correct the lesions. But you can do this: Take that temporal bone, and the occipital bone, and visualizing movement like the movement of the cap on a fruit jar, you can very gently turn the temporal bone in one direction and the occipital bone in the other, and hold gently while you direct the tide from the right frontal area. You are going to deal with many so-called traumatic injuries, and that is why we are stressing this directing of the potency of the fluctuation of the cerebrospinal fluid in diagnosis and technique. You are going to experience some revealing surprises under your gentle feeling-seeing-thinking-knowing fingers.

During the October session of 1947, we had an unexpected clinic. A boy of high school age, the son of an osteopathic physician, had a little scrap with another high school boy, and was taken advantage of in an unguarded moment. In fact, he was unconscious from the attack. The blow was somewhere here in the nasal area and the zygomatic on the left. His was a sadly disfigured face. You looked at it and thought the nasal bones were fractured, and he had a very serious syndrome in the left side of his head that indicated caution in treatment. We had here an indication of a frontosphenoidal lesion posterior on the left and an occipitomastoid lesion indicated on the left. That in itself is a serious condition. An occipitomastoid lesion is one of the most serious that you can encounter in your practice because it disturbs the normal fluctuation of the cerebrospinal fluid. We had to be very cautious as to how to proceed in this case, so we tackled it from the frontosphenoidal lesion on the left side. An assistant held the pterygoid [process], and another assistant was directed to use the "cant-hook technique"–with which he was familiar–on the frontosphenoidal lesion, just to lift it a little to free it from its articulation. Someone directed the fluid from the right occipitomastoid articulation diagonally over here to this [left frontosphenoidal] and things went into place easily and gently.

What did it? The releasing of the frontal bone from the greater wing of the sphenoid and the directing of the potency of the tide from the right occipitomastoid. No force was applied, but the tide–an unerring intelligent motive force–did the work.

At this time, a traumatic injury case–a war casualty–was discussed in which there had been trephining along the sagittal suture and also below, in which the parietal bone had been removed and reinserted.

Later, this case was treated cranially. By directing the potency of the tide, we changed the size of the trephine, and we removed a pressure from that side of the cerebral hemisphere. And where did we direct the tide from? Not from the left side, but from the right. It could be done from the right occipitomastoid articulation–it could be done from the right frontal over to that area.

Now, think–what is included in the primary respiratory mechanism as the cranial consideration goes? The fluctuation of the cerebrospinal fluid, the intraspinal membranes and the articular mobility of the sacrum between the ilia. The point of extreme caution in this case was on the left side of the skull. So–you go down here to the right side of the sacrum and direct diagonally to the left side of the skull, directing the potency of the cerebrospinal fluid fluctuation by way of the sacrum. It is the same fluid, is it not? We have also, when indicated, directed this tide down to the spinal area from the cranial mechanism.

Not long ago I had occasion to examine a traumatic injury, and the patient asked, "How did you know there was a restriction on this side and none on that?" He had felt the movement of the tide on his own frontal area and thought I must be psychic to know where the trouble was by simple pressure elsewhere. No, nothing psychic at all. I knew there was restriction and where because there was a little hesitancy in the fluid in fluctuating to the left side. He felt the restriction in the fluctuation in the left side and the freedom with which it moved to the right. Simply a principle of diagnosis–the directing of the potency of the fluctuation of the cerebrospinal fluid with no blind force from the outside. This is not an idle dream. You will find "the proof of the pudding" during your practice session. Thank you.

5. "Bent Twigs:" Infants and Children

April 16, 1948.

On display was Dr. Sutherland's collection of infants' and children's skulls, ranging from four fetal months to ten years. These were closely examined and studied.

On the board you will see the subject, "Bent Twigs." I am sure you are familiar with the quotation, "As the twig is bent, so the tree inclines." In other words, the osseous tissue may become bent way back in the prenatal stage, with resulting irregularities which must be taken into consideration in diagnosis of cranial lesions. Dr. Rebecca Lippincott will tell you in her talk how some of these things occur prenatally, natally and postnatally.[21] So it is not necessary for me to go into details.

As you know, in the prenatal stage and on up to the fifth and sixth years, our cranial structure is not operating with articular gears. Some of the osseous tissues have a membranous interlacing or contact, while

---

21. Rebecca C. Lippincott, D.O (1894-1986: Philadelphia College of Osteopathy, 1923) was a member of Dr. Sutherland's teaching staff. She co-authored *A Manual of Cranial Techniques* with her husband, Howard, and together they conducted an active study group in Moorestown, New Jersey.

those at the base of the skull have cartilaginous interunion. So during that stage, the structure is operating without any mechanical gears, excepting at one place–at the junction of the condylar parts of the occiput and the atlas.

You will notice that the condylar portions have a little protuberance, even on that skull as early as the fourth month, that fits into a concave surface on the atlas bone, known as the facets of the atlas. These condyles converge anteriorly and diverge posteriorly, and also converge inferiorly. So, supposing you have the head resting in the pelvis and you have a force like a labor pain, and the amniotic fluid coming right down over the top of the skull–right directly over what? The contact on those condyles in the fulcrum of the atlas–that is a bony contact at that age, the only bony contact you have between the bones of the skull at that age. A fulcrum–a force driving down and driving those condyles into the concavity of the atlas. And if you have the force back here [*demonstrating on infant skull*], it would drive them forward. Or, if here, drive them backward. Condylar portions that have a cartilaginous union, and forming the lateral borders of the foramen magnum. Back of that is the squama [of the occiput] with a cartilaginous union between it and the condylar portions, and anteriorly you have another cartilaginous union between the condylar portions and the basilar process of the occipital bone. Now then, what happens when a force with a bony contact–the only bony contact that you have in that period with the condyles of the condylar part and the facets of the atlas–you have all seen the subluxation of the ulnar bone and the radius–that is an illustration of what takes place. Often times, through trauma over the top of the head, at the back of the head, or the front of the head, prenatally, postnatally, and sometimes during the normal passage of the babe through the birth canal wherein in the normal passage the parietal bone molds over the frontal bone, and molds over the squama of the occipital bone, so that the little head can pass normally through the pelvis, and after passing through neglects to return to its normal position.

Along about the fourth year perhaps, little horn-like protuberances begin to come out on the ossification centers of the parietal bone. Why?

Because the parietals still lap over the squama [occiput] and the frontal bones–a normal lapping that neglected to go back to normal position following birth. You call it a birth injury? No. The spank on the sacrum, the cry of the babe, and the fluctuation of the cerebrospinal fluid usually bring the bone back into place. But, not always. When this is indicated, we find that our cranial technicians, if given opportunity, do bring it back into place at the time of normal delivery.

No, not birth injuries, although improper application of the forceps can cause birth injuries. As in one case that came under my care. A young woman at the age of 25, with a forceps mark right down the cheek. One frontal bone was down, the other up. Double vision, at the age of 25. One orbital cavity looking up this way and the other down that way. I am happy to say that she no longer sees double and is able to drive a car. So, harm can be done, although we find more abnormalities occurring during normal deliveries than you will find through the application of forceps when properly applied.

Then a little child learns to creep, and to walk. He falls over on the back of his head. A little bump to which no attention is paid. On a mechanism still without its articular gears. You have learned something about sidebending-rotation in the cranium. Ever stop to think that could be a bent twig? Take a rotation of the squama of the occiput, and another there, the membrane. So, starting with the sidebending-rotation, you have an abnormality in the adult skull that started way back there in the infant–the bent twig. Likewise, you can also have a torsion, or an extreme flexion or extension, as a bent twig. You may have irregularities in the frontal process of the maxilla–bent– and continuing to grow until it is so inclined. You see some bent twigs here in these skulls at the age of ten. These things must be taken into consideration in the diagnosis of any cranial lesion. Bent twigs, abnormalities, the tree inclined, and so on into adult life.

Dr. Kimberly asked me a question the other day about the mandible. You can have a bent twig in the formation of the mandible. One-half of the mandible may, in its formation, grow longer than the other. This must be taken into consideration in diagnosing by the mandible. There may be a difference in the size of one zygoma from the other. I am not telling this to discourage you but to point out bent twig influences. I think this is enough to give you the picture I want to get across right now. You will be told about some of the things that start from the bent twigs prenatally, natally, and postnatally.

6. Final Lecture

April 25, 1948.

What I am about to say is not a religious talk, although it may appear to be. You have observed the case in which several reductions were made and the ease with which I made a diagnosis. You have heard a great deal about Dr. Still and his diagnoses and reductions. Through the years, I have endeavored to think osteopathy with Dr. Still. Consequently, I am able to practice osteopathy to a certain degree. I agree with Dr. Harry L. Chiles who said: "If one thinks osteopathy he will practice osteopathy."

A few weeks before we came down here to Des Moines, we had a visit from a young lady, a ballet dancer whose name is well known on Broadway. In our living room, she gave a dramatic and reverent dance interpretation of the biblical saying, "Be Still and Know that I am God."[22] In her impressive presentation, we could see that she lost all awareness of the physical senses. "Be Still" these physical senses and get as close to your Maker as you can–closer than breathing. Where you realize what is meant by the Breath of Life, not the breath of air–the breath of air being merely one of the material substances which man utilizes in his walkabout on earth.[23]

---

22. "Be still and know that I am God . . ." Ps. 46:10, King James Version.

23. For a fuller discussion of Dr. Sutherland's use of the Breath of Life see article 23, "Untitled Talk 1944." Cf. "And the Lord God formed man of the dust of the ground, and breathed into his nostrils the breath of life; and man became a living soul." Gen. 2:7, King James Version.

Have you ever sat by the bedside of a departing patient with your hand upon the squama of the occiput in an endeavor to ease and realized that the patient in that final moment was closer to his Maker than breathing? My experiments have not been confined to the mere correction of a temporal bone, etcetera. It has been my endeavor to get as far away from the physical senses as I possibly could, that is, to a point where one begins to experience, to realize, "Be Still and Know." That is why I have so much to say about information gained solely through laboratory tests and experiments and information often gained through the application of erring or unreliable physical senses. How many of you have the same degree of vision? The same degree of touch? You saw me making that diagnosis during the application of seeing-feeling-thinking fingers–fingers that endeavor to get away from the sensation of physical touch, wherein you have the knowing touch. In many instances, you then place your hands right upon the lesion. But, as I said before, this is not intended as a religious subject.

One time when called to a neighboring town for consultation, I arrived at the home of the patient to find about 14 persons gathered in the parlor waiting sadly for the patient to die. His condition had been diagnosed as heart pathology and the time limit had been given also. He was near the borderline. I walked into the room with the realization that the patient was closer to his Maker than breathing, but I had been called in as a consultant for a serious condition and I had to do something. I sat down at the bedside and my fingers went right up here in the area of the third rib on the left side. My fingers held there for a minute, and next thing I knew, I did that. [*Illustrated with a quick movement.*] That took place about 30 years ago. The patient lived, married and the last I knew was pitching in the hay field. Thinking-feeling-seeing-knowing fingers. By *knowing*, I mean not information gained by physical senses but a knowledge that comes from getting as far as one can from the physical sense. So, along the way I have been searching here and there.

At one time I had the opportunity to have "class instruction" in

Christian Science by one of Mrs. Eddy's first students.[24] I am not a Christian Scientist. But we were taught the truth that man is made in the image and likeness of God, the Creator. I think that Dr. Still saw that man; I think you will find him pointing to that man if you will get between the lines and get his thought. That is what I mean by thinking osteopathy, not thinking osteopathically.

Osteopathy is here to stay. Osteopathy is a science. The cranial concept is osteopathy. It therefore is a science. It is not an integral part of osteopathy, it is osteopathy. It is not a "therapy." That is why I feel so intensely about the term "therapy." For this is a science that deals with the natural forces of the body. You have seen evidence of this this week in the application of diagnosis and in the application of techniques. Was this a "therapy?" No! It is scientific knowledge and it is what Dr. Still endeavored to leave with us. As Dr. Agersborg said, "Stay osteopathic." Many medical men see more in osteopathy than do some in our own profession. Yet, we imitate them, while on the other hand, they wish they had our knowledge of science dealing with the natural forces of the body. That is enough to give you my thought. Thank you.

---

24. Mary Baker Eddy (1821-1910) was the founder of the Church of Christ, Scientist.

26. Philosophy of Osteopathy and Its Application by the Cranial Concept

Given at the second annual convention of the Osteopathic Cranial Association, Boston, Massachusetts, July 18, 1948.

The assignment of this task takes me back to the time when Dad assigned to my elder brother and me the job of digging potatoes in the garden patch. We dug potatoes in our own original way. Dad looked over the patch the following morning and said, "Boys, go dig again." He sent us back to the job three times, and at each occasion we found a generous supply of potatoes, including quite a number of little seedlings. Through that boyhood experience, I found that it pays to dig, even in an original way.[1]

Years later I began digging in Dr. Andrew Taylor Still's science of osteopathy. In that intensive study, I discovered an abundance of little things which Dr. Still called the big things in his philosophy. These remind me of the little seedlings in that hill of potatoes.

Among many interpolations contributed by members of the profession to the text of *The Cranial Bowl* is one by Dr. Asa Willard, known everywhere by his hat and his utmost enthusiasm for the science of osteopathy: "Along in 1874, after years of independent thinking, there came to Doctor Still the conception of the basic principles of a great truth."[2]

I like that thought: "there came to Dr. Still." We need not know

---

1. This is the idea Dr. Sutherland is alluding to when he uses the phrase "digging on."

2. Asa Willard, D.O. (American School of Osteopathy, 1900) was president of the American Osteopathic Association in 1925.

from whence it came. It is sufficient to understand that it came during a sad period in the Founder's life, a time when a devout prayer went out to his Maker with Whom, it has been said, he lived closer than breathing.[3]

The concept of osteopathy lies deeper than the usual material interpretation and it recalls to mind a thought expressed by the late Dr. Harry L. Chiles, "If one can think osteopathy one will practice osteopathy." In my interpretation *thinking* osteopathy means thinking with Dr. Still, and in so doing one may think between the lines of his printed texts, *Research and Practice* and *Philosophy of Osteopathy*. It is *thought between* that should be included in our understanding of the basic principles of the osteopathic concept.

It was through this interpretative interlinear thinking that my attention was drawn to view that potent fluctuant liquid, the cerebrospinal fluid, which is now emphasized as of fundamental importance in the cranial concept. To illustrate that interlinear view, may I call attention to several extracts from *Philosophy of Osteopathy* [p. 39]:

> Another period of observation appears to the philosopher.... His mind will explore the bone, the ligament, the muscle, the fascia, the channels through which the blood travels from the heart to local destiny, with lymphatics and their contents.... It...does obtain blood abundantly to and from the heart, but the results obtained are not satisfactory, and another leaf is opened of why no good results are obtained and *where is the mystery*...?
>
> ...A thought strikes him that *the cerebrospinal fluid is the highest known element in the human body* and unless the brain furnishes this fluid in abundance a disabled condition of the body will remain.

---

3. In the spring of 1864, spinal meningitis killed three of Dr. Still's children despite the best efforts of both preacher and physician. It was a time of great spiritual crisis for Dr. Still, the resolution of which resulted in the birth of the science of osteopathy ten years later. See Still, *Autobiography*, pp. 87-88, 303-304.

> He who is able to reason will see that *this great river of life must be tapped* and the withering fields irrigated at once or the harvest of health will be forever lost. [Emphasis added.]

Thus have we been thinking between the lines with Dr. Still in an endeavor to tap "this great river of life," the cerebrospinal fluid; and we trust that you may understand how the cranial concept became a contribution of thought directing attention to hitherto unexplored areas or channels in the science of osteopathy. It is in no way an idea apart. The main thought expresses the significant recognition of Dr. Still's philosophy. The cranial concept, as I endeavor to teach it, is the science of osteopathy as envisaged by Dr. Still.

I do not consider this contribution of thought mine. I call it a guiding thought; and where it came from no one knows. It came while a student, thinking in the channel of Dr. Still's philosophy, back there in the early days at the American School of Osteopathy. It was while viewing the intricate bevel-articular surfaces of the greater wings of the sphenoid and the squamous portions of the temporal bones. The thought was as follows: Beveled, like the gills of a fish, and indicating an articular mobile mechanism for respiration. One might say that this, too, was thinking osteopathy.

As one continues thinking in this osteopathic channel, the attention is drawn to another golden vein: Dr. Still's reference to the "irrigation of withering fields" of the body system through the "waters of the brain." The following are more extracts from *Philosophy of Osteopathy*:

> The brain flushes the nerves of the lymphatics first, and *more than any other system of the body.*
>
> The lymphatics consume more of the *finer fluids of the brain* than the whole viscera combined.
>
> Finer nerves dwell with the lymphatics than even with the eye.
>
> ...all...nerves...drink from the waters of the brain.[4]

This thought carries one into deep water, figuratively speaking,

---

4. These four quotes are found respectively on pp. 109, 104, 104, and 105; emphasis added.

and into the studious consideration of that highest known element, the cerebrospinal fluid, the element that is thought by the cranial concept to provide nourishment to the brain cells with consequent *transmutation* of the element throughout nerve fiber to terminal. Perhaps this transmutation is the nerve force to which Dr. Still referred. In reality, one knows about as much about this element as do recognized authorities who seem inclined to wind up their summaries: "In conclusion, there is no conclusion."[5]

The cranial thought views the cerebrospinal fluid as *fluctuating* rather than circulating, as other fluids in the body system do. "Fluctuation" according to Webster's medical definition reads: "The motion of a fluid contained in a natural or artificial cavity, observed by palpation or percussion."

The cerebrospinal fluid is contained within a natural cavity and its motion, or fluctuation, is readily observed by palpation as reported from the experience of cranial technicians in daily practice. If I interpret correctly, fluctuation of the cerebrospinal fluid now has evidence from the laboratory experiments outlined by Speransky in his book, *A Basis for the Theory of Medicine.*

It is possible to make this assertion without hesitation: The fluctuation of the cerebrospinal fluid may be controlled in its rhythm by thinking-feeling-seeing-knowing fingers to a degree where all the fluids of the body have a rhythmic-balance-interchange. Ample clinical proof of the statement lies in various tests in general use before and after application of the maneuver. Some of these are the recording of temperature, pulse and respiration, as well as blood pressure readings and analysis of blood chemistry. Observation of the tone of any or all tissues is clearly revealing. The cranial technician is learning how to irrigate Dr. Still's withering fields.

Members of the publication committee of The Osteopathic Cranial

---

5. A.D. Speransky began the final chapter of *A Basis for the Theory of Medicine* with these words. He was a Russian scientist who conducted a wide variety of experiments, including those on the nature of the cerebrospinal fluid.

Association have been requested to analyze the concept of the *primary respiratory mechanism* so as to offer an interpretation understandable to the scientist.[6] Such an analysis would require the presence of the scientist and an intensive study as cranial students now pursue, including attendance at graduate courses explicative of the subject.

According to the authority of the scriptural record, the *Breath of Life*, not the breath of material air, was breathed into the nasals of a form of clay and man became a living soul.[7] If this record may be considered as literally true, then it agrees with the hypothesis of a *primary respiratory mechanism*–an involuntary mechanism that includes fundamentally that highest known element, the cerebrospinal fluid, within which dwells that invisible Breath of Life.

The primary mechanism consists of the fluctuation of the cerebrospinal fluid within and around the brain and spinal cord, fundamentally. The motility of the brain and spinal cord, the mobility of the cranial bones and the sacrum between the ilia, and the intracranial and intraspinal membranes, functioning as reciprocal tension agencies between poles of articular attachment, are also included. The mobility of the sacrum between the ilia is an involuntary movement and is to be differentiated from the postural mobility of the ilia upon the sacrum. There are no muscular agencies directing cranial mobility, and there are no muscular attachments between the sacrum and the ilia. The cranial bones and sacrum function as a unit in involuntary mobility during periods of primary respiration.

The hypothesis recognizes the information gained from authoritative anatomical texts: "All the physiological centers, including that of

---

6. The Osteopathic Cranial Association was organized as an affiliate of the Academy of Applied Osteopathy in July, 1947. The name was changed in 1960 to The Cranial Academy.

7. "And the Lord God formed man of the dust of the ground, and breathed into his nostrils the breath of life; and man became a living soul." Gen. 2:7, King James Version.

respiration, are located in the floor of the fourth ventricle."[8] This indicates a primary physiological center of respiration that controls secondary respiratory activities of the heart, lungs, diaphragm and so forth.

Understand that the cranial concept is not the head to osteopathy. Far from it. Osteopathy is the head, while the cranial idea might be called the "tail" to the "body" of Dr. Still's symbolic "squirrel within the hole in the tree," the cranial thought being only a "breech presentation" with perhaps a firmer grip on the "tail."[9] The idea simply "draws aside a curtain," opening an invitatory and studious pathway on which the osteopathic physician and surgeon may continue the study of the science of osteopathy as envisaged in the writings of its founder.

What is the significance of this thought?–"The brain is God's drugstore having within all drugs, lubricating oils, opiates, acids and every quality of drug that the wisdom of God thought necessary for human happiness and health."[10] Does it mean that someday the osteopathic physician will become sufficiently skilled in the art of a technician so as to be able to assume the role of the pharmacist, filling the prescription from the "drugstore?" Perhaps the rhythmic-balance-interchange between all the fluids of the body, secured by compressing the fourth ventricle, is coming close to the art of releasing these bodily "drugs."

Compression of the fourth ventricle applies to the contents of the ventricle and not to the medulla oblongata, nor the floor of the ventricle. During inhalation periods of respiration, the ventricle dilates, in common with all the other ventricles, while during the exhalation peri-

---

8. "In the floor of the fourth ventricle....are situated certain important centers, i.e. cardiac, vasomotor, respiratory, vomiting, and deglutition centers." Wright, *Applied Physiology*, p. 108.

9. Dr. A. T. Still presented osteopathy as a science, a philosophy and an art whose potential was not fully realized, much as a squirrel only partially seen within a hole in a tree would not be fully visualized. He stated that only the tail of the squirrel was currently in view.

10. Still, *Autobiography*, p. 182. Note that in the 1908 revised ed., Dr. Still changed the word "brain" to "body;" cf. the original 1897 ed., p. 219.

ods, the fourth and all the other ventricles return to contraction. There is a corresponding change occurring in the fluctuation of the cerebrospinal fluid tide that affects normal nourishment to the physiological centers.

The cranial technician has learned a specific method of compressing the fourth ventricle, and through this gentle technique, restriction in the fluctuation of the cerebrospinal fluid tide is accomplished until it reaches a brief rhythmic period in its functioning. This is not an idle statement. The method can be demonstrated. Immediately, at this brief rhythmic period, a rhythmic-balance-interchange occurs between all the bodily fluids. Because of this physiological effect, physicians are told: "If you do not know what else to do, compress the fourth ventricle." It is far-reaching in its physiological effects.

The method has not only been demonstrated by licensed physicians but also by a patient who had gathered a bit of knowledge about the treatment that had been applied to his own head. This young man evidently entertained confidence in his own ability to offer aid to a case of transverse myelitis, a so-called incurable case that had reached an advanced stage with complications of diverse extensive bedsores during long weeks in the hospital. Among other serious complications, there was a profuse bleeding at the toenails. When I was on the Pacific Coast, this young man begged me to see the patient. I found that the bedsores had healed in a rather short time and that the bleeding at the toenails had ceased. I asked the young man, "What have you been administering as a treatment?" He replied, "Compressing the ventricle." There are many other such tales that might be related in evidence.

I have permission to quote Dr. Howard A. Lippincott, one of my associate instructors in the cranial concept[11]:

> It is hard to appear conservative in considering the uses of ventricular compression because this potent fluid, activated

---

11. Howard A. Lippincott, D.O. (1893-1963: American School of Osteopathy, 1916) was a member of Dr. Sutherland's teaching staff. He became president of the Sutherland Cranial Teaching Foundation following Dr. Sutherland, wrote several

> by the technique, produces results that justify enthusiasm.
>
> There is a beneficial effect upon the entire circulatory system with reduction of congestions, ischemias and edemas, such as is in the realm of possibility without surgical interference.
>
> Metabolic processes are improved, including nutrition to the tissues and the gradual absorption of fibrous and calcium deposits that are not physiological or compensatory.
>
> It enhances organic function, and in the presence of infection, immunity is increased through effects upon the spleen, pancreas and liver.
>
> The endocrine system is regulated to the immediate needs of the body.
>
> The cerebrospinal fluid is in command of the metabolism, much of the involuntary operation and the autoprotective mechanism of the system.
>
> Dr. Sutherland calls attention to the fact that secondary osteopathic lesions become less perceptible under the influence of ventricular compression. So it is of value in determining the primary lesion.

It is well to add to that last quotation that the cranial concept does not overlook spinal lesions. In fact, techniques that apply to the entire body and its mechanical problems are demonstrated at courses of instruction in cranial technique.

The third and lateral ventricles, as well as the cerebral aqueduct and the spinal canal, also possess motile physiological activities in connection with the fourth chamber during alternating periods of respiration: dilating during inhalation and contracting during exhalation, with corresponding changes in the fluctuation of the cerebrospinal fluid tide. The control of the tide of fluctuation within the fourth ventricle includes that in the third and laterals as well as that in the fluid surrounding the brain and spinal cord. It is within the province

---

publications regarding osteopathy in the cranial field, and conducted an active study group with his wife, Rebecca, in his home in Moorestown, New Jersey.

of the cranial art to control the tide by way of the lateral ventricles, the third or down at the sacrum.

In this fluctuation of the cerebrospinal fluid tide, the cranial concept recognizes a potency that may be utilized effectively in diagnosis and treatment. This potency does not function blindly, as is common to force applied from outside the cranium.

Authoritative writers on the subject of cerebrospinal fluid call attention to an interchange with the arterial blood at the choroid plexuses. We are inclined to reason that the interchange could not occur without some degree of motility within the plexuses. The cranial thought calls attention to an accommodative mechanism as follows: The choroid plexuses have their location within the walls of the ventricles and not within the chambers. Motility, common to the walls, necessarily occurs throughout the structural form of the plexuses. During the exhalation period, while the walls function in contractile motility, the plexuses take on a *short* formation and present the irregular or bunched appearance visualized in inanimate specimens of the anatomical laboratory. During the inhalation period, as one should visualize in the normal animate functioning brain, while the walls dilate in motility, the plexuses stretch out into a *long* formation.

Authorities hesitate to make an absolute assertion as to what actually occurs through this mechanism of physiological interchange between the cerebrospinal fluid and the blood. Yet the cranial thought presents an elucidative picture of how the mechanism possibly functions in the physiological interchange.

The pituitary body, riding so majestically in the sella turcica of the sphenoid bone, has an important physiological act in the cranial drama. It is strapped down in its saddle and attached to the floor of the third ventricle by the infundibulum. This "body" is the leader of the endocrine system. Imagine a leader without activity. Motility is essential in its physiological functioning. Otherwise there might follow a lack of secretory elements to feed the "flock." A pulsing motility, as well as a ridable mobility during the alternating movement of the sphenoid, occurs with the periods of respiration.

Apparently, the pituitary body is governed by the nervous system through a cable of multitudinous nerve fibers in the infundibulum with cell centers in the hypothalamus. These cells would receive nourishment from that highest known element, the cerebrospinal fluid, according to the cranial thought.

In the intracranial picture of the concept, the difference between the walls of the main venous channels within and the walls of veins without the skull is recognized as significant. The construction of the walls within the dura mater offers no means of propelling the movement of venous blood unless a mechanical factor can be found. This factor is provided by the accommodative movement of the cranial bones. Restriction of this movement leads to serious pathology in the brain.

The jugular foramina are also of utmost importance to the venous drainage of the cranium. These are formed by the articulation of two bones, the occiput and the temporals, and the strained relations that may occur between them can modify the shape and size of the foramina so as to restrict the venous flow. In contrast to the possibilities that may restrict the movement of venous blood, the main arterial supply enters the interior through individual channels in bones and other protected avenues. The arteries within the skull have the same type of walls as arteries without.

There is much more to be said concerning the interior respiratory mechanism, but time forbids it. And we should give you a brief picture of the mechanics of the osseous shell that is operated by the mechanism within.

The picture begins in the prenatal commencement of man's walkabout on earth. At this stage, the cranial bones lack articular contact with each other. This arrangement permits an adaptation of the head for convenient passage through the birth canal. The occipitoatlantal joint is the one established articulation in the region.

Furthermore, the several parts of most of the cranial bones are separated by the cartilaginous matrix in which they have been developing. At birth, these cartilaginous unions may be subjected to luxations. They are analogous to the epiphyseal union elsewhere. The four parts of the occiput that form the margin of the foramen magnum are united by cartilage at birth and are located in an area where luxations of a serious nature frequently occur. The shape of the foramen magnum may be studied by X-ray. Cranial technicians have learned to recognize problems in this area and give them skillful attention. The cartilaginous unions between the parts of the occiput do not fuse completely until the third to fifth years. On the principle of the saying, "As the twig is bent, so is the tree inclined," it can be seen why the shape of heads varies so much. The majority of adult skulls observed in our anatomical laboratories are pathological specimens that point to luxations of the intercartilaginous unions back in early life.

The union between the basilar part of the occiput and the body of the sphenoid presents a modified intervertebral disc. This union does not ossify until the twenty-fifth to thirtieth years.

The bones of the cranial vault develop in membrane instead of cartilage and are free of articular contact with each other within this membranous connection. Under these conditions it seems impossible to question movement of the bones of the cranium by interior respiratory agencies at this early period of life. The question of articular mobility arises at a later period, after the bones have grown outward from ossification centers and are forming articular contact with one another.

My own thinking entertained considerable doubt back there in the early days, and I started out to prove that there could be no mobility between the separate bones of the skull. In that fruitless endeavor, I found many mechanical features upon the articular surfaces indicating a design for mobility. The following are a few of the mechanical features that I found:

Beveling, both internal and external, with opposite articular contact, signifying gliding mobility.

Corrugations, running transversely, diagonally and so forth, picturing: worm gears, cone gears, compensative gears, cryptic gears, friction gears, and screw gears. Ball and socket, ball bearing, ball crank, box coupling, pintle, pulley, countershaft and even a cradle. Equalizing bars, escapements, feather keys, flexible shafts, force pumps, governors, jiggers and fulcrums.

The proof of articular mobility came about through digging to prove otherwise, which reminds me of a quotation by a philosopher: "To the dreamer who will work and the worker who will dream, life surrenders all things." To this I might add: To the digger who will take time to dream and the dreamer who will wake up and dig, Dr. Andrew Taylor Still's science of osteopathy will unfold into a magnitude equal to that of the heavens.

27. The Core-link Between the Pelvic Bowl and the Cranial Bowl

This brief talk, with technique demonstration, was given at a meeting of the International Society of Sacro-Iliac Technicians in St. Louis, Missouri, in July 1949, during the annual convention of the American Osteopathic Association.[1]

During the meeting of this Society in this city of St. Louis back in the year 1940, it was my privilege to give a talk on the subject: "The Core-link Between the Cranial Bowl and the Pelvic Bowl." Dr. Goode has asked me to say a few words again today relative to my "pet subject."[2] Well, my pet subject is the science of osteopathy. Inasmuch as that early-day talk gave the first boost to the cranial concept, I have decided to turn the subject upside down. Instead of "The Core-link Between the Cranial Bowl and the Pelvic Bowl," we will consider "The Core-link Between the Pelvic Bowl and the Cranial Bowl." It matters not which is up nor which is down.

The intimate correlation between the two bowls is such that there is much difficulty in deciding which is first and which is last, or which is top and which is bottom. The bottom doth affect the top and the top doth affect the bottom. On the other hand, the bottom may effect to the top and the top may effect to the bottom. An anterior *sag* of the promontory or base of the sacrum becomes a *drag* on the intraspinal membranes and effects abnormal disturbances to the top. On the other hand, an elevation of the sphenobasilar symphysis may

---

1. The International Society of Sacro-Iliac Technicians was an informal organization of osteopathic physicians who met annually to explore new viewpoints and concepts in the field of osteopathy.

2. George W. Goode, D.O. (American School of Osteopathy, 1905) was president of the International Society of Sacro-Iliac Technicians at that time and had been president of the American Osteopathic Association in 1922.

become a pull on the intraspinal membranes effecting abnormal disturbances to the bottom. Or, the pull of the elevation of the sphenobasilar symphysis may affect the bottom with resulting effecting reflexes to the top. Is it a wonder that we ponder: Which is affect and which is effect?

So it seems that this core-link function of the intraspinal membranes, as I emphasized in my talk in 1940, is the important link to be considered between top and bottom, or bottom and top. This core-link hath attachments to the foramen magnum and the second cervical vertebra and then hangs like a tube, without other firm attachment to bones, until it reaches the sacrum.[3] It functions with the falx cerebri and tentorium cerebelli as a reciprocal tension mechanism between the articular movements of the cranial structure and that of the sacrum between the ilia. Disturbance to this physiological functioning signifies disturbance likewise to the normal fluctuation of the cerebrospinal fluid within which we find that "highest known element in the human body."[4]

There are *mental* disturbances resulting from sags of the sacrum. Today I wish merely to leave with you my contribution of technique that I have found effective in some of these mental cases.

The patient sits on the end of the table while the physician sits on a stool facing the patient. The operator's thumbs travel gently along the inside of the crests of the ilia to their posterior areas. The patient

---

3. Subsequent anatomic studies have demonstrated that the dura mater is attached to the vertebral canal in the lumbar region. The anterior attachments are short and strong while the posterior attachments are weaker and longer. The anterior and anterolateral connective tissue bands attach to the posterior longitudinal ligament. The bands are strongest at the L5-S1 level and less strong in the upper lumbar region. The dural nerve root sheaths are also attached to the posterior longitudinal ligament anteriorly and to the periosteum of the inferior pedicle laterally. Cf. Parkin and Harrison, "The Topographical Anatomy of the Lumbar Epidural Space," *Journal of Anatomy* 141 (1985):211-217, and Spencer, Irwin and Miller, "Anatomy and Significance of Fixation of the Lumbosacral Nerve Roots in Sciatica," *Spine* 8, no. 6 (1983): 672-679.

4. Still, *Philosophy*, p. 39.

is then requested to tip the body first to the left and then to the right. This side-tipping tends to gently facilitate further movement medially by the operator's thumbs along the soft tissues until they reach the proximity of the alae of the sacrum. The patient then leans forward and places hands upon the operator's shoulders. He exhales and raises up with the following inhalation. In the meantime, the operator's thumbs are *holding* the alae of the sacrum. Back goes the sacrum without a pop or an unnecessary thrust.

28. Obtaining Knowledge Versus Information

This lecture relates to early experiments in the cranial field of the science of osteopathy. It was written at Carmel-by-the-Sea, California and presented at the fourth annual meeting of the Osteopathic Cranial Association in Chicago, Illinois, July 16, 1950.

Obtaining knowledge rather than information began in the days of early childhood. One memorable event occurred when Dad, in parental affection, placed my pelvic bowl in a prone position across his knees and spanked the sacrum. Thus I obtained a knowledge rather than mere information of *how* sacral technique effects a fluctuation of the cerebrospinal fluid and changes one's personality. I am grateful to Dad for that early instruction by parental affection.

There were various other events which left important impressions that gave knowledge of the potency of the "tide." My older brother, three years my senior, took great delight in climbing aloft some high building and teasing me to follow. Then Steve would leap and light safely upon nimble feet, leaving his wee brother to jump and land *athump* on his tuberosities. During another stunt, Steve ran swiftly down a steep hill while roly-poly Bill reached bottom by rolling rapidly, in the manner of a barrel, bumping boulders here and there along the way. This experience may have been obtaining knowledge that later became helpful in the formulation of the technique now known as the alternating lateral fluctuation of the "tide." On yet another occasion Steve, showing off, closed his eyes and walked safely across the rail of a bridge. Bill, lacking Steve's extraordinary skill, fell off the bridge into deep water below to be carried by the current to the opposite shore. This was a valuable experience in obtaining knowledge of the necessity of being able to "paddle one's own canoe."

As this talk relates to the experimentation conducted upon my own skull to obtain knowledge, rather than information gathered from others, we leave childhood days to report some serious recollections. I have frequently mentioned that the thought that came to me back in 1898 was not mine. The thought of beveled articular surfaces in the skull and their indication of respiratory articular mobility seemed at the time as irrational to me as it does to many physicians in our profession today. However, there seemed to be a Presence near by, the Creator of the cranial mechanism, whom one might think of with the endearing term of "Dad." To me, the term "Dad" is not irreverent but tends to bring one into a closer understanding of a Heavenly Father. I like to think of the thought of cranial articular mobility as coming from Dad. In such understanding it became a personal task to prove this thought, otherwise, as Dad was ever present, He might in parental kindness place my pelvic bowl across His knees as did the earthly parent in childhood days.

Through this interpretation it became my personal mission to *dig* and *dig* for an intimate acquaintance, or knowledge, with the articular surfaces upon the disarticulated bones of the skull that would further indicate a mechanism for respiratory physiological functioning. This knowledge was not obtainable in authoritative anatomical texts, and many of the available specimens were pathological "bent twigs."[1]

That continual search revealed:

Beveling, both internal and external, with opposite articular contact, signifying gliding mobility.

Corrugations, running transversely, diagonally and so forth, picturing: worm gears, cone gears, compensative gears, cryptic gears, friction gears and screw gears. Ball and socket, ball bearing, ball crank, boxcoupling, pintle, pulley, countershaft and even a cradle. Equalizing bars, escapements, feather keys, flexible shafts, force pumps, governors, jiggers and fulcrums.

Convincing indications were thus found upon the articular surfaces:

---

1. The term "bent twigs" refers to the saying, "As the twig is bent so the tree inclines."

picturing the thought of cranial articular mobility as *not an idle dream* nor an irrational notion. But–*where* were the indications for a primary respiratory mechanism? Such a mechanism would necessarily include *motility* of the central nervous system and *motion* of the cerebrospinal fluid. During a diligent search for this information, an authoritative text furnished the following cue: "All the physiological centers, *including that of respiration*, are located within the floor of the fourth ventricle."[2]

The same text referred to the medulla oblongata as the "floor" and the cerebellum as the "roof." So, in accordance with the cue of gathered information, I reasoned: If one were able to enter within the cranium and compress the cerebellum in the manner utilized in compressing the bulb of a sphygmomanometer, it would effect motility in the walls of the fourth ventricle with subsequent motion of the cerebrospinal fluid–a motion that would be continuous within the other ventricles and the subarachnoid space surrounding the brain and spinal cord. I also reasoned that the compression would affect the physiological centers in the medulla oblongata, and in consequence, the secondary physiological activity throughout the body systems.

As the fourth ventricle lies somewhat anterior to the supraocciput, my personal knowledge of the occipital articulations became pertinent to the problem. I had found that below a point in the lambdoidal sutures where the beveling changes, the articular surfaces of the occipital squama are beveled externally. This fact would provide an accommodation for specific compression of the supraocciput that would have a similar effect on the walls of the fourth ventricle. That is, by springing the supraocciput or compressing it, I could effect a compression of the walls of the fourth ventricle. Thus it became necessary to find a suitable appliance with which to make a compression upon the supraocciput specifically.

---

2. "In the floor of the fourth ventricle....are situated certain important centers, i.e. cardiac, vasomotor, respiratory, vomiting, and deglutition centers." Wright, *Applied Physiology*, p. 108.

A visit to a sports supply house led to the purchase of two well-padded baseball catcher's mitts. These were laced together at one end of each with shoestrings, in order to make the mechanism adjustable to the correct fitting contacts at the lateral edges of the supraocciput. An adjustable strap was attached to the opposite end of one mitt and a buckle to the other. This mechanism was so devised to provide adjustable leverage with which to secure a desirable amount of compression upon the lateral edges of the supraocciput. With some sense of taking a step into the unknown as well as a clear mental picture of the procedure I wished to carry out, I placed my head within the V-shaped apparatus much in the manner in which it might rest in the V-shaped head rest of a dental chair. I gradually increased the compression by the adjustable strap and buckle until my senses reached a stage of almost complete inanimation. Then followed an *intense sensation*, as though someone was milking or stripping the digits of my feet and hands toward the hips and shoulders together with a similar sensation throughout the entire body, organic and osseous.

It is well to pause at this point in relating the experiment to quote from a pamphlet that was sent as a birthday remembrance on the occasion of my seventy-seventh milestone. Why the pause? Because one is quite apt to find himself rather close to the Maker of the human body at this stage of obtaining knowledge versus information.

> The great secret, you see, is not to think of yourself, of your courage or your despair, of your strength or your weakness, but of Him for whom you journey. Then you will understand that He cannot show you a task without making you capable of fulfilling it–not send you a trial without also giving you means of surmounting it. Knowing yourself upheld by His strength, you will be no longer concerned about your own, either to doubt it or be proud of it.
>
> By Phillippe Vernier, *With The Master*[3]

---

3. Vernier, *With the Master: Short Devotional Studies.*

Strange to relate, but nevertheless true, without material strength of my own apparently left, I managed to release the buckle of the leverage strap. The release was immediately followed by a sensation of warmth at the area of the cisterna magna and fourth ventricle and a remarkable movement of fluid became noticeable up and down the spinal column, throughout the ventricles and surrounding the brain. I interpreted this movement of fluid as respiratory fluctuation of the cerebrospinal fluid–the terminology "fluctuation" being defined by Webster as: "The movement of a fluid contained within a natural or artificial cavity, observed by palpation or percussion." To this terminology I added the statement:

The arterial stream *is* supreme *but* the cerebrospinal fluid is in command; and its fluctuation within a natural cavity *can be* and *is* observed by palpation in cranial technique.

While this fluctuation became noticeable, there was also an apparent movement of the sacrum between the ilia that was rhythmical with a definite movement of the bones of the skull. As the cranium changed its shape alternately between what is now known as flexion and extension, a movement in the orbital cavities and eyeballs was included. I also sensed an active motility of the brain and spinal cord, the latter shortening, drawing upward like a tadpole's tail, followed by a reciprocal downward lengthening.

The apparent movement of the sacrum between the ilia needed an interpretation, as such a movement had not hitherto been considered in connection with the thought of cranial articular mobility. This led to special study of the pelvic bowl, particularly the L-shaped articular surfaces of the sacroiliac joints. Reference to anatomical texts failed to reveal muscular attachments from the sacrum to the ilia but gave vivid description of transverse and oblique ligaments that hold the joints together. The same texts referred to these joints as synarthroses, meaning immovable. But Dr. A. T. Still had proven them to be movable. It was now my mission to also prove that the cranial articulations possess articular mobility.

One could reason: The two types of ligaments not only hold the articulations together but also regulate a normal range of mobility, as do the various types of ligaments functioning in connection with spinal articular mobility. But–down here at these sacral articulations–muscular agencies are lacking, and the same can be said in relation to articular mobility of the cranial bones. In fact, at a later date one comment was made about the cranial concept to that very point in constructive criticism of one of my early papers.

At this early stage of progress in the endeavor, the effort was to *think osteopathy* (not merely thinking osteopathically or in an osteopathic manner) and Dr. Still's Ram of Reason[4] began to *bump* my frontal lobes with the following thought: If the cranium is a primary articular mechanism, it does not require muscular agencies to activate its own mobility. It could have an intracranial reciprocal tension arrangement functioning between various poles of articular attachment to regulate the range of mobility.

Then began a period of deeper study into the arrangement of the falx cerebri and the tentorium cerebelli as well as the connection with the sacrum by way of the intraspinal dural membrane. This study indicated: The cranial bones and the sacrum function together as a unit in a primary respiratory mechanism.

The next experiment was made to learn whether it is possible to restrict the sacrum from moving between the ilia. A small leather pad was constructed to fit snugly at the base of the sacrum while lying on one's back. This contact held the sacrum in the extreme extension position and especially restricted fluctuation of the cerebrospinal fluid, as cranial technicians have exemplified. The restriction resulted in a dull heavy sensation in the area of the cisterna magna. It seemed likely that through a depressed or forward position of the base of the sacrum, a predisposing etiology to some mental problems might be seen. A clinical study could well be made in mental hospitals to find how common this one factor is among the patients. Other experiments

---

4. Ram of Reason: Still, *Autobiography*, pp. 355-356, 362-363.

were made with the pad resting beneath the apex of the sacrum and also with a small round appliance to function transversely as a fulcrum at the second sacral segment.

Following the sacral experimentation, baseball-mitt compression was applied to the sides of the cranium that changed my skull to the extension shape. In this experiment, a facial mirror was used to observe any changes that were likely to occur in the skull and the facial area. There was a gradual but extensive change to the longer, higher and narrower shape of the skull that is characteristic of extension at the cranial base, including a narrowing of the orbits and apparently elongated eyeballs. "Apparent elongation" means that the elongation was indicated through the necessity of drawing the mirror closer for clear observation.

The experiment led to a deeper study of the facial osseous mechanism to obtain knowledge that: The maxillae, while functioning as a unit with the basilar articular mobility, lacked direct articular contact with the cranial base. The sphenoid articulates first with the palatine and zygomatic bones and they with the maxillae; the temporal bones first with the zygomatics and they with the maxillae.

This, too, was obtaining knowledge rather that information, for the important interosseous mechanical device through which the cranial base influences the face had no previous written record in any authoritative text. It was knowledge interpreting: a mechanism providing narrowing-widening orbits and narrowing-widening eyeballs to accommodate important physiological changes occurring during respiratory periods. It was likewise knowledge obtained indicating: a physiological function molding the eyeballs; showing how restriction in the articular mobility of the orbital cavities may account for the need of ocular lenses to provide proper vision.

The catcher's mitts, while applicable in securing compression, were useless in obtaining knowledge relating to a flexion type mechanism. This meant further consultation with Doctor Still's Ram of Reason. So, having read as text information that the bones at the base of the skull are formed in cartilage and those of the vault are formed in membrane, I connected the knowledge obtained in the study of articular surfaces with the information and reasoned thus:

> The bones at the base of the skull being formed in cartilage function in articular mobility, while the bones of the vault, having formation in membrane, function through especially designed sutural contacts as compensatory to the basilar mobility.

I had previously pictured the basilar bowl which resulted later in naming the text *The Cranial Bowl.* This bowl has a cap, and it would be impossible to have articular mobility of the bowl without compensation through the cap. Furthermore, it would be possible, as well as technically mechanical, to regulate the articular mobility of the bowl by lifting the components of the cap, as indicated by the osseous contacts.

So, another visit was made to the sport shop in search of a mechanism applicable for not only lifting the lateral edges of the vault cap but also suitable for drawing them laterally. This movement would simulate lifting the eaves of the roof of a barn and drawing them laterally, in which movement the top or central area of the roof would sag. A football helmet proved valuable as the mechanism for the application of the experiment. The ear appendages were cut off to avoid compression at the lower area of the vault cap.

Then we went on a hunt for a chamois skin of a texture that would not stretch but would also have a soft surface to avoid pinching or creasing the skin. From the chamois skin, we cut a bandage about two inches in width with length suitable for fastening around the skull, leaving two appendages of two-inch width to pass upward over the helmet resting on top of the vault cap. Then the bandages around the skull were fastened together with a hemostat, which also served in rolling the ends of the bandage to secure the proper lifting contact to the vault. The ends of the appendages passing over the helmet were also fastened with a hemostat and rolled in a similar manner. Now view the bandage around the head as making the skull contact and the appendages over the helmet in the act of lifting the middle areas of the contact upward and laterally, and you have the picture of the early experiment. In the picture it is well to include the sagittal suture as widening and considerably more lateral movement of the parietals at their posterior inferior angles.

The same mirror was used to provide suitable observation of the changes occurring. The view pictured wide orbits with wide and forward eyeballs in a shorter, wider and lower head, the flexion shape that is characteristic of flexion of the cranial base. As all cranial technicians know, this experiment placed the sphenobasilar symphysis into flexion position while the compression experiment carried the symphysis into the extension position.

The changes occurring in relation to the orbital cavities, the eyeballs and the contour of the skull in flexion and extension experiments naturally stimulated *a habit of observation* of all faces and heads of persons with whom one came in contact. In many of these individuals, the observation pictured wide orbits and wide eyeballs on one side while on the opposite side they were narrow and elongated. Having gathered this information through observation of others, it now became the task to obtain knowledge through further personal experimentation upon my own skull.

In the experiment, the appendages of the bandage were placed in a diagonal direction, instead of passing laterally over the helmet, with bandage-lift contacts near the frontal bone on the right side and near the mastoid angle on the left. The mirror observation pictured a wide orbit and eyeball on the right and a narrow orbit and elongated eyeball on the left. During the experiment I sensed what seemed to be a twisting movement at the sphenobasilar symphysis. The diagonal lift was then changed to the opposite side of the skull which resulted in the view now known as torsion, with the greater wing of the sphenoid high on the left. In both of these tests, we noted a uniformity in the skull contour from the anteroposterior diameter.

Observation of other individuals gathered further information that showed a type with a difference in the skull contour either side of the anteroposterior diameter. That is, one side of the head was long and convex while the other was shorter and concave in contour. In these people there were wide orbits and wide eyeballs on the concave side, while they were narrow and elongated on the convex side. The picture was similar in many respects to the torsion experiment, the most striking difference being the contrast in the contours of the skull from front to back. This required another conference with Dr. Still's Ram of Reason.

As an aid to the reasoning, we picked up an articulated spinal column and bent the ends toward the right. The middle area rotated markedly toward the left. The whole column was convex on the left and concave on the right. Then we bent the ends to the left and noted the rotation of the middle area to the right with the whole convex on the right and concave on the left. We also learned from this picture that the vertebrae tipped upward on the concave side and downward on the convex side. This information indicated what was likely occurring at the sphenobasilar symphysis in the concave-convex type of skulls. The next step was to invent an apparatus with which to bend the frontal and occipital ends of the skull in the same direction. The helmet mechanism was not applicable to the experiment.

In the search for suitable material from which to fashion an apparatus, we found an old-style wooden butter bowl that had been used by a farmer's wife for molding butter after churning the cream. The butter bowl was cut with a hacksaw down to near the size of the helmet and recut to a concavity on one side, leaving the other convex. This mechanism was placed on the top of the skull with its convexity on the left and the concavity on the right. The chamois skin bandage was place around the skull and the ends fastened together with the hemostat on the right side instead of in front. The appendages were placed so as to pass longitudinally over the skullcap mechanism and fastened securely. The ends of the bandage were rolled with the hemostat on the right side, thus drawing the frontal and occipital ends to the right with resultant concavity on the right and convexity on the left. The mirror observation pictured a wide orbit and eyeball on the right and a narrow orbital cavity and elongated eyeball on the left. Throughout the experiment we easily sensed a rotation of the sphenobasilar symphysis to the left.

The mechanism was then reversed to change its concavity to the left side by turning it end to end. The bandage ends were then rolled together on the left side with mirror observation viewing a wide orbit and eyeball on the left with the narrow orbit and elongated eyeball on the right. This time the concavity of the skull contour was on the left side and the convexity on the right. We also sensed the rotation of the sphenobasilar symphysis to the right.

Throughout all these experiments we sensed the reciprocal tension movement of the flax cerebri and tentorium cerebelli and the automatic shifting in the area where the falx adjoins the tent. This area has come to be known as the "Sutherland Fulcrum" since Dr. Harold I. Magoun called it that.[5]

These experiments were repeated from time to time to determine the activity of the petrous portions of the temporal bones. On each occasion, the petrous portions rotated externally when the motion of the sphenobasilar symphysis carried it into flexion, and into internal rotation during sphenobasilar extension. In the torsion and sidebending experiments, the petrous portions were found to rotate internally whenever the basilar process of the occiput tipped upward on its side, and to rotate externally whenever the basilar process tipped downward on its side. The result is the now familiar rule: Whenever the basilar process is tipped downward *on that side*, the petrous portion will always be found in external rotation. Whenever the basilar process is tipped upward *on that side*, the petrous portion will always be found in internal rotation.

During the repetition of these experiments, considerable attention was given to sensing the movement of the reciprocal tension membrane, especially at the area where the falx cerebri adjoins the tentorium

---

5. Magoun, *Osteopathy in Cranial Field*, 1st ed., p. 39. Harold I. Magoun, Sr. (1898-1981: Andrew Taylor Still College of Osteopathy and Surgery, 1924) was a member of Dr. Sutherland's teaching staff and one of the founders of the Sutherland Cranial Teaching Foundation. He compiled and edited the first edition of *Osteopathy in the Cranial Field* and authored its two subsequent editions.

cerebelli. It was necessary to formulate a mental picture of a *balance point* or fulcrum that regulated the various articular movements of the cranial bones. As an aid to reasoning, I stood on my head up against a wall and visualized the falx as suspended from the tent. In the upright posture, the tent is suspended from the falx. When lying on one side, one half of the tent was suspended from the other half and the falx. Understand the picture as centered on a suspension area hanging in the middle and not from the attachments of the dura mater to the sagittal suture and other distal points. The resemblance of each half of the tentorium to the falx contributed to the view of three sickle-shaped membranes meeting in the area of the straight sinus. For my own convenience I came to think of the tent as the *falx* tentorii, with a sickle on each side. This helped with the visualization of an automatic-shifting-suspension fulcrum that included the area where the three sickle shapes adjoin.

A fulcrum is a *still* mechanism over which a lever moves and from which it gets its power. In the use of a fulcrum, it may be changed to various areas beneath the lever, but it remains a *still balance mechanism* over which the lever operates and secures its potency. When the cranial technician visualizes this mechanism in its operation clearly and senses the important *knowing feel*, he will have a picture that will come alive as it did for one who wrote as follows:

Now I *know* what you mean by a suspension fulcrum. Whew! How those membranes swing. Somehow I am reminded of the caller at a square dance: "Swing your partners to the left, everyman." What rhythm in them thar membranes.[6]

Our associate instructors frequently have difficulty in explaining the *balance-tension-point* in cranial technique. Perhaps the visualization of this automatic-shifting-suspension fulcrum in its rhythm will aid in a clearer understanding. It is not the visualization of a point relative to one falx or another but the balance point where the three sickles adjoin.

---

6. Edith E. Dovesmith, D.O. (1895-1970: American School of Osteopathy, 1918).

Thus far we had been experimenting with appliances adaptable to the use of external force in establishing cranial articular mobility–a force lacking the intelligence of thinking-feeling-seeing-knowing fingers. This was not in accordance with *thinking osteopathy*, with considering inherent agencies more dependable than external agencies. After learning of the usual method of disarticulating the cranial bones for anatomical specimens by filling the cranium with dry peas and water to provide a pressure from within, when the peas swelled, Dr. Still's Ram of Reason called attention to the potency of the cerebrospinal fluid. This potency might be considered as a fundamental principle in the functioning of a primary respiratory mechanism. This reasoning meant a beginning of experimentation with feeling-seeing-thinking-knowing fingers.

The first experiment commenced with the movement in connection with the basilar process and the petrous portions of the temporal bones. In the application, a modification of Dr. Still's wrist technique was devised–that is, to use only the flexor digitorum profundus and flexor pollicis longus muscles as agencies for initiating movement. The thenar eminences made gentle but firm contacts in the convenient grooves behind the ears on the temporal bones with the fingers clasped together beneath the supraocciput. The first three fingers of each hand acted as agencies to initiate external rotation of the petrous portions while the two little fingers initiated circumrotation of the occiput. Understand that we merely initiated movement, and with all contacts still in position, as means of observing through the sense of touch, waited for the potency of the cerebrospinal fluid to carry the mechanism into the limit of its normal range.

In this experiment, recognition was made of the fact that while the supraocciput was circumrotating in one direction, the mastoid portions and processes of the temporals were turning in an opposite direction. This interprets the convex shape but sagittal plane of articular contact of the mastoid portion, with the concave shape and sagittal plane of the lateral border of the occiput posterior to the jugular process. It indicated a ball-and-socket movement, or the cap-and-fruit-jar mobility to which I have frequently called attention. As the majority of anatomical specimens available for the study of articular surfaces are pathological "bent twigs," this normal movement is not readily recognized.

In the experiment of initiating extension mobility of the occiput and the consequent internal rotation of the petrous portions of the temporal bones, the contacts were made in the same manner as when initiating flexion. In this instance, the first three fingers of each hand acted as agencies in directing the mastoid processes laterally while the two little fingers initiated the occiput into the circumrotation movement of extension. In this movement the concave lateral surfaces of the occiput rotated or turned in a posterior direction, while the convex mastoid portions rotated anteriorly and the mastoid processes moved forward and laterally.

The next experiment was the vault-lift initiation into the flexion and extension positions at the sphenobasilar symphysis. With the palms resting upon the parietal bones and the fingers laced together above the vault, it was easy to initiate the mobility at the sphenobasilar symphysis. This was accomplished by drawing the inferior borders of the parietals laterally and upward for flexion, and then drawing the parietal edges medially for extension. A similar contact was applied to the frontal bones in such manner as to lift the angles forward for flexion and medially for extension, thus widening the ethmoidal notch posteriorly in flexion and narrowing it posteriorly in extension.

There were many other experiments, with repetitions along the way, besides these few that are presented today.

The remainder of this talk relates to some personal experiences with external traumatic agencies employed in producing cranial membranous articular strains. One of these was an endeavor to produce what is known as the occipitomastoid strain that occurs frequently through falls and other forces contacting the supraocciput. The resultant complications were exceedingly serious, and I trust that no one will repeat the experiment unless an expert cranial technician is nearby. In the experiment, we reconstructed the butter bowl mechanism by cutting out another concavity on the other side. The idea was to utilize the convex bottom surface for contacting the supraocciput specifically. Long straps were attached to the ends of the mechanism and then fastened securely to a hook in the wall, near the foot of the operating table that had been placed against the wall to provide pushing service for the feet. The straps led in an inclined direction to the mechanism situated at the head of the table.

Then, while lying on my back with the supraocciput in contact with the mechanism and holding the mastoid portions firmly with the palms of my hands, I gradually pushed with both feet against the wall. The experiment resulted in a typical occipitomastoid type of a membranous articular strain, *including the serious complications.* Yes, I began "seeing things!" In fact, I became a fit subject for commitment to a mental institution. The complications continued for several days. Thus, by experiencing it myself, I obtained knowledge rather than simply the information that would come from the experiment performed upon a colleague.

The knowledge obtained from this experimentation with thinking-feeling-seeing-knowing fingers in connection with the occipitomastoid articulation quieted my fears of becoming an inmate in a mental hospital. The strain was reduced briefly and easily in the following manner: The same position was assumed upon the table with a small pad placed beneath the apex of the sacrum, to hold it in the flexion position and thus direct the tide to the occiput. The fingers were interlaced beneath the supraocciput with thumbs contacting along the mastoid processes. The fingers circumrotated the supraocciput gently toward the direction in which it had moved during the production, while the thumbs eased the mastoid portions laterally until the desired balance at the automatic-shifting-suspension fulcrum was sensed; and then the tide came in by dorsiflexing the feet. This experiment is an example of the many that were made in producing and correcting cranial membranous articular strains on myself.

There was an accidental experiment that occurred through neglect to stoop and lower the head while entering a basement. A rather severe ramming on an overhead beam forced the frontal bones posteriorly at their articulations with the greater and lesser wings of the sphenoid and disturbed the area of reasoning. This was followed by the tendency of the eyeballs to roll backward.

There was one experiment in which the dental surgeon provided the traumatic agency for producing the strain and resulting complication. It concerns the successful extraction of an upper molar tooth. Although the desensitization with novocaine freed me from any pain during the extraction, I sensed what seemed like a separation occurring between articular contacts farther back. For two weeks I suffered from what the dental surgeon called a "dry socket." This was a sufficient period of obtaining knowledge of pain and sleepless nights to stir Dr. Still's Ram of Reason into calling attention to the sensation of separation. I thereupon placed an index finger back upon the pterygoid process of the sphenoid and held the contact firmly and tipped my skull away from the contact. This provided immediate relief from all "dry-socket" complications.

Another personal experience that should be mentioned in this review was connected with an occupational task when serving as a printer's devil. Among the many duties was that known as "kicking" a Pearl job-press for hours at a time with the right foot moving up and down at each impression. This movement developed a depression of the right sacral ala forward from its contact with the ilium. Two types of drag affecting the area of the right cisterna magna and the normal fluctuation of the Tide subsequently resulted. One was through the intraspinal reciprocal membrane and the other was through the fascia. Through the recollection of this early experience, I developed the technique for contacting the sacral alae by the anterior approach.

A fellow's conscience, believe it or not, affects a disturbance to the fluctuation of the tide and secondarily effects physiological centers within the floor of the fourth ventricle. I learned of this fact while writing editorials on a daily evening newspaper. It was during the year when Bryan, with his silver-tongue oration, secured the democratic nomination for President. The paper with which I was employed decided to campaign for the democrats. In order to hold my job, it was necessary to fill the editorial column with arguments in favor of Bryan and free silver. Personally, I had always voted the republican ticket and was also covering the county for a republican paper, *The Minneapolis Journal.* Although an endeavor was made to ease the little voice of conscience by quoting many of the views of a democratic writer on another daily paper, I became aware of the balance point occurring in the lives of little men who walk about on earth. The resolution of the strain was found when I decided to study Dr. Andrew Taylor Still's science of osteopathy and forego a promising journalistic career.

29. A Thousandth of an Inch

November 18, 1950.

Prepared for the closing lecture at a course in cranial osteopathy in Des Moines, Iowa.

If we possessed that vision of the infinitesimal in the human mechanical structure that Dr. Andrew Taylor Still had, we might readily observe the multitude of "little things" as "big things" to be seen in the science of osteopathy. *Then* our vision of the possibilities might become enlarged to equal the magnitude of the heavens.

My attention has been directed recently, by a marked photographic reproduction presented by Dr. Joseph W. Peterson, to one of those visions of the infinitesimal found in Dr. Still's *Philosophy and Mechanical Principles of Osteopathy*. I quote in part:

> He [meaning the osteopath] must have brains...in osteopathic practice, curing disease by skillful readjustment of the parts of the body that have been deranged by strains, falls or any other cause that may have removed even a minute nerve from the normal, *although not more than a thousandth* of an inch.[1]

Think of that minute thousandth of an inch and you may find yourself *thinking osteopathy* with the Founder of Science. You may then have an inkling of Dr. Still's superior *mechanical* knowledge of the human body, a mechanism including fluids, soft tissues, cells, nuclei and electrons, as well as the mere osseous structure. Through that immense knowledge he was able to magnify the little things and interpret *how* they might alter affects and effects in physiological functioning. Listen to this thought from the same text [p. 33]:

---

1. Still, *Philosophy and Mechanical Principles*, p. 18; emphasis added.

> With anatomy in the normal properly understood, we are enabled to detect conditions that are abnormal.

Dr. Still's fundamental principle of anatomy in the normal, properly understood, should be of primary importance in teaching the science of osteopathy. I am sorry to learn from one of our prominent professors of anatomy in an osteopathic college that it has been suggested that instruction in applied anatomy be discontinued in order to devote time to other subjects now required in our college curricula. Fortunately, there are two colleges where the department of anatomy is headed by doctors of osteopathy. I have been assured by one that he will fight against this drifting away from a fundamental principle in our science, and I have confidence that the other will hold steadfastly to instruction in applied anatomy.

Now that I have expressed my feeling in this matter let us consider another significant statement in the quotation, viz.:

> It may be that by measurement we can discover a variation one-hundredth of an inch from the normal, which, *though infinitely small*, is nevertheless abnormal.[2]

Take note that here Dr. Still changes the vision, yet still infinitesimal in degree.

This reminds me of a flock of baby wrens, just out from their nest and learning how to utilize their wings. They flew into my garage. One little wren became alarmed by my sudden appearance and, in great fright, bumped its tiny head upon a beam in the doorway. The little babe fell to the floor, apparently lifeless. I lacked the anatomical knowledge of where and how to register the pulse, but the respiration was absent. Even the tiny head was less than two centimeters in measurement. I picked the baby up and very gently flexed the tiny head upon what were probably the facets of the atlas. There followed a tiny click, indicating something returning to normal position. I pictured this as a ligamentous reduction of what may have been an

---

2. Ibid, p. 33; emphasis added.

occipitoatlantal ligamentous articular strain.

The tiny wren regained consciousness and turned from its side to a sitting posture. The eyes opened and respiration became very apparent. Thirty minutes later our little patient flew away into the lilac bushes to join its flock without leaving even its tiny bill in return for professional services rendered. Yet, somehow I know that the tiny wren was grateful and may return in the springtime to build a nest in my backyard. I shall listen for its cheerful song and hear it say: "Even though a tiny wren fall by the wayside, the Father knoweth."[3]

In further connection with events in small dimensions, I would like to mention an interesting observation reported by a member of our own profession. It concerns a tiny ant busy dragging a long worm, ten times its own measurement, to a distant area. It dug a hole and placed the worm within, carefully covering the hole with earth and tramping it firmly. Later the ant returned, uncovered the hole, dug up the worm and dragged it to another distant area. Then it dug another hole and placed the worm within, covered it with earth and tramped the covering firmly. This narration is not a fable but a true story, reminding us of how big little things may be when seen by focusing one's visual lens to one-hundredth part of an inch.

To continue the last quotation from Dr. Still:

> If we follow the effects of abnormal straining of ligaments, we will easily come to the conclusion that derangements of *one-hundredth part of an inch* are often probable of those parts of the body over which blood vessels and nerves are distributed, whose duties are to construct, vitalize and keep a territory, *though small in width*, fully up to the normal standard of health.

His reference to the *abnormal straining of ligaments* in a derangement of one-hundredth part of an inch coincides with my view of spinal lesions as ligamentous articular strains and cranial lesions as

3. Cf. "Are not two sparrows sold for a farthing? And not one of them shall fall on the ground without your Father [knowing]." Mt. 10:29, King James Version.

membranous articular strains and also that ligamentous and membranous restrictions lead to pathological effects. In other words, ligamentous and membranous strains are the predisposing factors to which Dr. Korr referred in his lecture before the Academy of Applied Osteopathy, in Chicago, this past summer.[4] That terminology is not new to early students in the science of osteopathy. It was gratifying to hear Dr. Korr using it.

A case came to my attention recently that illustrates the predisposing factor. The problem required focusing one's imaginative lens to the perspective of one-hundredth part of an inch, as the usual gross palpation and motion tests were negative. The complaint, of long duration, had been diagnosed as a systemic infection, confirmed by ugly appearing sores. Its manifestation, however, was localized throughout the forearms and on the forehead and chin. To an old-timer, this local manifestation was a cue to a predisposing factor, of slight or larger degree, throughout the area of the upper dorsal region.

Our mechanical anatomical knowledge of "anatomy properly understood" visualized a possible one-hundredth part of an inch tension in ligaments related to the heads of the upper ribs, which effected disturbance to the sympathetic ganglia near them. This mechanical knowledge pictured the normal articular movement of the heads of the ribs in the following manner: rotating in a ball-and-socket action in the demi-facets of the vertebrae, externally and slightly posteriorly during inhalation (similar to the activity of the head of the femur in the acetabulum), and internally and slightly anteriorly during exhalation. In connection with the head-of-the-rib action, ribs also circumduct, much in the manner of circumducting a horseshoe in a game of quoits, and in the process the sternal ends, through intermembranous attachment, draw the sternum backward during

---

4. Irvin M. Korr, Ph.D. (Princeton, 1936) is a physiologist who has taught, researched and written extensively on the subject of applied physiology in relation to osteopathy. His work in the field began in 1947 when he joined the faculty of the Kirksville College of Osteopathic Medicine.

inhalation, and when they circumduct in the opposite direction during exhalation, through the intermembranous attachment, the sternum is drawn forward.

This view of normal rib action differs widely from the usual athletic instruction of how to expand the chest to fill the lungs with air during inhalation. This common exercise would likely handicap the normal descent of the diaphragm during inhalation. The same procedure might strain ligamentous tissue in connection with the heads of the ribs. In some cases, this exercise might account for round shoulders.

With this picture of the normal and the cue to where the strain might be in the case under discussion, the description of the application of the technique comes next. The patient sat in a chair facing me seated in another chair. My thumbs made gentle and firm contacts beneath the ventral surfaces, near the glenoid fossae, at the upper axillary borders of the scapulae to assume the *still* points of fulcrums. These fulcrum contacts on the scapulae were held slightly laterally. The patient was then instructed to throw her arms over my shoulders (or around the operator's body in some circumstances) as far as possible, and pull gradually forward. This facilitated a swinging action laterally, or outwardly, of the vertebral borders of the scapulae. In the picture you may view a relaxation of muscular tissue between the origin and insertion of the serratus magnus muscle, so important for securing specific action of the ligaments related to the heads of the ribs. It was gratifying to be able to sense the circumducting movement of the ribs as this simple technique operated true to form. It was encouraging to observe the immediate changes in color and texture throughout the local manifestation of the infection in the forearms. I am not saying that the case was cured. In my practice, cures were never promised nor miracles performed. Professional skill to the best of my ability was the only guarantee. However, this response to a technique based on the vision of a *predisposing factor* in the minute ligamentous tensions around the heads of ribs secured an encouragement where other methods had failed. Furthermore, as only one treatment had been applied, there is hope that with repetitions given over a sufficient length of time, the systemic infection may clear.

Great appreciation has been expressed by some members of the Academy of Applied Osteopathy for Dr. Howard A. Lippincott's article on "Ligamentous Articular Strains" that appeared in the 1949 *Year Book.*[5]

Dr. Lippincott, being an ardent advocate for detail in the plan for a reproduction of the technique in the coming text, *Osteopathy in the Cranial Field*, by Harold I. Magoun, D.O., suggested that a group of cranial technicians spend a few weeks in an anatomical laboratory.[6] A very profitable period, usually set aside for a summer vacation, was occupied in an endeavor to become more familiar with many of Dr. Still's visions of the infinitesimal. It was my pleasure to spend a week in observation of the work accomplished on two very interesting specimens.

One of these had been dissected down to the ligamentous tissue to free the articulations from all muscular influence, in accordance with the view of specific ligamentous reduction. This was exceptionally well demonstrated in the specimen throughout all the articulations, including the digits of the extremities, and photographic illustrations were made of the technique utilized in each. The specimen also included an exceptionally fine open-window exhibit of the cranial reciprocal tension membrane. Testing of the function of this membrane was very satisfactorily exemplified.

---

5. The Academy of Applied Osteopathy, originally the Osteopathic Manipulative Therapeutic and Clinical Research Association (established in 1937 and granted affiliation with the American Osteopathic Association in 1938) is the forerunner of the modern American Academy of Osteopathy.

Howard A. Lippincott, D.O. (1893-1963: American School of Osteopathy, 1916) was a member of Dr. Sutherland's teaching staff. He became president of the Sutherland Cranial Teaching Foundation following Dr. Sutherland, wrote several publications regarding osteopathy in the cranial field, and conducted an active study group with his wife, Rebecca, in his home in Moorestown, New Jersey.

6. The first edition was edited by Dr. Magoun and approved by Dr. Sutherland. Drs. Howard and Rebecca Lippincott, along with Dr. Paul Kimberly and others, contributed substantially to this text. Subsequent editions were rewritten by Dr. Magoun.

The work on the other specimen brought forth convincing testimony regarding our reference to the intraspinal membrane as a continuous reciprocal tension agent from the occiput and upper cervical down to the sacrum. The specimen revealed a firm osseous attachment to the second sacral segment so firmly attached that it might have been possible to couple up two or three other cadavers with it and drag them by the membrane from Chicago to New York. An observer, who wandered in, thought the attachment might be an anomaly. But somewhere he had read about an attachment of the membrane to the posterior longitudinal ligament of the spine. The following day he returned with an authoritative reference by Trolard. I had heard that same statement made by a member of my audience many years before. This specimen provided an opportunity to find out, and the dissection was continued through the posterior arches. The attachments to the posterior longitudinal ligament were verified, one at each segment of the spinal vertebrae. But! these attachments to the common ligament were of *sufficient length to allow freedom* of movement between the occiput and the upper cervical and the firm osseous attachment at the second sacral segment. The Trolard attachments are for a purpose and, as I see them at present, coincide with my concept of forward-bending of the entire body as flexion.

Among other events at the laboratory was a discussion of the manner in which the cranial nerves go through the dura mater. Dissection of the trigeminal ganglion appeared to bear out an indication that the three branches from it that are considered in tic douloureux carry with them a sleeve of dura. The ganglion lies on a layer of external dura and one of internal dura. It is covered by two layers of internal dura. Histological studies are needed to determine how far the nerve carries its sleeve with it. This calls attention to another one of Dr. Still's visions of the infinitesimal, in which a minute nerve may have disturbance, "though not more than a *thousandth of an inch*."

The interosseous membranes outside the cranium received special study as well as the intracranial and intraspinal membranes. The radioulnar interosseous membrane, or middle radioulnar union, cooperates with the ligaments of the proximal and distal radioulnar joints and aids greatly in ligamentous reduction of radioulnar strains. When this mechanical feature is properly understood, the "jerk" method now commonly used will be discarded. The mechanical function of this interosseous membrane confirms my statement that not one of the radioulnar joints can be deranged separately; a derangement affects the movement at both the proximal and distal ends of the forearm.

The interosseous membrane connecting the tibia and fibula, or the middle tibiofibular ligament, may also be considered an aid in ligamentous reduction, as both ends of the fibula are in derangement rather than one.

While the obturator membrane that almost fills the obturator foramen does not connect bones that move in relation to each other, it is similar in mechanical function because it possesses partial origins of muscles on each side–the obturator internus on its pelvic surface and the obturator externus on its exterior surface. This membrane reminds one of a drumhead, with the muscle action pulling in opposite directions. It is quite subject to strains. I have known of such derangements that affected a small branch of the sciatic nerve and an arterial vessel on their way through the obturator canal to reach the interior of the acetabulum. This area and its problems picture another place where Dr. Still's vision of the infinitesimal should have deep study in complaints pertaining to the hip joint.

My article, "Grandfather's Bootjack Remedy in Flat Foot," was reprinted in *The Osteopathic Physician*, published by my classmate, Dr. Henry S. Bunting. Bunting's editorial column was headed by the following quotation: "Hew to the line, let the chips fall where they may."

During this period of time the American Osteopathic Association became interested in a little gadget for the reduction of the third cuneiform bone in the foot. It was a thrust type of technique and rather severe. Consequently, a few old-timers were "hewing to the line" and the chips were falling. My feature article was a "chip from the Old Block." Because: Grandfather was never troubled with flat feet. He wore long-legged, tight-fitting boots requiring the aid of a bootjack in removal at bedtime. The bootjack drew the calcaneus inwardly beneath its articulation with the talus. When the bootjack was not available, Grandfather would place his leg across the opposite knee, grasp the boot heel with one hand and the toe with the other, and accomplish the same simple technique.

Technique *is* simple if anatomy is "properly understood." That is why a special observation was made in the laboratory to study the movement of the talus upon the calcaneus as well as the grooves on the under surface of the talus and the upper surface of the calcaneus. Within this groove is the interosseous talocalcaneal ligament, the mechanism of which, in connection with the bones, will simplify the technique when properly understood.

Another study of important problems was that concerning fascial drags from the pelvis that affects the physiological functioning of the cranial primary respiratory mechanism. This study centered on the diaphragm, which is regulated in its secondary activity by nervous impulses originating in physiological centers located within the floor of the fourth ventricle. There was specific manipulation of the central tendon of the diaphragm which disclosed a response at the sphenobasilar symphysis. The movement at the sphenobasilar was flexion and extension and also internal and external rotation of the petrous portions of the temporal bones. The fascial connections between the external surface of the head and the central tendon of the diaphragm were also studied. As the pharynx is suspended from the pharyngeal tubercle on the underside of the basilar process of the occiput, and the pharyngeal raphe on the petrous portions of the temporal bones and the sphenoid, and as the accompanying cervical fascia connects with the central tendon of the diaphragm, we have a possible interpretation of the problem of how fascial drags affect the physiological functioning of the cranial primary respiratory mechanism.

The distal sacral region of the craniosacral primary respiratory mechanism had profitable observation, especially including the sacroiliac ligaments in their regulation of movement. The problem of the forwardly depressed derangement of the sacrum with the consequent drag by way of the intraspinal dura mater was closely analyzed. This drag undoubtedly affects the fluctuation within the area of the cisterna magna as is frequently indicated by the complaint of a dull heavy sensation in that region. I visualize a deranged position of the cerebellum, its hemispheres bending back and down to crowd the cisterna beneath. Occipitomastoid membranous articular strains have the same consequences.

Your studies of the past two weeks have introduced you to the various pictures of the infinitesimal to be seen in the mechanisms in the cranial field. In this talk, I have merely pointed out to you a few places in other areas of the body where Dr. Still's vision of derangements of one-thousandth of an inch are applicable.

30. The Lighthouse Beam

'Tis the mortar in *the space between the bricks* that holds a structure together.

As usual, some member of the Associate Faculty blossomed out with a bright idea. He suggested issuing a publication medium at the Sutherland "Fulcrum" occasionally, thus keeping the faculty members linked together.[1] The thought kindled into enthusiasm and the presentation of a mimeograph at the convention in Milwaukee.

This *Beam* is our first attempt in operating the mechanism. So, read the *space between* both the lines of smudge and the print.

Also read the *space between* the physiologic centers within the floor of the fourth ventricle.

In reading between the lines, we suggest the mental vision through the small end of the microscope followed by the view through the big end of a telescope to observe the material elements disappearing into *endless space.*

By none other than...W.G.S.

1. August 4, 1951

We live close to the lighthouse by the sea and view the water of the Pacific day by day; and even when we do not see the sea, we *feel its presence.*[2]

---

1. The "Fulcrum" was the name Dr. and Mrs. Sutherland gave to their home in Pacific Grove, California.

2. The Sutherland's home in Pacific Grove was across the street from the Coast Guard station at Point Pinos and light from the lighthouse would come into their home on a regular basis, a phenomenon which Dr. Sutherland enjoyed very much.

We have been told that the pleasant land about us is only a *side-show* so far as life and action on this planet goes and that *the main arena is the sea.* According to Rachel L. Carson, in *The Sea Around Us* [p. 51]:

> There is no drop of water in the ocean, not even in the deepest parts of the abyss, that does not know and respond to the mysterious forces that create the tide. No other force that affects the sea is so strong.

We have read in another text that *the waters were divided and the earth appeared,* and that the material body had its form from the *earth.*[3] We, living close to the lighthouse by the sea, visualize great heaps of sand dunes and solid rock disintegration as differentiations in formation of the earth from which the material body hath its form. We visualize *the space between the grains of sand* and *know* that the solid rock is crumbling back into sandy grains.

We, living close to the Lighthouse by the Sea, *feel the Presence* of the fluid tide, day by day.

We are looking forward to the study of another text, known as *The Science of Osteopathy in the Cranial Field,* wherein anatomy-properly-understood invites intelligent application.

–W.G.S.

2. September 1951

At the Fulcrum, 53 Asilomar Boulevard, Pacific Grove, California.
To: The Association Faculty.

Without a *pause-rest* between notes there could not be a musical tone.

---

3. "And God said, Let the waters under the heavens be gathered together unto one place, and let the dry land appear: and it was so." Gen. 1:9, King James Version. "And the Lord God formed man from the dust of the earth…" Gen. 2:7, King James Version.

Without a *pause-rest* between shutter openings of the camera there could not be a motion picture.

At long last the text, *Osteopathy in the Cranial Field* by Harold I. Magoun, D.O., will be ready as a valuable aid in the continued progress in teaching.

One of our problems has been: teaching the *feel* of the fluid. It might be more effective if the instructor called attention at first to the *feel* of the "juices" rather than fluid.

Credit for this thought goes to four-and-a-half year-old Joe Franz, an intelligent son of Dr. Ruth Franz of Pittsburgh. Joe surprised Dr. Ruth, while being treated, with the question: "Mommy, do you feel the juices flow?" Mommy, in relating the incident, said that she could not recall describing the action to Joe at any time–the question evidently cropping forth because of his own sense of feeling.

The definition of *fluctuation* as applied to the cranial concept should be given occasional stress: the movement of a fluid contained within a natural or artificial cavity, observed by palpation or percussion.

Finger contacts should be *firm* and *gentle*, applied like the bird's digits in contacting the bark of a twig on a tree–alighting gently and gradually increasing firmness without injury to the bark.

–W.G.S.

3. October 1951

53 Asilomar Blvd., Pacific Grove, California.
To: The Associate Faculty.

The Talk at Milwaukee

Dr. Still's vision of the infinitesimal, the incalculably small, is especially useful in the study of the science of osteopathy in the cranial field. For cranial strains in many instances correspond in minute measurement to the dimension of the injury to the baby wren. In that little bird tale, the adjustment required specific mechanical knowledge mentally viewed through the small end of the microscope.[4]

Consider that small point in the sphenosquamous suture where the beveling changes, often referred to as the sphenosquamous pivot. The motion mechanism at that point is very minute, yet it affords a wider range of movement of the temporal bone at the upper and lower areas of the squamous portions as well as a greater range in the external and internal rotation of the petrous portion. An infinitely small strain at the sphenosquamous pivot can change the position of the mandibular fossa, with consequent abnormal alignment in the articular contact by the head of the mandible, thus causing the jaw to click and jump forward to the embarrassment of the patient.

Consider another picture of the infinitely small type of cranial strain, the sleeve of dura mater that extends out along the branches of the fifth cranial nerve as they leave the trigeminal ganglion. In cases of tic douloureux, where rotation of the petrous portion of the temporal bone has increased tension in the local dura mater, it is well to focus attention on an infinitely small strain of the dural sleeve. Imagine a man's sensitive and irritating discomfort when wearing a tightfitting shirtsleeve and cuff. It is an appropriate illustration comparable to the sensitive facial discomfort experienced in tic douloureux.

Another infinitely small cranial abnormality to be considered in tic douloureux is a specific *stretching strain* of the infraorbital nerve. The stretching may occur along the nerve pathway, from a tightfitting dural sleeve, around the small groove on the minute orbital process of the palate bone and on around through the groove within the orbital area of the maxilla to reach its exit beneath the zygoma. This type of strain, that is of nerve stretching in a specific place and mechanism, may be illustrated in a larger nerve, the sciatic. The method for demonstrating sciatic nerve stretching is simple: While the patient rests comfortably on the table in the supine position, bend or flex the entire lower extremity toward the head, being careful not to bend or

---

4. Dr. Sutherland tells the story of adjusting the neck of an injured bird; see article 29, "A Thousandth of an Inch," note 3.

flex the knee, and then dorsiflex the foot. A rather painful sensation usually follows throughout the sciatic nerve pathway. We advise thorough attention to possible *infinitely small* palatine and maxilla strains in some cases of tic douloureux.

When focusing on this same infraorbital nerve, include a view of the Creator's suspension mechanism for the sphenopalatine ganglion in your mental field. Two suspension fibers drop down from the area of possible nerve stretching and afford swinging activity in accommodation to movement of the sphenoid and palatine bones.

There are other rather interesting arrangements common to the physiologic functioning of cranial ganglia and bulbs to focus the mental microscope on for the view of the infinitely small. Look at the trigeminal ganglion near the tip of the petrous portion of the temporal bone. See the roly-poly action during petrous rotation. Look at the olfactory bulbs on the cribriform plate of the ethmoid and see the rocking movement. Then see the suspension sway of the ciliary ganglion. The *motion-vision* of nerve fibers and ganglia is quite important in our cranial problems. This motion-vision should include the nerve tracts forming the walls of the cerebral aqueduct, such an important area to normal fluctuation of the cerebrospinal fluid from the third to the fourth ventricles and vice versa.

Dr. Still's reference to "*finer nerves* dwelling with the lymphatics than even with the eye" requires hours of study through the small end of the mental microscope in order to understand the interpretation.[5] It is also wise to interpret a noted pathologist's reference to "forty thousand nerve fibers passing from the hypothalamus via the infundibulum to the pituitary." This latter reference becomes more difficult in interpretation since the experiment on a porpoise by a prominent anatomist at a Texas medical school. He was quoted in the press as follows:

> The experiment proved that the master gland does not have nerve fibers going directly to it from the brain or central nervous system, as previously thought. We are as certain now as any

5. Still, *Philosophy*, p. 104; emphasis added.

> scientific experimentation can let us be that there is some other means of control of the central nervous system.... There is good evidence that there is another means of control which, if we find it, will lead to correction of many disorders caused by man's nervous system.

A member of a class in cranial instruction brought me a small section of a coaxial cable that likely aids in a theoretical interpretation of Dr. Still's reference to "finer nerves than those of the eye," as well as the reference by a pathologist to "forty thousand nerve fibers" passing via the infundibulum. The cable contains a number of copper tubes. Each tube is insulated from a wire passing through the center. The wire is said to carry the electrical potency from which many messages may be transmitted at the same time through the copper tube.[6] By centering our mental vision at the small end of the microscope, one may theoretically visualize the infundibulum as the copper tube over which forty thousand nerve impulses might be conveyed from the hypothalamus via the infundibulum and vice versa. Scientists have also referred to nerve fibers as being hollow, and one might visualize theoretically one minute hollow nerve as a copper tube conveyor, possessing finer nerve impulses than those of the eye.

A Thought Here and There

A continuation of "The Talk at Milwaukee."

When we commence to *think osteopathy with Dr. Still* and perhaps understand his frequent reference to the "little things" as the "big things" in the science of osteopathy, it brings us closer to a possible interpretation of his thought that the *buzzard*, living on dead matter, is the largest type of microbe in existence.

---

6. A coaxial cable is composed of an insulated central conductor with tubular stranded coppper conductors laid over it concentrically and separated by layers of insulation. This arrangement allows the cable to simultaneously transmit thousands of telephone, radio or television signals while preventing a loss of signal strength from outside electrical interference.

From visualizing the normal articular movement of the heads of the ribs and the effect a minute strain would have in effecting disturbances in the sympathetic ganglia near them, we can read between the lines and see a larger picture as follows:

In connection with the head-of-the-rib activity,

Reading between the lines, one may

the ribs circumduct much in the manner corresponding

view the thoracic cage functioning in

to circumduction of a horseshoe in a game of quoits.

a spiral movement like the main-spring

During the procedure in inhalation, the sternal ends,

of the balance wheel of the enlarged

through intermembranous or cartilaginous attachments,

watch observed at the New York Grand Central

draw the sternum backwardly; and during exhalation,

Station in New York City.

the ribs circumduct in the opposite direction, drawing the sternum forwardly.

This viewpoint differs widely from the athletic instruction of expanding the chest during inhalation that likely handicaps the normal descent of the diaphragm. The same procedure might strain ligamentous tissue in connection with the heads of the ribs. It appears that I am not alone in my thought, according to the quotation of a prominent surgeon of Dallas, Texas in the Associated Press. The following is the quotation in part:

For generations we have all been harped at to throw our shoulders back, throw out our chests and sit perfectly straight in chairs...From old military circles of the past we've inherited the ideas that throwing out the chest and assuming a strut attitude is representative of good posture...But actually, these postural habits have been devastating because they *disregard anatomical facts....*

The next thought concerns the two occasions (in 1940 and 1949) when I was invited by Dr. George W. Goode to address the International

Society of Sacro-Iliac Technicians, convening in St. Louis, Missouri. On both occasions the subject concerned the connection between the cranial bowl and the pelvic bowl. In 1949 I reversed the title of the talk given in 1940. Bottom side up, it was "The Core-Link Between the Pelvic Bowl and the Cranial Bowl." In this presentation, my technique using the anterior sacral contact was demonstrated publicly for the first time. This technique applies to the specific type of sacral *strain* commonly existing in many patients throughout hundreds of mental hospitals in the United States. It will be demonstrated later on in the program by one who has become especially proficient in its application.

Now: All this introductory thought leads up to the importance
By specific study between
of study in relation to the various minute differentiations
the lines one may observe
common at the sacroiliac articular surfaces.
an anterior convergence
Then, perhaps, you may entertain a different understanding
with a consequent divergence
in differentiating the anterior, or forward, sacral strain
posteriorly at one important
from the usual postural sacral strain.
area of the sacroiliac articular
The anterior, or forward, sacral strain initiates a drag upon
surface, so arranged by The
the intraspinal section of the reciprocal tension membrane,
Architect of the mechanism to
or the core-link between the pelvic bowl and the cranial
accommodate the respiratory articular
bowl, affecting, or rather, effecting disturbance to the fluctuation
movement that is differentiated from
of the cerebrospinal fluid within the cisterna magna.
the postural movement.

Editor's Note: See illustrations of coronal sections of anterior, middle and posterior sacral segments in Gray's Anatomy of the Human Body, *26th edition, 1954, p. 351.*

Dr. Still's parable of "The Goat and the Boulder" brings forth *a thought of great importance* in our study of the science of osteopathy in which his vision of the *infinitely small* beholds a predisposing factor developing gradually into cardiac valvular pathology.[7]

In the parable, the goat represents the *heart*, the pathway down the mountain the *descending aorta,* and the boulder, the crura of the *diaphragm*. The goat comes down the mountain pathway and gives the boulder quite a *bump*, without securing movement, *but* the goat's tail flops up. The goat then *backs up* the mountain pathway to secure additional momentum for another bump. Still the boulder refuses to move. This time *both the tail and the hind heels* flop up. The goat, being a determined little bumper, then *backs up* to the top of the mountain to secure greater power and speed. Still the boulder remains rigidly motionless, but this time the *tail*, the hind *heels* and *the entire works flop up*.

The next time a patient complains of palpitation, remember Dr. Still's vision of the area where the abdominal aorta passes through and under the crura of the diaphragm. Also review your knowledge of *anatomy-properly-understood* in relation to the cisterna chyli into which the lymphatic stream enters before being carried upward through the thoracic duct to empty into the left subclavian vein. Some marvelous results have been accomplished in cardiac and lymph disorders by attention to the crura of the diaphragm. The application of applied anatomy is *skilled* attention. The technique becomes *simple* when one's knowledge of the lumbocostal arches, or ligamenta arcuata, interna and externa, is properly understood. The ligamentum externum, having its lateral attachment on the tip and lower margin of the twelfth rib, is of easy access by the insertion of a finger beneath the rib, affording

---

7. See Dr. Sutherland's rendition of Dr. Still's parable in Sutherland, *Teachings*, p. 214.

gentle movement upward and laterally. This draws the ligamentum externum laterally, and it in turn draws the ligamentum internum laterally and *frees abnormal tension strain at the crural area.*

I might continue on and on with other *thoughts* applicable to the importance of centering one's mental vision at the *small end* of the microscope as well as of a *reversal* to the *big end* of the telescope to *simplify* technical skill. However, this is the end of today's talk. Thank you.

31. The Science of Osteopathy

Presented to the members and guests of the Osteopathic Cranial Association meeting in Atlantic City, New Jersey, July 1952. This talk also was used to make a special recording at Pacific Grove, California, March 9, 1953.

In his lectures and writings, Dr. Sutherland made noticeable use of "we" and "our" in telling of his cranial findings and experiments. It is an editorial habit that persisted from his earlier years as a newspaper man. Actually, his entire research project was carried on in solitude.

According to Dr. Andrew Taylor Still, "no human hand has framed the laws" pertaining to the science of osteopathy.[1] It has proven to be an inviting, intriguing and profitable trip through the years gone by to learn a *few* of those laws governing an anatomical-physiological mechanism created by a Master Mechanic for the maintenance of man's progressive walkabout on earth. In consequence, I now possess a firm conviction that these God-given laws coordinate with a *true* science–or, with a *truth* revealed to Dr. Still as were "other truths that came to benefit mankind."

In my personal interpretation, the God-given laws apply specifically to a non-incisive surgical art. That thought will be a continual theme throughout my talk. To emphasize the theme, I quote a statement by Dr. Asa Willard in *The Cranial Bowl*: "Along in 1874, after years of independent thinking, there came to Dr. A.T. Still a conception of the basic principles of a *great truth*."[2]

In my interpretation, a *great* truth signifies an art greater than mere

---

1. "I do not claim to be the author of this science of Osteopathy. No human hand framed its law; I ask no greater honor than to have discovered it." Still, *Autobiography*, p. 302.

2. Asa Willard, D.O. (American School of Osteopathy, 1900) was president of the American Osteopathic Association in 1925.

structural manipulation. Thinking osteopathy between the lines *with* Dr. Still has aided immeasurably in acquiring an intimate knowledge of the laws which the Founder frequently expressed in parables and analogous illustrations that necessitated interpretation.

One of these remarkable analogous illustrations was found in an unpublished manuscript entitled "The Pig's Snout." It required considerable analytical thought. In it he referred especially to the importance of primary concentration on the study of the snout before seeking an introduction to the remainder of the pig anatomy. This differed quite materially from the method of commencing anatomical study with an extremity. Naturally, the pig snout analogy coordinated with the thought of the primary respiratory mechanism in my analysis. As in the human specimen, the pig snout possesses apertures for the intake of material air, so necessary to man's first function in beginning life on earth.

Analytical study of the snout revealed maxillae, palatines, zygomatics, lacrimals, nasals, the vomer and ethmoid–all these bones together with all their anatomical-physiological minutiae that now have so much significance to innumerable possibilities in the healing art. For instance, I am reminded of a simple technique applied to the primary respiratory mechanism by Dr. Still by the mention of minutiae.

In *Research and Practice* [p. 57 (n. 125)], he describes it thus:

> Pterygium–I have treated many cases of pterygium removing the growth and leaving the eye in its original condition. In all cases of pterygium I go to the nasal bones which you know are situated just a little below the bridge of the nose where the spectacles cross the nose. I place my thumbs on both sides of the nose on the upper part of the nasal bones and gently but firmly push the nasal bones down towards the eyeteeth. I do this in order to get a free circulation of the fluids and let them pass out of the pterygium. By so doing I have succeeded in removing them. In a few weeks, two to four, the pterygium has generally passed away under the treatment just indicated.

It should be noted that the main thought in the technique is to secure a *free circulation* of the *fluids* and to allow the *fluids* to *pass out of the pterygium*. The cranial technician visualizes in the application of the technique the fact that the two small nasal bones articulate in the midline with the perpendicular plate of the ethmoid, which is one of the bones of the cranial base.

It is easy to picture that when the two nasal bones are pushed downward, the push initiates movement of the ethmoid with consequent membranous-articular mobility of the other bones of the base because the ethmoid is a unit of mechanical operation of the whole. In connection with this fact, visualize important changes occurring within the orbital cavities, including deepening of the lacrimal ducts, widening of the sphenoidal fissures (considered as the gateways of venous drainage from the orbits to the cavernous sinuses), and a narrowing of the sphenomaxillary fissures in accommodation of elongation of the orbital cavities–and all movement being in unity *to secure a free circulation of fluids*.

We recognize in this technique the *non-incisive surgical art* taught by Dr. Andrew Taylor Still. I stress the fact that his contact on the osseous parts of the mechanism was gentle and firm. The fingers should alight like the digits of a bird, gently on a twig, and *then* gradually securing firm contact so accomplished as not to injure the bark of the twig. This is not what is commonly known as "manipulative therapy" but a demonstration of our theme: *non-incisive surgery*.

Another feature of the Boulder-in-the-Path-of-the-Goat analogy comes to mind because it brought forth concentrated attention concerning the anatomical-physiological law governing the function of the ureters.[3] This came about following a failure in a written examination

---

3. For a description of "The Goat and the Boulder" see article 30, "The Lighthouse Beam," note 7; also see Dr. Sutherland's rendition of Dr. Still's parable in Sutherland, *Teachings*, p. 214.

4. John Martin Littlejohn, D.O. (1865-1947: American School of Osteopathy, 1900) was born in Glasgow, Scotland. Resigning as president of Amity College in Iowa,he began a series of visits to Dr. A. T. Still for relief of physical ills in the late 1890's. In 1897 he became a lecturer in physiology at the American School of Osteopathy

given by Dr. J. Martin Littlejohn when he was professor of physiology at the American School of Osteopathy.[4] Fortunately, I was granted an oral examination and could substitute the fluid-drip through the ureters for the constant-flow theory as stated in the written test. I had missed Dr. Littlejohn's lectures on kidney function, having been absent earning a few necessary pence in a print shop where I composed his text in physiology into long-primer type. This fact was unknown to him. In the end, perhaps, I learned as much about the physiologic laws concerning the kidney as the average student, and it was sufficient to keep me digging deeper and deeper.

I feel free to join with the late pioneer osteopath, Joseph H. Sullivan, D.O., in the following thought: "If you cannot comprehend osteopathy, step aside, and allow the real science to pursue its progressive march."

Since that early day, the Mayo brothers of Rochester, Minnesota, near my field of professional activity, evolved a method of diagnosis in ureteral complaints–a ureterogram–that is now employed successfully by our own osteopathic surgeons.[5] The method of diagnosis, as well as the treatment, is rather painful for the patient. So, I evolved a method, in my early years in practice, that is suitable for application by a non-incisive surgeon. It requires a trained and skillful tactile sense coupled with physiological-anatomical knowledge. A successful technique was also devised for attention to the abnormal kinks often found present in ureters, kinks which back up the normal drip of urine from the kidney into the renal pelvis, with consequent pathology.

(ASO), enrolled as a student in 1898 and was appointed dean of faculty and professor of physiology shortly thereafter. He graduated in 1900 and established the American College of Osteopathy and Surgery in Chicago, Illinois with his two brothers (also prior faculty members at the ASO) in that same year. In 1913 he returned to England and founded the British School of Osteopathy. See Berchtold, *History of the Chicago College*.

5. Charles H. Mayo, M.D. (1865-1939), an American surgeon, and his brother, William J. Mayo, M.D. (1861-1939), established the Mayo Clinic in Rochester, Minnesota in 1889.

The technique necessitates personal cooperation by the patient. The patient makes a mental effort to move the lower ribs laterally while inhaling, rather than anteroposteriorly. During this assistance, the non-incisive surgeon gently and firmly draws the ribs in the same lateral direction. This physiologic procedure not only secures greater excursion for the function of the diaphragm up and down but also reaches the lumbocostal arches, or ligamenta arcuata, externa and interna. It succeeds in removing Dr. Still's analogous "boulder," frequently found restricting the pathway of the abdominal aorta, with resultant pathology in the cardiac valves.

A larger picture that considers factors which may restrict the normal ureteral drip recognizes that the ureters lie anterior to the fascia of the psoas muscles, that the sigmoid flexure on the left and the caecum on the right lie anterior to the ureters. These relations may involve the ureters in the consequences of an external rotation strain of the head of the femur in the acetabulum. This type of strain occurred often in the early days of making professional visits when the roads were not as passable as they are today. Perhaps when pushing a car out of a mudhole, the tendon of the psoas major muscle undergoes severe traction from origin to insertion, on the lesser trochanter of the femur. This strain pattern would include the lumbocostal arches.

With this enlarged picture in mind, the non-incisive surgeon enters the problem with simple, effective, gentle skill as follows: The patient reclines comfortably on the back. The operator's trained index finger or thumb is passed medially along the psoas tendon over the brim of the pelvis. The leg is flexed on the trunk (without bending the knee) to secure a necessary relaxation of muscle tension in its function of flexion. The flexion also allows the finger or thumb contact to drop further downward, medial to the tendon. The leg is then drawn across the other leg which allows the finger or thumb contact to drop laterally beneath the tendon, near to its insertion upon the lesser trochanter. This contact then operates as a fulcrum beneath the tendon as the leg is rotated into external rotation to secure balance in ligamentous tension and is immediately followed by ligamentous reduction of the head of the femur in the acetabulum.

In connection with the above problem related to the abdominal and pelvic areas, it is advisable to stress the need for attention to fascial drags. Considering the multitude of lymph nodes abounding amidst this fascial area, it is well to emphasize that their pathway leads to the cisterna chyli.

This receptor might be called a decomposition station, providing necessary physiologic dissolution of some elements before the lymph passes on upwardly through the thoracic duct to empty into the venous channel. The thoracic duct, like the abdominal aorta, passes through the area of Dr. Still's analogous boulder. Restriction at this area leads to retardment of lymph flow as well as restriction of arterial circulation leading to cardiac pathology.

As a non-incisive surgeon with over 50 years of professional experience, good and bad, I desire to stress the importance of this simple psoas major technique. It has possibilities for the successful care of cardiac valvular, pyloric, hepatic, renal, bladder and prostatic complications.

The human structure as a whole unit, including the cerebrospinal fluid drive, is a mechanism governed by laws "not framed by human hand" yet a mechanism from which man has taken mechanical patterns to make inventions, including fluid control.[6] In connection with the abdominal and pelvic areas, look at the thoracic cage with its physiological spiral movement from which many of man's inventions have been patterned. Although this spiral movement has already been mentioned, special emphasis is essential. This cage, with its lungs, heart, liver and spleen, is a secondary respiratory mechanism and one of great importance in the regulation of normal air intake, circulation of the blood and lymph streams and the chemistry of the body. In my interpretation of anatomical-physiological laws not framed by human

---

6. Reference is being made to Dr. Still's words: "I do not claim to be the author of this science of Osteopathy. No human hand framed its law; I ask no greater honor than to have discovered it." Still, *Autobiography*, p. 302.

hand in contradiction to laws evolved by man's mistaken understanding, the sternum recedes backward during inhalation and moves forward during exhalation. In other words, the common exercise of throwing out the chest to secure a breath of fresh air handicaps the normal physiologic mobility of the thoracic cage.

I made a working model from an anatomical specimen in order to study this mechanism. I began by suspending the articulated spinal column separately from a standard. I also remodeled the thoracic cage by substituting flexible bands for the rigid wire connections. Then it was suspended separately from an adjoining standard. The two standards were so arranged for close study of the articular contact of the heads of the ribs in the demi-facets of the vertebrae as to allow raising and lowering of the specimens as needed.

In this study, we readily interpreted external rotation of the rib heads in the demi-facets during inhalation, or what might be termed a ball-and-socket mobility like that of the femoral head in the acetabulum and an internal rotation of the rib heads during exhalation. The sternal ends of the ribs receded and drew the sternum inward during inhalation and just the opposite during exhalation. Through the membranous and cartilaginous interconnections, this circumductory or spiral mobility of the ribs adds up to the changes that occur in the thoracic cage as a whole.

As this interpretation was in contradiction to common professional thought, like that of the cranial concept, there was hesitation in making a general statement of it to the profession. Now that I am joined in this interpretation by a Texas surgeon, I will append a quotation from an Associated Press article:

> For generations we've all been harped at to throw our shoulders back, throw out our chests and sit perfectly straight in chairs. From old military circles of the past we've inherited the idea that throwing out the chest and assuming a strut attitude is representative of good posture. But actually, these postural habits have been devastating because they disregard anatomical fact.

I will add to the surgeon's statement that these postural habits also disregard a physiological law not framed by human hand. The habits disregard the downward movement of the diaphragm during inhalation and handicap respiration through tension on the fascia all the way upward from the diaphragm to the neck and head.

My frequent reference to non-incisive surgery is not a criticism of surgery as a science and an art. It is an endeavor to call attention, step-by-step, to the fact that the charter of our first osteopathic school read: "...to improve our present system of surgery, obstetrics, and treatment of diseases generally, and place the same on a more rational and scientific basis, and to impart information to the medical profession."[7]

Frankly, the science of osteopathy is a system of surgery, and whether we practice major, minor or non-incisive surgery, we are skilled surgeons. The surgeon prefers to demonstrate artistic skill through an operation rather than "manipulation." Music is one of the arts and the pianist prefers to demonstrate the application of artistic talent, expressive of tone modulation, rather than "manipulation of the keys." Our beloved Louisa Burns corrected one of our technicians when asked if "manipulation" in the upper dorsal cured the cataract by replying: "When the lesion in the upper dorsal was *corrected.*"[8]

The practice of the science of osteopathy is one of the greatest arts and I prefer: *Motivating an expression of non-incisive surgical skill to secure balance in the laws attributive to the mechanism.*

This seems more in rhythmical accordance with the following statement by the late Dr. Dwight J. Kenney: "If you *comprehend* osteopathy, you will realize that you have a system that is vastly superior to any other now in use, and you will have implicit faith in its improved efficiency for the future."

---

7. Still, *Autobiography*, p. 142.

8. Louisa Burns, D.O. (1870-1958: Pacific College of Osteopathy, 1903). Dr. Burns (who pronounced her name Lou-Isa) contributed significantly to the body of osteopathic research in her 50 years of work. See the 1994 *Year Book* of the American Academy of Osteopathy which is dedicated to her work.

Now to a few special remarks relative to the cranial field in the science of osteopathy. Not many years past, the Mayo brothers, surgeons, were quoted by the Associated Press as saying that they commenced their art of surgery in the abdominal and pelvic areas of the body and gradually progressed towards knowledge and perfection, finally reaching the realm of the brain. Perhaps they might have made greater progress had they realized the full importance of an early anatomical statement reading as follows: "All the physiological centers, including that of respiration, are located within the floor of the fourth ventricle."[9]

Our own profession, also overlooking its full interpretation, began and followed their practice in the territory below the brain. When the idea of a primary respiratory mechanism suggested control of the fluctuation of the cerebrospinal fluid through the non-incisive surgical art of compressing the fourth ventricle, it became possible to reach the physiologic-center connections that secure an immediate interchange between all the fluids of the human body. There are now some three to four hundred non-incisive surgeons who are following the suggestion. A statement made in the preface to *Osteopathy in the Cranial Field* [p. xii], edited by Harold I. Magoun, D.O., reads as follows:

> The conception of the primary respiratory mechanism, with its possible lesioning, goes far towards a satisfactory answer to the problems of cerebrospinal fluid stasis, cerebral edema, retarded venous drainage, congestive states, altered chemistry, accumulation of metabolites, "withering fields" along perivascular and perineural channels and cellular pathology leading to both local and remote disease.

Dr. Still's own view of osteopathy in the cranial field has an indicative picture that is found in *The Philosophy of Osteopathy* [pp. 38-39]:

> Another period of observation appears to the philosopher.... His mind will explore the bone, the ligament, the muscle, the

9. "In the floor of the fourth ventricle....are situated certain important centers, i.e. cardiac, vasomotor, respiratory, vomiting, and deglutition centers." Wright, *Applied Physiology*, p. 108.

> fascia, the channels through which the blood travels from heart to local destiny with lymphatics and their contents.... It...does obtain blood abundantly to and from the heart, but the results obtained are not satisfactory, and another leaf is opened of why no good results are obtained and where is the mystery, what quality and element of force and vitality has been withheld? A thought strikes him that the cerebrospinal fluid is the highest known element that is contained in the human body, and unless the brain furnishes this fluid in abundance, a disabled condition of the body will remain. He who is able to reason will see that this great river of life must be tapped and the withering fields irrigated at once, or the harvest of health be forever lost.

This thought carries on into deep water, figuratively speaking, and into the studious consideration of that highest known element, the cerebrospinal fluid, the element that is considered by the cranial concept as providing *nourishment* to the brain cells with consequent *transmutation* of the element throughout the nerve fiber to its terminal. Perhaps this transmutation is the *nerve force* to which Dr. Still referred in *The Philosophy and Mechanical Principles of Osteopathy*. In reality, one knows as much about this element as do recognized authorities.

Our knowledge is like that of the electrician who merely *knows* that the potent current, or M-element, is present and that he is learning *how to utilize its force.*[10] We, too, merely *know* that the cerebrospinal fluid is present and contains the "highest known element" and that we are now learning, through the cranial concept, *how to utilize its force* in behalf of the ills of mankind. We know that the fluid is replenished from time to time, but as to *where from* and *how*, it is not necessary to know.

However, the cranial thought views the cerebrospinal fluid as

---

10. M-element: An electrical term for expressing the amount of mutual inductance. Inductance is the property of an electric circuit by which a varying current in it produces a varying magnetic field that induces voltages in the same circuit or in a nearby circuit.

fluctuating, rather than circulating, as do other fluids of the system. Fluctuation, according to Webster's medical definition, reads: "The motion of a fluid contained in a natural or artificial cavity, observed by palpation or percussion."

The cerebrospinal fluid is contained within a natural cavity and its motion, or fluctuation, is readily observed by palpation, according to the experience of cranial technicians in daily practice. Furthermore, it is possible, without hesitation, to make this assertion: The fluctuation of the cerebrospinal fluid may be controlled in its rhythm by thinking-feeling-seeing-knowing fingers to a degree where all the fluids have a rhythmic-balance-interchange. Tests made before and after treatment in the feel of the tissues, blood pressure readings, laboratory observations and so forth provide ample clinical proof of the statement. Through this method the cranial technician is learning how to *irrigate* Dr. Still's "withering fields."

During the interchange between all the fluids, an attenuation occurs equal to that of the penetrating oil used by all mechanics on rusty bolts to prevent injury to the articular threads. This rhythmical fluctuation to the fluid-balance-interchange is valuable in the reduction of old chronic vertebral lesions, as these not only become easier in reduction, but there is also less injury to what may be called "rusty threads" within the articulations.

Venous drainage from the head is also emphasized in the cranial concept, especially that through the sinuses formed by membranous walls. The great difference between the intracranial membranous venous channels and venous channels without the cranial mechanism is especially important in our consideration of the anatomical-physiological laws "not framed by human hand." The application of these laws provides the reason for my terminology: "cranial membranous articular strains" and "vertebral ligamentous strains." Such strains in the *membranous* walls of the venous channels frequently retard the venous flow as well as the fluctuation of the cerebrospinal fluid. In some instances even the arterial stream, due to the backup of the venous circulation, may lose its supremacy and seek anastomotic detours, often found ineffectual.

Were it possible for Dr. Still to make a visit here today, I feel that he would be pleased with our endeavor to interpret his early vision of the place of the cranial concept in osteopathy.

Yes! Doctor Still's non-incisive surgical art is an *improvement in the systems of surgery*. Furthermore, it is also an improvement in *obstetrics.*

Among many letters arriving at my desk, there are expressions of deep gratitude for instruction received in the cranial non-incisive surgical art with which many in the profession have been able to provide immediate skillful attention to complications occurring in condylar compression in the newly-born. Without question, this skillful art may be considered as the greatest *improvement* in obstetrical practice.

It is a great improvement in the care of the expectant mother and in the skillful delivery of the infant. It is another great improvement that indicates a large decrease in the multitude of unfortunate babies whose parents have been confronted with the verdict: "Nothing can be done for your baby but to place it in an institution."

In conclusion, and in verification of this greatest improvement in obstetrical practice, it is a pleasure to quote an interesting testimonial from Dr. Robert B. Bachman, our own obstetrical surgeon, from whom many in the field of practice have received instruction. I have his permission to quote the following letter:

Dear Dr. Sutherland:

I am most happy to give in writing the gist of the comments I made to Dr. Anna Slocum of Des Moines, Iowa, about my experiences with cranial osteopathy and newborn infants.[11]

Over a period of thirty-five years as an obstetrician and director of obstetrical clinics and head of the department of obstetrics and gynecology in osteopathic institutions, I have been confronted with newborn babes with varying degrees of central nervous system disturbances. Some of these disturbances were transitory

---

11. Anna Slocum, D.O. (1903-1988: Des Moines Still College of Osteopathy, 1938), a member of Dr. Sutherland's associate faculty, provided osteopathic service to the newborns in the Des Moines hospital.

and others had a tremor when moved. Some appeared in a semi-torpor, some had convulsions or convulsive movements, others had a projectile type of vomiting. These cases were carefully observed and a few select ones with major evidence of disturbance, especially the projectile type of vomiting, gave evidence of intracranial pressure. On these select cases, a spinal tap was made and a few cubic centimeters of spinal fluid drained off; sometimes clear and at other times bloody. In every instance it was noted that there was immediate relief of projectile vomiting with rarely a recurrence and lactation could be carried out with very little interruption. When cranial osteopathy was first called to my attention, I reasoned that it should be of unusual value in these particular cases.

As soon as technicians were available, their services were employed and treatment was given to all babies that showed the slightest symptoms that can be ascribed to cranial distresses, either as a molding problem or pressure reactions during the course of labor, whether delivery was a normal one or completed by forceps, versions or breech extractions.

Since I have used the services of trained technicians in cranial osteopathy, I have not made a lumbar puncture for relieving cranial pressure. It was noted that projectile vomiting could be definitely controlled after one or two treatments. Irritation tremor of the extremities or evidence of discomfort on handling the child as noted by crying or facial expression was markedly reduced or relieved after a series of two or three, occasionally more, cranial osteopathic treatments. Babies with convulsions or convulsive movements showed varying results. In my opinion, all babies were benefited with cranial osteopathy. I consider this form of treatment most valuable for postnatal care of infants and it had been a standing order for baby care in the nurseries that were under my supervision until I went into semi-retirement one year ago.

I highly prize the time I have spent with you, limited as it was, and feel that due credit is not given to the possibilities of cranial osteopathy in the care of newborn babes. If occasion presents itself that my comments may be of interest to others you have my consent to quote these statements because the results that I have observed are nothing short of spectacular.

Yours sincerely,

Robert B. Bachman, D.O.

July 10, 1952

Yes, indeed! The science of osteopathy does offer a magnificent multitude of possibilities in behalf of the ills of mankind. I thank you.

32. Talks at the Clinical Conference: Kirksville, Missouri

January 5-9, 1953.

1. The Fascial Drag and the Fulcrum

My search for a perfect human specimen, either animate or inanimate, ended finally in a fruitless endeavor, with the conclusion that there were only two: Adam and Eve. Perhaps they, too, lacked perfection...having erred, according to historical record. Therefore, my talk this morning is subject to the verdict encountered by Speransky: "in conclusion there is none."[1]

Much information has been presented in past and present publications relative to fascial tissues. I have found it to be a rather interesting experience to observe the various differentiations made by authors.

The description of the deep fascias as given by Gerrish in 1902 is adaptable to my reasoning:

> The typical deep fasciae are *close sheets of fibrous tissue*, in which the white variety exists in an almost unadulterated form. On account of this histological composition these fasciae are pearly white, *flexible*, *strong* and *inelastic*. Their structure and physical qualities immediately bring to mind the characteristics of *ligaments* and *tendons*, which have identical structure; and the suggestion is especially apt for the reason that some fasciae are really *inter-osseous ligaments*, and a number are properly to be regarded as tendons. Moreover, the employment of the word "fascia" is often arbitrary, as, for example, in the case of the transversus abdominis muscle whose tendon or origin is almost

---

1. A.D. Speransky began the final chapter of *A Basis for the Theory of Medicine* with these words. He was a Russian scientist who conducted a wide variety of experiments, including those on the nature of the cerebrospinal fluid.

> always described as a layer of lumbar fasciae and whose tendon of insertion is conventionally dubbed an aponeurosis, although in both instances the tendons are sheet-like expansions which serve for the ensheathing of muscles. In this connection it is interesting and useful for the student to observe anew the continuity of the fibrous membranes...ligaments, tendons and fascial blending with the periosteum, tendons, and fascia serving as ligaments, tendons losing themselves as fascias, tendons of some muscles acting as fascias for other muscles and so on.[2]

This description by Gerrish and another by Cunningham fit into my subject of "The Fascial Drag and The Fulcrum." It is well to interpret my use of the word "drag:" "To drag is to draw with difficulty against active or passive resistance."

One of the frequent fascial drags occurs at the upper dorsal region, an area that became designated as the "old-age center" during the early presentation of the science of osteopathy. It is an area with problems that confront one in daily practice today. One with which we all are familiar. Therefore, my subject will have its commencement relative to the "old-age center."

The Cunningham description of *deep prevertebral cervical fascia* especially adapts in the presentation: "The prevertebral fascia extends from the *basilar part of the occipital bone* into the thorax where it *blends with the anterior longitudinal ligaments*."[3]

Note that no mention is made of a blending with the anterior longitudinal ligament in the cervical area, where it is supposed to form the posterior limit to the fibrous compartment containing the larynx, trachea, thyroid gland, pharynx and esophagus, as well as a section for the scaleni muscles, having insertion with the first and second ribs, and conducting important vascular channels and nerves. This posterior limit to the prevertebral fascia somewhat resembles an

---

2. Gerrish, *Textbook of Anatomy* ; emphasis added.

3. Cunningham, *Textbook of Anatomy* ; emphasis added.

origin and insertion of a muscle–visualized with specific origin of the basilar part of the occipital bone and insertion into the anterior longitudinal ligament near the upper dorsal "old-age center."

So, in visualizing the extension of the posterior limit of the prevertebral fascia and its blending with the anterior longitudinal ligament after entrance into the thorax, we may picture a lesion at the "old-age center" initiating a drawing or dragging by the fascia and encountering difficulty in active resistance at the fascial attachment to the basilar part of the occipital bone. Then, in secondary compensation, or complication, affecting the intracranial reciprocal tension membrane, with consequent shifting of the fulcrum at the junction of the falx cerebri with the tent[orium cerebelli]. Thus we provide the picture adaptable to our subject: "The Fascial Drag and the Fulcrum."

Inasmuch as the anterior longitudinal ligament extends downward to the sacrum, we may also picture similar drawing or dragging, by way of the fascial-ligamentous blending, that encounters difficulty through active resistance at the basilar part, through the initiation by a sacral lesion. Such dragging would likewise effect compensation or complication to the reciprocal tension membrane and a shifting of the fulcrum.

In this picture, we may also visualize compensation or complication shifting the pineal shifting mechanism that functions between the cerebellar and the cerebral motility as a possible automatic slack-tension regulator. The intracranial picture is important in all cases and the location of the little pineal body is as important in visualization as is the pituitary body. This little cone-form body is situated near the posterior area of the third ventricle, within the dorsal aspect of the neural tube, or what may be pictured as the gate entrance, or exit, to the cerebral aqueduct. Were one able to crawl within an animate cranium, with an index finger passed over the cerebellum, very likely he would find the pineal protruding into the superior cerebellar cisterna and that a slight pressure upon the protuberance might initiate motility of the brain structure as a whole.

I visualize the *little* pineal mechanism as becoming of *great importance* in our study of Dr. Still's science of osteopathy, with possibilities encouraging in the treatment of epileptic seizures. Its indicative mechanical slack-tension functioning is especially important to the normal fluctuation of the cerebrospinal fluid through the cerebral aqueduct, as well as to the normal venous flow through the straight sinus, or fulcrum area of the reciprocal tension membrane, or the junction of the falx with the tent.

Osteopaths, as we old-timers enjoyed being called in the days of "early osteopathy," are familiar with recurring occipitoatlantal and upper dorsal lesions. As skillful non-incisive surgeons and cranial technicians, who emphasize the thought that our concept is not a separate unit in the functioning of the body mechanism, we have observed recurring occipitoatlantal lesions being controlled through attention to the cranial area. There are similar possibilities in connection with recurring upper dorsal lesions, through lifting of the posterior-inferior angles of the parietal bones.

We are not forgetting the lateral, medial and intra-limitation boundaries to the deep prevertebral fascia which possess a greater extension and blending to facilitate freedom of muscular movement, vascular circulation and nerve impulse in the neck region below the chin. In this area we are apt to encounter a twisting-entanglement of fascial boundaries obstructing vascular and nervous channels and especially restriction in muscular activity.

This brings to memory a statement made by Dr. Still indicating that the Parkinson syndrome is "a condition that the muscles labor to overcome, a condition that will produce shaking palsy."[4] We might reason along that line of thought regarding a case of occupational upper dorsal lesions that came under my observation. A member of our profession, carrying a heavy practice, decided that a year's vacation would be a pleasant event. Not wishing to be entirely idle, he secured

---

4. See Still, *Research and Practice*, pp. 190-194 (nn. 439-454) for a description of shaking palsy.

a position as a traveling salesman for the Appleton Book Company. This is recorded as early history when automobiles were nonexistent and salesmen traveled by railroad accommodation. The doctor's occupational habit involved the carrying of two heavy grips containing medical books and considerable climbing of stairs. In consequence, he developed a typical postural habit and gait similar to that observed in the Parkinson syndrome. He also developed the syndrome. The upper dorsal postural lesion presents the picture of the twisting complication of fascial boundaries below the chin, with consequent restriction to muscular activity and disturbance to normal circulation as a predisposing factor leading later to the Parkinson syndrome.

The deep fasciae of the midriff, or diaphragmatic region, are especially important in our study of fascial *dragging* or *drawing, with difficulty against active resistance*. In this area we find the ensheathing accommodation for the psoas major muscle apparently descending from the muscle's origin above and below the lumbocostal arches to the insertion of the tendon at the lesser trochanter of the femur. The fascial accommodation associates with a blending with the medial lumbocostal arch and also with the transversalis, iliac, true pelvic, obturator and the rectovesical fasciae. Then, later, continuing on down the lower extremity in blending association through the popliteal space, the fascia finally attaches to the end of the digits of the foot.

Before venturing further in our midriff reasoning, it may prove advantageous to "think osteopathy" relative to Dr. Still's parable of The Goat and the Boulder.[5] The "boulder" at the midriff is a predisposing factor leading to cardiac valvular pathology as well as to pathological disturbances resulting from restriction of lymphatic drainage through the thoracic duct. This area might be considered the specific region of active resistance encountered by the fascial drag from below.

---

5. For a description of "The Goat and the Boulder" see article 30, "The Lighthouse Beam," note 7; also see Dr. Sutherland's rendition of Dr. Still's parable in Sutherland, *Teachings*, p. 214.

Our study that developed into the psoas major technique began during a three-month winter vacation in Florida in 1946. The study might be called: "Observation of habitual posture by shell hunters along a seven-mile sandy shore." Instead of stooping to pick up a specimen, these local hunters would bend the entire body with especial care in not bending or flexing the leg upon the thigh. Vacationers on the beach began to follow the example, finding that picking posture easier and less tiresome than the stooping method. Several of the vacationers wore abdominal supports because of pendiculous proportions and weight. They found the new posture beneficial, losing weight and discarding the suspension supports. This interprets the necessity of not bending the knee during the administration of the "fiddle-string" technique in behalf of psoas major muscular strains that always include drags upon the fasciae–drags with difficulty against a resistance at the midriff region.

2. Fascial Strain and the Sacrum

The subject this morning may be said to have problems in close association with two different types of sacroiliac lesions:

1. Craniosacral, or respiratory, of the sacrum *between* the ilia;
2. Postural, or iliosacral, of the ilia *upon* the sacrum.

It therefore becomes important in our discussion of "Fascial Strain and the Sacrum" to view *two* separate areas relative to the sacral articular surface designed to facilitate the two separate types of movement. Otherwise, the mechanism would not be clearly seen and our interpretation would be subject to considerable criticism.

The articular surface which provides the functioning of the craniosacral or respiratory type may be confined to a rather *small* area, another one of the significant small features with magnitudinous import in "thinking osteopathy" with Dr. Still.

This small articular area functions as a fulcrum, affording the flexion and extension movement of the sacrum in unity with the flexion and extension mobility at the sphenobasilar symphysis of the cranium. This area is located at the second sacral segment and is found, on the normal specimen, converging anteriorly and diverging posteriorly. [*See Fig. 388, coronal section of middle sacral segment in Gray's Anatomy of the Human Body, 26th ed., 1954, p. 351.*] It is well to note the difference between this area and the posterior sacral segment where the divergence is anterior and the convergence posterior. The small fulcrum-like area provides rotative functioning to accommodate sidebending-rotation and torsion mobility of the cranium, in addition to flexion and extension, like the combined fulcra-pivotal mechanism of the jugular process in the cranium. The so-called long-and-short arm articular surfaces accommodate the movement of the sacral base posteriorly and the sacral apex forwardly during the respiratory flexion period, and vice versa during the extension mobility. The long-and-short arm accommodation surfaces may be pictured as functioning in the postural types as well.

The priority problem, relative to which came first, the egg or the bird, enters into the title of our subject, "Fascial Strain and the Sacrum." Therefore, I am turning the title around to read, "The Sacrum and Fascial Strain," in order to provide the picture of a *sag of the sacrum forwardly at the fulcra-pivotal area.*

This is the type that Dr. Anna Slocum of Des Moines prefers to designate as "anterior-sacrum" from the scientific viewpoint.[6] However, I prefer the *sag* description because the sacrum is suspended between the two ilia and relatively corresponds to another unit of the cranial-respiratory mechanism...the sphenoid bone which is suspended between and beneath two frontal bones. *Sag* also has my preference because there are no muscular agencies from the sacrum to the ilia to initiate articular mobility and none to be found from bone to bone in the cranial unit. Then again, sag rhymes with drag; and sags and fascial drags lead to chronic rags.

---

6. Anna Slocum, D.O. (1903-1988: Des Moines Still College of Osteopathy, 1938) was a member of Dr. Sutherland's associate faculty.

As an interlinear thought, my memory goes back a number of years to the period when one of my manuscripts advocating cranial articular mobility had consideration by the first American Osteopathic Association bureau of professional development. The late John E. Rogers was chairman of the board which had five additional silent members. One of the members responded by note with the comment that: "Muscular agencies were lacking in the cranial mechanism and without which cranial articular mobility would also be found lacking." Not knowing by whom the kindly comment was made, I was unable to retaliate in effective argument by calling attention to the lack of muscular agencies functioning between the sacrum and the ilia. However, that day has gone by and advocates of "osteopathy in the cranial field" are demonstrating mobility in the cranial mechanism. Otherwise this clinical conference would not now be in session at the "Cradle of Osteopathy."[7]

The *sacral fulcra-sag* type of strain is especially effective in relation to disturbances in the mentality. The many mental institutions of the world likely provide evidence of multitudinous sacral fulcra-sag types of strain.

It is not difficult to picture various *fascial strains* occurring throughout the pelvic realm that result immediately and secondarily in the excessive tension common to the sag of the sacral fulcra. In connection with these, nerve and vascular disturbances to the head follow and in themselves are of serious import.

Aside from this, participants in the cranial thought consider the traction, or drag, by way of the intraspinal membrane, in its function as a unit in the cranial respiratory mechanism with the cranial reciprocal tension membrane, to be a *specific* disturbing factor leading to mental complications. Etiological factors are many that lead to the production of this type of sacral sag and the resulting strain. Among them are factors incidental to the delivery of a child.

---

7. The "Cradle of Osteopathy" was a name often given to Kirksville, Missouri as the home of the American School of Osteopathy, the first school of osteopathy.

Well do I remember one early-day obstetrical mission, during a period when muddy-gumbo roads, buggies and runaway horses were involved in transportation. My mission, due to gumbo roads, necessitated a half day of travel to cover a comparatively short distance. While en route the spokes of the buggy wheels filled up with gumbo and an axle broke. So I straddled one horse and led the other. About a mile distant from the patient's farm home, I met the lady walking along the muddy road and noticed immediately the disturbed, or irrational, state of mind that occasionally follows birth delivery. In other words, I was behind time in my mission. However, I succeeded in placing the lady straddle-fashion upon the horse that I had been leading. Evidently the straddle-fashion position fixated the ischii to the horse's back, allowing the ilia to rotate laterally away from the sacrum, while the walking movement by the horse, and possible sacral fluctuation of the cerebrospinal fluid, reduced an indicated sacral fulcra-sag type of lesion to normal position. This was indicated by the change in the patient's state of mind from the irrational to normal during that eventful ride.

The early-day obstetrical mission led to the development of the *anterior sacral alae contact technique*. The technique is applied while the patient sits erect on the table or a chair, so that the ischia can function as fulcra to allow a lateral gliding away by the ilia from the sacral alae. The physician, sitting in front of the patient, passes thumbs along the crest of the ilia backwardly, near to the posterior iliac spines, and then drops the thumbs downwardly to contact the front of the sacral alae. The thumbs hold these contacts firmly while the patient bends forward, with hands resting upon the physician's arms. During this procedure, the ilia glide laterally away from the sacral alae. The patient is then instructed to resume the sitting posture, being careful not to extend the lumbar area. The ligaments thus draw the sacrum back into normal position and relieve the drag upon the intraspinal membrane. Secondary fascial strains usually receive relief at the same time. Yet they should be given attention or observation.

Dr. Anna Slocum, who has skillfully demonstrated the technique at various conventions and instruction courses, mentioned a *slight* push upon the sacrum also, which I have regarded as unnecessary. However, at Atlantic City or Chicago, in 1952, while giving her description of application, she mentioned the anterior contact as being on the ilia; and in this contact, the slight push would be on the ilia, rather than on the sacral alae. This might be considered an improvement in the application through its tendency to rotate the ilia in a gliding mobility laterally away from the sacral alae.

It was my honor to represent the Minnesota State Osteopathic Association in the first House of Delegates in the history of the American Osteopathic Association. That same year, 1920, Dr. H.Virgil Halladay's text, *Applied Anatomy of the Spine*, appeared in print. "Virge" placed on exhibition an animated lumbar-pelvic specimen in a room adjoining the assembly room where the delegates were in session.[8] This provided an opportunity, during recesses and lunch periods, to experiment with the specimen. Through that experimentation a very simple method, applicable in both diagnosis and administration of treatment, was developed.

In the diagnostic method, we placed the specimen in a sitting position so that the ischial tuberosities would be held in apparent fixation in order to function as fulcra for the accommodation of anterior and posterior rotation by the ilia. By rotating one ilium anteriorly and the other posteriorly, we found that the anterior ilium corresponded to what might be termed a "long leg" while the ilium in posterior rotation corresponded to the "short leg." This might indicate an iliosacral lesion of anterior rotation on one side and posterior on the other and could easily be observed by palpation with palms contacting the iliac crests.

In the development of technique, both extremities were lifted nearly

---

8. Virgil Halladay, D.O. (American School of Osteopathy, 1916) was a professor of anatomy at the American School of Osteopathy in Kirksville, Missouri. He developed a chemical process by which the natural flexibility of the ligaments in cadaveric specimens could be preserved. He prepared such specimens of the spine, rib cage and pelvis that were often called the "animated skeleton."

to the level of the table. The long leg or anterior iliac rotation was drawn forward while the short leg, corresponding to the posterior iliac rotation, was pushed backward. These positions were held while the lumbar spine and sacrum were rotated toward the same direction of the anterior iliac rotation. In the meantime, the ischial tuberosities functioned as fulcra to facilitate the anterior and posterior rotations.

I had the opportunity to apply this simple method when called in on consultation. The case concerned a rather definite fixation of several years with no success in reduction of an anterior iliac rotation on the left side. The sciatic pain had indicated a degenerated disc problem affecting the left side and surgery had been advised. Instead, non-incisive surgical skill was administered in the following manner: While the patient sat erect, we requested the physician in charge to raise both of the patient's legs nearly to the level of the table, draw forwardly on the left extremity and push backwardly on the right. Then we asked the patient to cooperate by rotating her body in the same direction as that occurring in left anterior rotation. This cooperation was obtained by simply reaching the left arm across the abdomen to rest upon the right hand, which was providing body support by resting on the table. At the commencement of the patient's cooperation, the surprising remark was made: "Why, I can feel my sacrum moving." Then, at the balance degree in ligamentous regulation, the patient merely rotated her body back to normal position.

A spectacular reduction? Decidedly not! Simply an application of skillful non-incisive surgery which requires knowledge of an intricate articular mechanism having two different types of movement: the craniosacral, or respiratory; and the iliosacral, or postural.

One may utilize the sitting ischial tuberosity fulcrum method in the sacral fulcra-sag strains. The patient sits on the table and both legs are raised to the level of the table to change the necessary rotation of the heads of the femurs within the acetabula, the means of pulling directly on the ilia. As the physician places finger contacts on the sacrum, to merely observe the progress of movement, the assistant draws both legs forwardly. This rotates the ilia anteriorly and laterally in gliding motion away from the sacral alae. The patient is then requested to bend the body forwardly. At the balance degree, the patient resumes the sitting posture, being careful not to extend the lumbar area.

3. Liquid Light

January 9, 1953.

This closing talk at the conference in Kirksville, Missouri was given spontaneously by Dr. Sutherland and recorded on tape by Dr. Kistler, who kindly transcribed it.

Is there any space to get into after that talk by Dr. Kimberly?[9] And the one by Dr. Della Caldwell, who really gave the closing lecture of this session? A chapter of experience, valuable experience, not found in the book. Let me say, Good Lord deliver us! He has done so with this item of news from the Monterey Peninsula which Dr. Margaret Barnes has just handed me. It is news from Pacific Grove, Point Pinos, the point on which I live in a house known as The Fulcrum:

> *Meteor Lights Up the Peninsula at Midnight*
>
> A brilliant silver-like meteor plunged into the sea off the California coastline early this morning after illuminating the Carmel Bay and Pebble Beach coastline. For from seven to fifteen seconds, thousands of persons saw the fiery spectacle in San Francisco and its shock waves rocked many homes there, the Associated Press reported.
>
> It was observed by residents within a hundred and fifty mile

---

9. Paul E. Kimberly, D.O. (Des Moines Still College of Osteopathy, 1940) was a professor of anatomy at the Des Moines Still College of Osteopathy. Beginning in 1944, he arranged for Dr. Sutherland to use the college facilities to conduct classes in "Osteopathy in the Cranial Field." At these courses Dr. Kimberly would extensively review the anatomy of the human head.

> area, from Carmel to Napa. A *Herald* reporter watched it from Carmel Beach. He said the entire sky lit up and reflected on the ocean at about 12:20 a.m. today. It was witnessed by plane pilots, airport tower operators and hundreds of San Francisco peninsula residents who flooded police and sheriff stations in that area with calls. Homes were shaken by the air waves. Dr. E.J. Lindsey, meteor research expert for the California Academy of Science and Meteors said, "Meteors sometimes push air ahead of them and set up shock waves." He also said, "they sometimes appear lower than they actually are.... "

A flash of light!–where did it come from?–*liquid light*!

We have historical record. The waters were divided when the earth appeared. From the earth *Man* was created.[10] The waters were divided! The fascia! Even the fascia is water, even the bony tissue is liquid... water...fluid...if you want to go back to historical record. Fluid! A fundamental principle in our cranial concept. Fluctuation of the cerebrospinal fluid. A motion like that of the tide of the ocean. Something that is governed by the same Intelligence that governs the tide of the ocean governs the rotation of the earth, the sun, the moon and all the planets.

Is there any space to get into after Dr. Kimberly's lecture? Yes! The fundamental principle in the cranial concept: the Breath of Life, not the breath of air. Another historical record: the Breath of Life, not the breath of air, was breathed into the nasals of this form of clay and man became a living soul to walk about on earth and utilize one of its elements...the breath of air.[11] This air is spoken of in relation to this meteor, the "push" on the air, material air. But the brilliancy of that

---

10. "And God said, Let the waters under the heaven be gathered together unto one place, and let the dry land appear: and it was so." Gen. 1:9, King James Version. "And the Lord God formed man of the dust of the ground..." Gen. 2:7, King James Version.

11. "...and breathed into his nostrils the breath of life; and man became a living soul." Gen. 2:7, King James Version.

light lit up the heavens, in the same way that sheet lightening lights up the clouds. I have often referred to that light, something which does not touch the cloud but lights up the cloud.

That is the picture I want you to see as the "highest known element" in the cerebrospinal fluid.[12] *An invisible element.* Something that may be illustrated in the potency that lights up the film in taking an X-ray picture. Something you do not see, but it lights up the X-ray film. It is not visible. You merely see the spark from the positive and negative poles–it jumps from one pole to the other. But you do not see the real element because you are the man formed from the earth and walking about utilizing this breath of air. If you recognized the real element, the breath of light in the fluctuation of the cerebrospinal fluid, I think you would begin to come closer to the success of Dr. Still in his knowledge of the human body. He had not only the material knowledge through his dissections etcetera of those early days but also his experience as an Army surgeon, the practical clinical experience. Beside that, he recognized a highest known element in the cerebrospinal fluid. You might say he was like the X-ray; he could look right through you and see things, and tell you things, without even putting his hands upon the body. I have seen him do that! Time and time again. When some of the early teachers had a clinic up before the class, hunting for the lesion, in would come the Old Doctor from the rear, "Here's your lesion."[13] How did he do it?

Someone has asked me to explain what I mean by the term transmutation. *Transmutation....* It is a change into another nature, substance, form or condition. It is not the same as...it is different from that transformer up there that you find in the electrical wire, the high tension wire, that brings the voltage down to 110, etcetera.... A transmutation changes something into another nature or condition. It is a term that is

---

12. Still, *Philosophy*, p. 39.

13. In his later years, Dr. A. T. Still was respectfully referred to as the Old Doctor.

used by others. Dr. Lustig, for instance, used it in the same way I do.[14]

Let us take that cable that goes across the ocean. In that cable you will find a number of copper tubes. In the center of each you will find a single wire passing through, carrying the potential, you might say, the electrical potential in that cable. In each copper tube. It is called a coaxial cable.[15]

You have read the statement by Dr. Still: "Finer nerves dwell with the lymphatics than even with the eye. The eye is an organized effect, the lymphatics the cause: In them the spirit of life more abundantly dwells."[16] Can you find those finer nerves? Can you find the 40,000 nerve fibers that are said to go between the hypothalamus and the pituitary body through the infundibulum? Think of the principle of the coaxial cable–how the copper tube may carry all those different messages at the same time. Anywhere you want, you can tune on that copper tube, not on the potential. Transmutation, an illustration of what is meant by transmutation. The potential in the center; the function, a different condition, in the copper tube.

Now we have hollow tube mechanisms in the nerves, and we have a hollow tube mechanism in the infundibulum. There is another in the pineal body. Can you see the potential, the highest known element in the human body, something that you cannot see materially? Neither can you see the element in the cerebrospinal fluid, the Breath of Life. But there is the function between the hypothalamus and the

---

14. Dr. R. T. Lustig, an authority on nuclear physics wrote: "With the opening of the Atomic Age we are getting a better perspective of energy, its sources and conversions....Sutherland's work....puts us on record as having recognized at an early date the interchangability of energy and matter as it relates to biology." Magoun, *Osteopathy in Cranial Field,* 1st ed., p. 15.

15. A coaxial cable is composed of an insulated central conductor with tubular stranded copper conductors laid over it concentrically and separated by layers of insulation. This arrangement allows the cable to simultaneously transmit thousands of telephone, radio or television signals while preventing a loss of signal strength from outside electrical interference.

16. Still, *Philosophy*, p. 104.

pituitary and the function of the nerves.

I have often said that we lost something in osteopathy that Dr. Still tried to get across. That was the spiritual that he included in the science of osteopathy. I don't mean the spirit world, no! I mean the *spiritual*, direct from his Maker, that came to him during one of the saddest periods of his life when a devout prayer went out to his Maker, not to the spirit world.[17] What came was the concept of osteopathy. What does he say? "It came as did other truths that came to benefit mankind." Read his *Research and Practice* and see how many times you can see the reference to his Creator, the Great Architect, etcetera. He is continually calling your attention to that.

If we want to *think osteopathy*, we have something that is a test tube that we can utilize in testing some of these so-called scientific tests and methods, which in themselves haven't been proven. We can use the science of osteopathy as a test tube, and we are doing it in our daily practice.

Do you ever think of what that great electrical wizard had to say? I have referred to it before. I repeat it again, as this may be the last time I appear before you. Dr. Steinmetz,[18] the eminent scientist, when asked what lies ahead in research, said:

> I think the greatest discoveries will be made along spiritual lines. Some day people will have learned that material things do not bring happiness and are of little use in making men and women creative and powerful. Then the scientists of the world will turn their laboratories over to the study of God and prayer and spiritual forces which as yet have been hardly

---

17. In the spring of 1864, spinal meningitis killed three of Dr. Still's children despite the best efforts of both preacher and physician. It was a time of great spiritual crisis for Dr. Still, the resolution of which resulted in the birth of the science of osteopathy ten years later. See Still, *Autobiography*, pp. 87-88, 303-304.

18. Charles Proteus Steinmetz, Ph.D. (1865-1923) was an engineer and mathematician who was regarded as a genius. Among his many endeavors, he developed a method for solving problems in alternating current circuits and experimented with artificially created lightning.

> touched or scratched. When that day comes the world will see more advancement in one generation than has been seen in the last four.

If we are going to think osteopathy with Dr. Still, we must utilize his science as a test tube for other scientific, so-called, ideas, many of then imperfect and undependable. How can anything be tested if the test tube itself is not perfect and hasn't been proven. Hasn't been proven! First, let's prove it. Just turn the thing right around and prove the test tube with the science of osteopathy.

The first school of osteopathy was chartered for the improvement of the present system of surgery. Do you realize the full meaning of that? You are not a manipulator of the human body, you are a non-incisive surgeon. This is not a criticism of major or minor surgery. No. I want to point out something here. You have something that is superior. When some big surgeon begins to boast, remember that you yourself have a superiority. You have an improvement in our systems of surgery because yours is non-incisive through the *thinking-feeling-knowing fingers*, through your absolute knowledge. No, I won't say absolute knowledge, but through the knowledge you have thus far obtained of this human mechanism.

You have been learning more about this improvement in our systems of surgery through the knowledge you have obtained in this summary of the fascia. The surgery that was performed by the late Dr. George M. Laughlin in congenital dislocations of the hip was called non-incisive surgery. The possibilities in Dr. Still's science of osteopathy are greater than the magnitude of the heavens. That statement can be proven, is being proven, by nearly every one present in this room and those who have been present here before.

What do you have when offering even encouragement to some of these unfortunate babes whose parents have been told, "Nothing can be done but to place your baby in an institution." What is it? Is it manipulation? No. Is it a special therapy by itself? No. It is the science of osteopathy. You don't need to add the words, cranial field. It's the science of osteopathy that understands the mechanism of that little unfortunate babe that later becomes the "bent twig" unless it has attention.[19]

Did you ever stop to think that your meeting together in study groups is to learn more about the mechanism, and one of the things about it is the study of the fluctuation of the cerebrospinal fluid? Knowing how to handle that cerebrospinal fluid and its fluctuation helps you to see the same principles in inventions that man has made patterned after this human mechanism, such as steering mechanisms and fluid drives.[20] When you are using these principles and powers, you not only offer encouragement, for in many cases you can say they are cured. Yes. And you are doing it yourself. When my brother and I went back to dig the potatoes, sometimes three times, we found, down on the bottom, some little seedlings. Little things that grow. That's what Dr. Still meant when he referred to the little things that are the big things in the science of osteopathy.

Scientists of today are looking out into space and we hear about atomic theory and nuclear scientists. Space. Ever try looking between the lines of a little thing with a high-powered microscope? Did you see the space between the lines as you find them there? Space. Do you think you can find any space between the lines in this fascial tissue? The fascia itself, with its white inelastic shape? Yes, you will find space between *if you have the vision to look in between.* A microscope powerful enough to see the space between.

Out on the ocean shore, you will see a big rock. Did you ever stop to think of the space between the layers of the rock itself? The solid rock? When the tide comes in and the waves roll over that rock, you will find it crumbling into sand as you find it along the shore, out along the Seventeen Mile Drive on the Monterey Peninsula. Sand! Rock! Those grains of sand have a lot of space between them. Out

---

19. The term "bent twigs" refers to the saying, "As the twig is bent so the tree inclines."

20. "Fluid drive" was a term used to describe the new type of automatic transmission then available in automobiles.

there, there is a processing plant that takes up that sand to send to glassmakers. This glass window that you are looking through came from that sand. Ever stop to think of what you are? Whether or not that earth from which you were formed was in the glass form of earth? Stop to think of that? The light from the sun passes through that glass. Does it touch that glass? It lights up this room and it is reflected.

Just for a moment, think of your body being formed from that glass. That you are a glass house through which this Breath of Life may be reflected. Not even touching your house, your glass house, but being reflected through and through. See that sun reflecting itself upon the moon and then see the reflection from the moon all through the ocean. Reflection that does not touch the moon, that does not touch the ocean, but lights them up. Makes a beautiful picture. Light! Liquid Light!

33. Special Recordings

The following five talks were recorded as a special project for the Sutherland Cranial Teaching Foundation at Pacific Grove, California. The recordings were subsequently produced as phonograph records.

1. The Primary Respiratory Mechanism

March 9, 1953.

The preparatory manuscript relative to *The Cranial Bowl* text, published in 1939, contained considerable detailed description in its presentation of the cranial concept, necessitating a rather large and bulky volume. We found it advisable to reduce the descriptive material several times in our eventful venture to secure the desirable attention of the osteopathic profession. Otherwise, the text might soon have been found in a hidden nook on a bookshelf resting silently and gathering the accumulative dust of time. This is the reason why the text dwindled to a mere presentation of the idea in a "nutshell."

We likewise found brevity advisable in the use of descriptive nomenclature pertaining to what was then, and continues to be known as, *the primary respiratory mechanism*. Apparently this brevity, as presented in two lectures given before the Eastern States Osteopathic Association in April 1943, was not sufficiently satisfactory and brought forth a request for an analysis. These lectures became copyright property of the *Journal of the American Osteopathic Association* and received special editorial attention by the late Dr. Ray G. Hulburt [1884-1947: American School of Osteopathy, 1920] in conjunction with Dr. R.C. McCaughan [American School of Osteopathy, 1914] with publication in April 1944.

The brief summarization read as follows:

> We take into consideration a *mechanism* which includes *motility* of the brain, intracranial membranes, fluctuation of cerebrospinal fluid and articular mobility of the cranial bones; and

also motility of the spinal cord, intraspinal membranes, again the fluctuation of cerebrospinal fluid and the articular mobility of the sacrum *between* the ilia.

In our analysis of the summarization, we said that the terminology "primary respiratory" was chosen because of specific accordance to an early anatomical text statement which read as follows: "*All the physiological centers*, including that of *respiration*, are located within the floor of the fourth ventricle."[1] This statement specifically calls attention to *primary respiration* as commencing in the central nervous system, and, in our interpretation, indicates both *primary* and *secondary* respiration in the human mechanism.

In addition, the nomenclature has been given interpretative description in the recent text, *Osteopathy in the Cranial Field* [1st ed., p. 16], by Dr. Harold I. Magoun, Sr.:

> Primary: first or principal.
>
> Respiratory: Relating to respiration. Physiological respiration is metabolism, the giving off of waste material and the formation of new by the cellular protoplasm. Metabolism is further defined as a tissue change, the sum of the chemical changes whereby the function of nutrition is effected. It consists of anabolism and catabolism.
>
> Mechanism: An arrangement or grouping of the parts of anything which has a definite action.

The mechanism consists of several units in its physiologic-operative function. First of all, coordinating with up-to-date terminology, it has a "fluid drive" through the activity of the cerebrospinal fluid.[2] It has a *tension mechanism*, necessary in alternative to-and-fro articular

---

1. "In the floor of the fourth ventricle....are situated certain important centers, i.e. cardiac, vasomotor, respiratory, vomiting, and deglutition centers." Wright, *Applied Physiology*, p. 108.

2. "Fluid drive" was a term used to describe the new type of automatic transmission then available in automobiles.

movement required in alternative respiratory changes from inhalation to exhalation. It has *articular mobility* throughout the skull and of the sacrum between the ilia. And there is a *primary respiratory physiological center* within the floor of the fourth ventricle.

The cerebrospinal fluid, with its "highest known element," is considered as the *fundamental unit* in the functioning of the mechanism.[3] I have frequently referred, during class instruction, to Dr. Still's highest known element as a *primary* Breath of Life that was breathed into a form of clay, according to scriptural record, and emphasized the thought that it was *not* the breath of material air utilized in man's walkabout on earth.[4] In another symbolic illustration, this was likened to a liquid-within-a-liquid. The element has also been symbolized in its function as like that sheet-lightening which *lights up* the cloud in brilliant array, though invisible as is the X-ray.

The fundamental unit of the cerebrospinal fluid with this element has been compared, in principle, to a coaxial cable with the copper tube on the outside and the insulated central conductor, or wire, and the electrical potential which builds up in the space between them. This cable is said to be capable of carrying thousands of messages at the same time, but only due to the electrical potential generated in the space, or field, between the two metallic elements. I have also used the coaxial cable illustration as an interpretation of Dr. Still's reference to "Finer nerves dwell with the lymphatics than even with the eye,"[5] as well as in connection with a statement in an authoritative pathological text that refers to "forty thousand nerve fibers passing from

---

3. Still, *Philosophy*, p. 39.

4. "And the Lord God formed man of the dust of the ground, and breathed into his nostrils the breath of life; and man became a living soul." Gen. 2:7, King James Version.

5. A coaxial cable is composed of an insulated central conductor with tubular stranded copper conductors laid over it concentrically and separated by layers of insulation. This arrangement allows the cable to simultaneously transmit thousands of telephone, radio or television signals while preventing a loss of signal strength from outside electrical interference.

"Finer nerves dwell....," Still, *Philosophy*, p. 104.

the hypothalamus to the pituitary."

From the viewpoint of the cranial concept *the artery remains supreme*, but the cerebrospinal fluid is considered to be *in command.*[6] The fluid does not circulate like the blood stream but *fluctuates* in its activity. Fluctuation is described by Webster as: "The movement of a fluid contained in a natural or artificial cavity and observed by palpation or percussion."

It is common practice to feel the pulse in observing the rhythm of the blood stream. The rhythmical fluctuation of the cerebrospinal fluid is now readily and intelligently observed through palpation by skillful non-incisive surgeons who include the cranial field in their practice of the science of osteopathy. Palpable observance of the fluid rhythm is useful and dependable in diagnosis of cranial membranous articular strains, and its *rhythmic potency* might be described as the *only* motive force necessary in the reduction thereof. Its *potency* has been likened to that of the ocean-sea-around-us as it is a constant body of fluid rhythmically moving into the ventricles of the brain and ebbing therefrom during periodic respiratory alternative changes. A quotation relative to its innate intelligence from *Osteopathy in the Cranial Field* [1st ed., p. 59] reads as follows:

The fluid possesses an innate intelligence which molds the head of the newborn and often reduces the traumatic lesions encountered in childhood and later.... In this occurrence we take it for granted as part of the Infinite Wisdom that shapes our ends.

I consider this functioning to be in accordance with the physiological laws "not framed by human hand" to which Dr. Still frequently referred.[7] There are special methods utilized in influencing the fluctuation and in controlling it. These will be taught at the tables.

---

6. Reference is being made to Dr. Still's principle that the rule of the artery is supreme and Dr. Sutherland's addition that the cerebrospinal fluid is in command.

7. "I do not claim to be the author of this science of Osteopathy. No human hand framed its law; I ask no greater honor than to have discovered it." Still, *Autobiography*, p. 302.

The second unit of the primary respiratory mechanism is represented by the intracranial and intraspinal membranes and will be discussed in another talk as the *reciprocal tension membrane*. This is a mechanical feature necessary in the operation of to-and-fro movements in all such mechanisms and is especially important relative to the to-and-fro articular movement of the cranial bones.

The third unit in the mechanism is known as *motility* of the brain and spinal cord, affording dilation and contraction of the ventricles that occur during alternate respiratory periodic changes. In an early description of this motility, we likened the motility of the spinal cord to that of a tadpole, with its tail drawing upward during swelling of its body and dropping downward as the body swell receded.

The fourth unit concerns the articular movement of the cranial bones and of the sacrum *between* the ilia. When I began digging into Dr. Still's science of osteopathy, I gained considerable information relative to the *shape* of the cranial bones, all about angles and surfaces and that they joined one another. But no information was given concerning the articular surfaces so important in the headpiece of a human body mechanism. Nor could I find reference thereto in any anatomical text. Thus it became my task to "go dig again" as I had learned to do in my early boyhood experience with potato digging.[8] In that digging, I found many little mechanical features upon the articular surfaces indicating a design for articular mobility. These little mechanical features, like the seedlings in the hills of potatoes, reminded me of Dr. Still's reference to the little things with the big significance in the science of osteopathy.

Among the indications was the *beveling* upon the greater wings of the sphenoid bone articulating with differentiative contrast *beveling* of the squamous portion of the temporal bone and bringing out the

---

8. The phrase "digging on" represents Dr. Sutherland's own approach to his study and the approach he encouraged others to follow. For his telling of the boyhood story that inspired this, see article 26, "Philosophy of Osteopathy and Its Application," note 1.

thought: Beveled like the gills of a fish and indicating a mechanism for respiration.

Due to the limited space on the record, the remainder of today's talk will merely outline the movement of the cranial bones to be observed during respiratory periods as follows.

Inhalation

During the inhalation period of respiration, the sphenoid bone circumrotates, or revolves like a wheel, anteriorly.[9] The L-shaped articular surfaces of the greater wings (converging anteriorly and diverging posteriorly) in their functioning turn the inferior angles of the frontal bones laterally, the middle area of the frontal bones receding posteriorly, while the ethmoidal notch widens at its posterior area. At the same period, the pterygoid processes of the sphenoid bone in articular contact with the palatine bones (with double grooves diverging posteriorly and converging anteriorly) rotate posteriorly and thus turn both the palatine bones and the maxillae laterally at the posterior borders, or areas. In connection, the incisor teeth recede posteriorly and the anterior borders of the nasal processes rotate medially, and the posterior borders laterally. The sella turcica of the sphenoid, in conjunction with the basilar process of the occipital bone, elevates into flexion position. At the same period, the occiput circumrotates, or revolves like a wheel, posteriorly, and the basilar process, in conjunction with the sella turcica, elevates into flexion position. During the same period, the petrous portions of the temporal bones rotate laterally, or externally, and the sacrum moves into flexion position between the ilia.

Exhalation

During the exhalation period of respiration, the sphenoid bone circumrotates, or revolves like a wheel, posteriorly. The L-shaped ar-

---

9. Illustrations of this general concept may be found in Sutherland, *Teachings*, pp. 26, 29.

ticular surfaces of the greater wings (diverging posteriorly and converging anteriorly) in their functioning draw the inferior angles of the frontal bones medially while the middle area of the frontal moves anteriorly and the ethmoidal notch narrows at its posterior area. At the same period, the pterygoid process of the sphenoid bone, in articular contact with the palatine bones (with double grooves converging anteriorly and diverging posteriorly) rotate anteriorly and thus turn both the palatine bones and the maxillae medially at the posterior borders, or areas. In connection, the incisor teeth move anteriorly while the anterior borders of the nasal processes rotate laterally and the posterior borders medially. The sella turcica of the sphenoid, in conjunction with the basilar process of the occiput, undulates downward into the extension position. At the same period, the occiput circumrotates, or revolves like a wheel, anteriorly, and the basilar process, in conjunction with the sella turcica, undulates downward into the extension position. During the same period, the petrous portions of the temporal bones rotate medially, or internally, and the sacrum moves into the extension position between the ilia.

2. The Reciprocal Tension Membrane

March 9, 1953.

One meets with frequent difficulty in the search for suitable terminology when preparing a talk new to the profession, like that relative to the cranial concept in the science of osteopathy. It became my good fortune to have the volunteered assistance of the late Dr. Ray G. Hulburt, editor of the *Journal of the American Osteopathic Association*, during the writing of *The Cranial Bowl* text.

I remember one especial difficulty very well. It concerned the falx cerebri and the tentorium cerebelli functioning as cooperative balance agencies in the delicate and intricate mechanism of cranial membranous articular mobility. We found considerable *information*, even in that early day, descriptive of the intracranial membranes as functioning in the act of shock absorbers, stress bands and partitions to prevent the cerebral hemispheres from bumping together. It is quite true that these intracranial agencies can function as stress bands, shock absorbers and partitions, but their function, according to physiological laws "not framed by human hand," had a *deeper significance.*[10]

After considerable discussion in correspondence, we finally agreed upon the terminology of: *the reciprocal tension membrane.* It should be remembered that the cranial articulations have no intermediate muscular agencies for operation. However, through the falx cerebri and tentorium cerebelli, the cranial bones possess a special membranous tissue that functions, not only as an intermediate agency, but acts also as a reciprocal tension agent limiting the normal range of their articular mobility. This tension tissue agent functions somewhat like the function of the tension spring to the balance wheel of a watch which regulates or limits the to-and-fro movement of the balance wheel. The term reciprocal tension membrane was chosen in relation to the function of the intracranial membranous tissue in accommodating to the to-and-fro movement of the cranial bones that must occur during respiratory periods. Attention is called to the specific poles of articular attachment of the falx cerebri and tentorium cerebelli that are especially adapted to maintain the normal range of movement of the basilar articulation.

There is an anterior-superior articular pole upon the crista galli of the ethmoid bone and an anterior-inferior pole upon the clinoid processes of the sphenoid bone. There are lateral poles of attachment upon the superior borders of the petrous portions of the temporal bones and posterior poles upon the occipital bone. In respiration, during the period of inhalation, the anterior-superior pole at the ethmoid spine of the sphenoid swings, or circumrotates, relatively forward, downward and backward while the anterior-inferior pole at the clinoid processes of the sphenoid swings, or circumrotates, backward

---

10. For the full quotation, see note 7 in this article.

and upward. At the same period, the lateral poles move upward while the posterior poles move forward. During the period of exhalation, a reverse movement occurs at the various poles of attachment.

Or we might say that, during the period of inhalation, the reciprocal tension membrane allows the ethmoidal spine of the sphenoid to drop downward while it draws the clinoid processes of the sphenoid backward and upward, the petrous portions of the temporal bones upward and the occiput forward.

During the period of exhalation, the reciprocal tension membrane allows the clinoid processes of the sphenoid to drop downward and forward, the petrous portions of the temporals downward and the occiput backward while it draws the ethmoidal spine of the sphenoid upward. Or, to make it simple, we might say that, relatively, the reciprocal tension membrane moves in an anterior-superior direction during the period of inhalation and in a posterior-inferior direction during the period of exhalation.

Knowledge of the direction of movement is quite important to the cranial technician in securing *balance in the tension* necessary in cranial reduction. Perhaps the "moving picture" will be easier to obtain by consideration of the terminology of "falx" in conjunction with cerebri, as "falx cerebri," and then by changing tentorium cerebelli to "falx tentorium" or "falx cerebelli." Falx, in definition, refers to a sickle and the falx cerebri was so named because of its sickle form. It does not require a stretch of one's imagination to visualize two additional sickle forms in the tentorium cerebelli. The three sickles join together at the area of the straight sinus, the junction which was so kindly christened the "Sutherland Fulcrum" by Dr. Harold I. Magoun, editor of the text, *Osteopathy in the Cranial Field* [1st ed., p. 39].

Neither is it necessary to swing a scythe in order to understand the simple mechanism of a sickle cutting grass, wherein one observes the sickle moving in a circular manner with its anterior end moving posteriorly while, as a whole, moving anteriorly. Consequently, as the reciprocal tension membrane moves in an anterior-superior direction, the end of the falx cerebri moves posteriorly and draws the crista galli of the ethmoid posteriorly. And, in conjunction, the two sickle forms of the tentorium cerebelli draw the clinoid processes of the sphenoid backward and upward while also moving in an anterior-superior direction. All of this relative movement occurs during the inhalation period and accounts for the receding movement observed at the metopic suture. By observing a reverse movement of the reciprocal tension membrane, during the exhalation period, one may picture the three sickle forms circling in the opposite direction, with the anterior ends moving forward and accounting for the prominence at the metopic suture as well as dropping down and forward at the clinoid processes of the sphenoid.

It is necessary to stress the importance of the Sutherland Fulcrum, where the falx adjoins the tent, in our study of the reciprocal tension membrane. The Fulcrum is the still leverage junction over or through which the three sickles function physiologically in the maintenance of balance in the cranial membranous articular mechanism. Like all fulcrums, it may be shifted from point to point, yet it remains *still* in its lever functioning. The fulcrum in relation to the reciprocal tension membrane is a *still leverage* point from which the three sickles are suspended. It also has provisional *automatic shifting* accommodation to the periodic respiratory changes occurring in the cranial mechanism, accommodation of what are known as torsion and sidebending sphenobasilar movements, as well as various malpositions occurring in cranial membranous articular strains.

Once again, we ran into difficulty in search of descriptive terminology. This still leverage point is now described as the *suspension-automatic-shifting fulcrum.* It describes our view of the reciprocal tension membrane as being suspended from a shifting fulcrum located in the center of the skull and having attachment to the various osseous articular poles, instead of being suspended from the osseous articular poles and having attachment at the fulcrum. Thus it becomes physiologically adaptable in postural changes. In the posture of standing on one's head, we would find the cerebral portion of the reciprocal tension membrane being suspended from the two cerebellar sickles, or portions. By lying on the left side, the left cerebellar sickle, or portion, would be suspended from the right and the cerebral portions, while the position of lying on the right side would assume the opposite in suspension. During the standing position, the two cerebellar portions would be suspended from the cerebral portion.

The mechanism is very simple, as is common to all physiological laws not framed by human hand. When properly, or intelligently, understood it is the key to simple reduction in cranial membranous articular strains. As an example pertaining to intelligent workable knowledge, permit a quotation from Dr. Edith E. Dovesmith [1895-1970: American School of Osteopathy, 1918]:

> Now I know what you mean by a "suspension fulcrum!" How those membranes swing. Somehow I am reminded of the caller at the square dance: "*Swing* your pardners to the left, every man." What rhythm in those membranes!

I like the thought of "rhythm in the membranes." It brings forth the necessity of recognizing tone quality with tactile sense rather than the mere "manipulation" of tissues–that is, a tone quality obtained by motivating an expression of non-incisive surgical skill to secure balance in the laws attributive to the mechanism. A bumper as a shock absorber or stress band may be necessary equipment on an automobile, but it has no physiological importance in relation to the laws governing the motivation of the mechanism. Similarly, there are many features in the living body that have no physiological importance to laws attributive to the physiological functioning of the suspension-automatic-shifting fulcrum operating in connection with the reciprocal tension membrane during rhythmic, or periodic, respiratory changes.

Possibly the Creator of the cranial mechanism solved a problem of available space by including an additional function to the reciprocal tension membrane, namely, by including the membranous walls of the venous sinuses as agencies for the motivation for the movement of venous blood. For these walls are materially different from the walls of venous channels outside of the cranium. These intracranial channels are frequently subject to cranial membranous articular strains so as to effect retardment of the flow of venous blood. This effect is now considered to be a grave predisposing factor leading especially to pathology in the central nervous system.

The superior and inferior sagittal sinuses, the transverse and straight sinuses, the superior and inferior petrosal sinuses and the cavernous sinus are important venous channels that should now have judicious consideration in the study of central nervous system disturbances. The straight sinus, passing through the automatic-shifting-suspension fulcrum, commences at its junction with the great cerebral vein and should have careful consideration in venous retardment. The straight sinus empties into the transverse sinuses which lack sutural accommodation in their course across the occipital squama. They do pass directly over the junction of the postero-inferior angles of the parietals with the mastoid portions of the temporals, a fact which indicates special attention in cases of venous retardment. Abnormal rotation of the petrous portions of the temporals indicates possible retardment to venous flow over the superior and inferior petrosal sinuses. Abnormal inactivity of the sphenoid bone mobility is indicative of venous retardment in the cavernous sinus and thus from the eye.

Disturbances in the normal fluctuation of the cerebrospinal fluid should also have our attention in connection with abnormal motivation of the reciprocal tension membrane, especially in cases of meningeal shocks that act like airbrakes and lock the cranial motivation as a whole. An early experience with meningeal shock will bear repeating as an example. It is told in *The Cranial Bowl* [p. 54] how this man, who had been drinking a poor brand of liquor, waded out into Lake Erie to go swimming but collapsed where the water was just above his waistline. He might have drowned had not a companion grabbed and dragged him to shore, a distance of two blocks or more. Upon reaching shore, helping hands tried various resuscitation methods, but he failed to revive. By the time I reached the scene, he was practically gone. His body was as blue as a whetstone, as stiff as a cadaver and without a sign of respiration. I did not pause to examine the pulse as the seconds were precious for success. I clasped my hands beneath the occiput with fingers locked to secure leverage through the flexor digitorum profundus and flexor pollicis longus muscles. With thenar eminences upon the mastoid portions and thumbs along the mastoid processes, as cushion contact points, I sprang the mastoid processes inward and posteriorly. Holding that position a second, I then sprang the mastoid portions inwardly. Almost immediately, a sensation of warmth occurred in the area of the lower occiput and the mastoid portions. It was followed by respiration. As soon as I released the technique, the respiration ceased. After an intermission of three or four seconds–while listening to a bystander cry, "Why doesn't somebody send for a doctor?"–I again applied the technique, but with greater force than was given in the first instance. This was followed by the same sensation of warmth at the lower occiput and the mastoid–and the return of respiration. His head gave a sudden jerk to the side, then back to normal range and he spoke a few words that were a great relief to a distracted sister by his side. A lady offered a flask of brandy, but a cup of hot coffee brought by another lady was the medicinal prescription given and all ended well.

Respiration in this case was initiated by placing the temporal bones in external rotation, wherein the attachment of the tentorium cerebelli upon the petrous portions carried the cranial mechanism into the inhalation period. The movement of the reciprocal tension membrane assisted in the return to respiration by fluctuating the cerebrospinal fluid.

During the commencement of initiation of respiration, one's acute tactile sense observes the suspension-automatic-shifting fulcrum commencing to shift its position, as well as the sensation of warmth due to the fluctuation of the cerebrospinal fluid. The dural intraspinal membrane, with osseous attachment around the foramen magnum and one or two upper cervical vertebrae, hangs down the spinal column to another osseous attachment at the second sacral segment and is considered a unit in functioning with the reciprocal tension membrane.[11] Moving the sacrum into flexion position is one of the possibilities for initiating respiration in cases of this nature. In fact, one may control the fluctuation of the cerebrospinal fluid in its fluctuation as well as initiating fluctuation when indicated. The sacral fluctuation of the cerebrospinal fluid is recommended in cases of possible cranial bone fracture.

3. The Cranial Articular Surfaces

March 10, 1953.

During our early teaching of the cranial concept, specific attention was given to introductory study of the articular surfaces of the skull bones and interpretation of indications of cranial membranous articular mobility.

Enlarged graphic chart illustrations were prepared by Adah M. Sutherland as an effective aid in the introductory study.[12] These lithographic and pen views have hung upon classroom walls where classes of cranial teaching have been in session. The charts were prepared from *normal* cranial bone specimens and differ materially from the

---

11. Subsequent anatomic studies have demonstrated that the dura mater is attached to the vertebral canal in the lumbar region. The anterior attachments are short and strong while the posterior attachments are weaker and longer. The anterior and anterolateral connective tissue bands attach to the posterior longitudinal ligament. The bands are strongest at the L5-S1 level and less strong in the upper lumbar region. The dural nerve root sheaths are also attached to the posterior longitudinal ligament anteriorly and to the periosteum of the inferior pedicle laterally. Cf. Parkin and Harrison, "The Topographical Anatomy of the Lumbar Epidural Space," *Journal of Anatomy* 141 (1985):211-217, and Spencer, Irwin and Miller, "Anatomy and Significance of Fixation of the Lumbosacral Nerve Roots in Sciatica," *Spine* 8, no. 6 (1983): 672-679.

12. Adah Strand Sutherland (1889-1976) married William G. Sutherland, D.O. in 1924. She acted as a "sounding board" for Dr. Sutherland, listening to his ideas and helping him to express them verbally, while also acting as secretary for early courses in Cranial Osteopathy. Her efforts to compile Dr. Sutherland's writings resulted in this text. She also authored *With Thinking Fingers*, a biography of Dr. Sutherland.

"bent twig" types common to the specimens found in our college laboratories.[13] Your attention has been called to this differentiation because of the importance it bears to the formulation of a mental picture relative to the normal specimen so necessary to one's understanding of the mechanism.

The early teaching included treks from coast to coast as follows: a number of classes at St. Peter, St. Paul and Minneapolis; one at Pittsburgh, with repetition the following year; another at the library of the Philadelphia college; two in New York City, followed by a third the next year; one each at East Orange, New Jersey and St. Louis; Mexico, Missouri; Des Moines; the Denver Polyclinic; Butte, Montana; Portland; Tacoma; Seattle; The Dalles, Oregon; The Drake and Stevens Hotels in Chicago; and in a log cabin at Saw Bill Lodge, 30 miles inland from the North Shore of Lake Superior. There was also a study group at the Lippincott's in Moorestown, New Jersey which was visited by Dr. Alfred Acton, the translator of Emanuel Swedenborg's anatomical texts.[14]

However, the specific attention in early teaching, relative to the articular surfaces in connection with the charts, seems to have fallen by the wayside at the time the Des Moines College sponsored the first class there. At this course, and others following, Dr. Paul R. Kimberly of the anatomy department at the Des Moines college devoted an entire week to review of the skull mechanism as found in all anatomical texts, which texts, even today, lack information concerning the articular surfaces so important in gaining the necessary mental picture required for understanding the cranial mechanism. Although these text reviews were valuable, the period of one whole week devoted thereto filled

---

13. The term "bent twigs" refers to the saying, "As the twig is bent so the tree inclines."

14. Emanual Swedenborg (1688-1772) was a Swedish scientist and mystic who studied anatomy in order to find the soul. His ideas blended spirituality with science and were incorporated into the Spiritualist movement in 19th century America, and are said to have influenced Dr. Still in his thinking. See Trowbridge, *Andrew Taylor Still.*

mental capacities to full and overflowing. Consequently, we found it advisable to discontinue the descriptive chart talk for the second week.

Recent requests from early students for a talk similar to that former one offer sufficient encouragement to make this recording today on the subject of "Cranial Articular Surfaces." Except for a few modifications, the talk will follow the early picture as given in two lectures before the Eastern States Osteopathic Association at New York City, which became the copyright property of the *Journal of the American Osteopathic Association*. Later it had special editorial attention from the late Dr. Ray G. Hulburt and Dr. R.C. McCaughan, with publication in April 1944.[15]

The cranial thought belongs to Dr. Andrew Taylor Still, founder of osteopathy, and provides an avenue for "digging on" through scientific research. We remember Dr. Still's dictum, "An osteopath reasons from his knowledge of anatomy. He compares the work of the abnormal body with that of the normal." And later, "...We must *know* the position and purpose of each bone and be thoroughly acquainted with each of its articulations. We must have a perfect image of the normal articulations that we wish to adjust."[16]

The cranium is an *intricate mechanism* and requires especial study of its complicated articular surfaces. For the perfection of skill required in cranial diagnosis and technique, it is necessary, primarily, to possess a perfect anatomical-physiological mental picture.

As a preliminary to further study, attention is called to these illustrations. Observe the L-shape of the superior articular surface of the greater wing of the sphenoid bone. There are two of these, one for each greater wing, articulating with L-shaped articular surfaces beneath the frontal bone. At birth there are two frontal bones, and in some adults the sagittal suture continues down to the ethmoidal notch. Inasmuch as there are two ossification centers, we may reason on the

---

15. This article was "The Cranial Bowl," (article 24).

16. Still, *Research and Practice*, p. 8 (n. 10) and p. 30 (n. 66).

basis of two frontal bones: the sphenoid being suspended by the L-shaped articular surfaces, between, or beneath them, as the sacrum is suspended by L-shaped articular surfaces between or beneath the ilia. Both bones, the sphenoid and the sacrum, have anterior and posterior rotation articular mobility as well as sidebending movement.

Now observe the little flat process upon the middle of the anterior superior area of the body of the sphenoid known as the ethmoid spine. This fits into a small groove upon the middle of the posterior superior area of the ethmoid. It provides the mechanical arrangement for movement of the ethmoid when the sphenoid moves downward. Immediately lateral to this process, on the superior articular surface of the lesser wings of the sphenoid, are two lateral beveled articular surfaces articulating beneath the two frontal bones lateral to the ethmoidal notch. These provide a mechanical arrangement for the accommodation of articular mobility between the lesser wings of the sphenoid and the frontal bones.

The beveled articular surfaces found on both lesser wings also have medial-lateral corrugations, indicating lateral movement during inhalation and medial activity during exhalation. This movement reminds one of a fellow traveler astride a Rocky Mountain burro on his way from Colorado Springs to the top of Pike's Peak. The burro had a stubborn habit of pausing to rest frequently, and when spurs stimulated movement ahead, the burro was inclined to bray loudly. It was observed that his ears moved laterally during the intake bray and medially during the expel bray, thus illustrating the movement of the lesser wings.

At the lower middle anterior area of the sphenoid is a beak-like process called the rostrum. Doubtless, the term was given by some anatomist because of its resemblance to the beak of a bird, which corresponds to the bird-like form of the sphenoid with its greater and lesser wings.

Next, we consider the vomer. It has a cup-like articular surface, a provision designed to fit over the beak, or rostrum. It provides a movement like that afforded by a universal joint. From that articulation, the vomer extends forward over the roof of the maxillae and palatine bones, which also have mobility. Down at this inferior area, we have rockers which are known as the internal and external pterygoid processes. They are convex in shape and beneath the bird-like, or boat-like, form from the bottom of the sphenoid. When the sphenoid rocks forward, these rockers rotate downward and backward. They articulate with double grooves within the little palatine bone.

Let us study this concave articular surface on the palatine bone in all its details and also the articular surfaces connecting the maxillae with the palatine bones. It almost calls for a magnifying glass to study the orbital surface that sticks up within the floor of the orbit.

The sphenopalatine ganglion lies between the palatine bone and the body of the sphenoid. Articular fixations commonly occur which crowd the palatine bone backward onto the ganglion, thus disturbing its functioning. The ganglion sends nerve fibers to the lacrimal gland, the turbinates, the nasal and paranasal areas and to the mouth of the eustachian tube.

The sphenoid does not articulate with the maxillae but does with the palatine bones. The palatine bones fit in between the sphenoid and maxillae and function as "speed-reducers" to retard the movement between the sphenoid and maxillae. The sphenoid also articulates with another equalizer in connection with the movement of the sphenoid and maxillae. This is the zygomatic bone, which articulates with the greater wing of the sphenoid *within the orbital cavity*. As the sphenoid rocks forward, the greater wing swings the zygomatic outward and widens the orbital cavity. As the anterior end of the sphenoid ascends ,the greater wing draws the zygomatic inward and narrows the orbital cavity. The zygomatic also articulates with the maxillary bone. Hence the movement of the sphenoid moves the maxilla through its equalizer, the zygomatic bone. The functioning widens and narrows the sphenomaxillary fissure within the orbital cavity. This fact is taken into consideration in the diagnosis of sphenobasilar lesions through observation at a glance. Wide or narrow orbital cavities provide clues which later may be verified by the skilled art of osteopathic palpation.

The orbital surface of the palatine bone is located immediately back of the maxilla, at the beginning of the sphenomaxillary fissure. The infraorbital nerve passes around the neck of that tiny orbital surface just before it enters a groove in the maxilla to find its way to the infraorbital foramen. Were it not for that especially designed little orbital surface, the maxillary bone might saw or wear the infraorbital nerve in two. The orbital surface of the palatine bone is an equalizer that removes the tension from the nerve.

The orbital cavity is not like the solid osseous acetabulum of the ilium but is formed by the articulation of the frontal bone, the maxilla, the orbital surface of the palatine, the zygoma and the greater and lesser wings of the sphenoid. It is a cavity designed for mobility. In addition, the origins of the extrinsic muscles of the eyeball were placed around the optic foramen, on the lesser wing of the sphenoid, with the exception of the one which was placed a little farther forward, arising from the maxilla.

As the sphenoid comes forward, the eyeball comes forward also. And, as the sphenoid moves backward, the eyeball moves backward. In addition to the infraorbital fissure, we observe another, the supraorbital fissure, which is formed by the greater and lesser wings of the sphenoid. The cavernous sinus leads from this fissure carrying its volume of venous blood that flows to the exit at the jugular foramen. The ophthalmic veins lead into the cavernous sinuses.

The maxillae hang by their frontal processes from the frontal bones lateral to the ethmoid notch. There is a gap between the frontal processes that is capped by the nasal bones. We may imagine the sagittal suture as continuing down to the ethmoidal notch, or ending between the frontal processes of the maxillary bones. The ethmoid lies beneath the frontal processes and nasal bones. It has processes known as the superior and middle turbinates. A lesion fixation of the frontal processes of the maxillae would crowd the turbinates. These fixations are quite common.

Our picture of the cranial articular surfaces continues with a view of the posterior articular surface of the greater wing of the sphenoid.

The upper half of its articular surface is beveled externally, and it articulates with an internally beveled articular surface upon the upper anterior half of the squamous portion of the temporal bone. At the halfway point lies a tiny niche, which articulates with a tiny projection on the squamous portion of the temporal bone. As we observe the lower half, we note that its articular surface has changed to an internal bevel and that it articulates with an externally beveled articular surface upon the lower half of the squamous portion of the temporal bone. These surfaces are designed especially for articular mobility.

Posterior to the squamous portion of the temporal bone, we find serrations running across the articular surface. These articulate with similar serrations that run across the articular surface of the posterior inferior angle of the parietal bone. These provide for a lateral movement between these bones, the temporal and parietal, inward and outward. At the inferior articular surface, on the mastoid portion of the temporal bone, we find the surface convex with what might be called a lateral surface. It articulates with a concave articular surface in the lateral part of the occiput in such a way that, while the convex surface of the temporal bone moves in one direction, the concave surface of the lateral part moves in the other. We have frequently likened this mobility to that of a cap and fruit jar movement–the cap revolving in one direction and the jar in the other. Just a little farther forward on the jugular process of the occiput is a small fulcrum which articulates with a groove beneath the petrous portion of the temporal. This fulcrum is immediately posterior to the jugular foramen and is known as the jugular process.

The basilar portion of the occipital bone anterior to the jugular foramen has a lateral ridge on its articular surface. This ridge articulates within a longitudinal groove on the petrous portion of the temporal. It is important to observe the peculiar shape of the temporal bone, that of a disk wheel, such a condition as sometimes occurs in the wheels of automobiles and causes them to wobble.[17]

---

17. It was popular to have disk, as opposed to spoke, wheels on one's automobile in the 1940's. If the disk warped, however, then the wheel would wobble.

The temporal bone was especially designed to wobble in order to accommodate the internal and external rotation of the petrous portions which, in my opinion, takes place with respiratory movements. When the mastoid portion is outward, the mastoid process will be inward; and while the mastoid portion is inward, the mastoid process will be outward. This feature of the wobbling of the temporal bone provides the means of diagnosing by palpation a sphenobasilar lesion, the mastoid portion being prominent in one type and depressed in another.

The cartilaginous portion of the eustachian tube is attached to the petrous portion. It is my belief that the petrous portion rotates externally during the period of inhalation, that the cartilaginous portion rotates externally also and that the mouth of the eustachian tube opens. Likewise, I believe that in exhalation the petrous portion rotates internally, that the cartilaginous portion rotates internally also and that this causes the mouth of the eustachian tube to close. In case of a lesion fixation in the movement of the petrous portion, the movement of the cartilaginous portion would be in the same fixation and the mouth of the eustachian tube would be either wide-open or closed.

The temporal bone, like the sphenoid, does not articulate with the maxilla. It articulates with one of the same equalizers, the zygoma, and the zygoma with the maxilla. This articulation is by way of the zygomatic process of the temporal. The articular surface is semi-oblique and overlaps the zygoma, providing an up-and-down movement as the petrous portion rotates internally and externally. One may take a disarticulated temporal bone and demonstrate the wobbling wheel motion by moving the zygomatic process upward and downward.

The bones at the base of the skull have their origin in cartilage, while the bones of the vault have their origin in membrane. Articular mobility occurs at the basilar area, in the bones having their origin in cartilage. The cranial structure is a *cranial bowl*, and we could not have articular mobility at the basilar area without compensation by the bones of the vault that are formed in membrane.

It is advisable to take a different view as to the structural consistency of the bones of the vault. We may reason that, having been formed in *membrane*, they remain as *membranous tissue* as long as the "sap" remains in them–like a soft-shelled egg, flexible throughout their structure as well as at their sutural serrations. The intracranial dural membrane has two walls, or sheets. The inner wall is smooth while the outer wall is rough. The diploe of the vault bones has two walls, an outer and an inner. Like the intracranial dural mater, the inner wall is smooth while the outer wall is rough. Why not call this diploe "membrane?"

One may pick up any inanimate skull in an anatomical laboratory and easily flex the structural portions of the vault bones. In the skull of the living human being, we are able to flex the vault tissues much more easily. In order to see the whole view of the response in the cranial vault to motion in the cranial base, it is useful to think of the dura mater and the bones formed in membrane together. As we have *mother* dura (dura mater) why not have *father* dura (dura pater)? Father dura is flexible throughout its structural portions as well as having special serrations along the sutural connections which provide sufficient compensation for the articular mobility of the bones at the basilar area of the skull.

Further provision was made in the outer wall serrations for compensation to articular mobility at the base of the skull. The serrations along the lower area of the occipital squama are externally beveled, while those on the parietal are internally beveled. In other words, the serrations of the parietal lap over those of the occiput at this area. At the upper area of the occiput, these serrations change to an internal bevel, while the serrations of the parietal change to the external. This signifies that the occiput laps over the parietal at the upper area–a special arrangement for compensation to articular mobility at the base of the skull. Other features of the vault sutures signifying the same function are the variations in the serrations in the sagittal suture and the change in beveling in the coronal suture. The serrations along the sagittal suture are coarser and further apart posteriorly than they are anteriorly. This provides compensation for a widening and narrowing at the posterior area of the sagittal suture as the bones move, upward and outward, and downward and inward. In the coronal suture, the frontal laps over the parietals at the upper area and fits in between them in the lower area.

The picture of the many changes occurring within the cranium is obviously so large a subject that is can be covered only sketchily in the space now available. We pass lightly over such dilation and contraction as may take place in the ventricles of the brain with movements of the sphenoid, and the effects upon the cerebrospinal fluid which Hilton, in *Rest and Pain* [p. 24], refers to as "a most beautiful, efficient and perfectly adapted water bed." We can but glance at the membranous walls with their content of venous blood, at the pituitary, the sella turcica, the infundibulum. We see the internal carotid artery with its branch which becomes the choroid plexus where, it is stated, an important interchange occurs between the cerebrospinal fluid and the arterial blood and note that movement, slight though it be, is essential to the freedom of that interchange.

As we look ahead of the cavernous sinuses, we see the supraorbital fissure of the sphenoid bone, the movements of which tense and relax the membranous walls of the sinuses, by way of which the venous blood passes. We observe also the ophthalmic veins entering the cavernous sinuses through this sphenoidal fissure. We likewise observe the oculomotor, trochlear and abducens nerves, as well as the ophthalmic division of the trigeminal passing through the same sinuses. Immediately anterior to the sella turcica, we note the optic chiasma and the optic nerves, together with the ophthalmic arteries, passing through the optic foramina in the lesser wings of the sphenoid bone.

Posterior to the sella turcica, we notice the junction of the sphenoid with the basilar process of the occiput and remember that up to the age of 25 to 30 years, in the average, there is a modified intervertebral cartilage present, and from then for a further period, mobility at the sphenobasilar junction is still present. Lateral to this junction, we note the foramina lacerum and see the internal carotid arteries passing into the cranium through individual canals in the petrous portions of the temporal bones. We take cognizance of the fact that these petrous portions extend diagonally forward and inward at their junctions with the basilar process of the occiput. We then remember that the cartilaginous portions of the eustachian tubes have their attachment to these portions, as already pointed out. Upon the apices of the petrous portions, we find the trigeminal ganglia embedded in dural membrane, having attachment upon both the petrous portions and the sphenoid. Then we see the ganglia sending out the branches of the fifth nerves, and further along we view the sphenopalatine ganglia in the pterygopalatine fossae. Is it not obvious that disturbances affecting their functions result from tensions in the membranes surrounding these ganglia, caused by lesions of the sphenoid and temporal bones?

Again we must hasten over a part of the picture, at this time giving less attention than should be paid to the fourth ventricle, the floor of which is occupied by various physiological centers, including that of respiration. We pass too rapidly over the dural and arachnoid membranes, the former carrying venous blood, over the superior sagittal sinus, into which empty the smaller cerebral veins, and the lateral sinuses.

However, in connection with my belief that normally there is movement in cranial articulations coincident with inspiration and expiration, I believe the venous blood is carried along by membranous activity to the exits at the jugular foramina. We keep in mind the fact that the main venous channels have walls decidedly different within the cranium than those without and that they find their way out of the cranium through exits formed by the articulation of two bones, the jugular foramina as examples. On the other hand, the arterial walls are the same within as without the cranium and have the same nervous systems. In addition, the arterial walls are protected on their way into the cranium by passing through individual canals in individual bones. Thus, we may reason that membranous restriction disturbs the venous flow and the fluctuation of the cerebrospinal fluid. While cranial lesions may be primary, the intracranial membranes are the real disturbing causative factors leading to disease of disturbed function of the brain.

The intraspinal membranes are included in the picture. They continue with the intracranial, being attached firmly to the foramen magnum, the second and third cervical vertebrae and without other firm attachment to bone until they reach the sacrum. In addition, I wish to call attention to the filum terminale as a unit in the functioning of the primary respiratory mechanism. The attachment to the first segment of the coccyx, where we have flexion and extension mobility at its junction with the apex of the sacrum, accommodates the motility changes occurring in the spinal cord during alternative respiratory periods. And, mention should be made relative to the animate structure of the sphenoid wherein its body, like that of a bird, apparently breathes by expansion and contraction–an important function necessary for an interchange of air within the sinus chambers. The maxillae also have similar animate functioning through the changes of shape of the maxillary sinuses. The vomer is a functional aid to the sphenoidal air interchange, its action being like that of a plumber's plunger directly upon the rostrum. The zygomatics function in a similar manner over the maxillary sinuses. Even the turbinates curl and uncurl during respiratory periods.

4. Types of Cranial Lesions

March 10, 1953.

Various types of cranial lesions are found in professional practice. Four of these are known as the sphenobasilar types: the sidebending-rotation, the torsion, the flexion and extension lesions. These occur at the junction of the sphenoid with the basilar process of the occiput and are quite common.

The sidebending-rotation lesion may be either to the left or right at the junction of the sphenoid with the basilar process of the occiput. If occurring to the left, the side of the basilar process will be tipped upward on the right and downward on the left, and the greater wing of the sphenoid will be upward on the right and downward on the left. Consequently, the right petrous portion of the temporal bone will be in internal rotation and the left in external rotation. Just the opposite will occur if the sidebending-rotation is to the right.

In the torsion type of sphenobasilar lesion, the sphenoid is twisted in one direction at the sphenobasilar junction while the basilar process is twisted in the opposite direction. In these, the side of the basilar process is usually tipped upward on the side on which the greater wing is tipped downward. As the petrous portion of the temporal is always found to be in internal rotation when the basilar process is tipped up on that side and in external rotation when the basilar process is tipped downward, it can be reasoned, for diagnosis, from the temporals what the position of the basilar process will be found to be.

During normal flexion and extension mobility at the sphenobasilar junction, the orbits widen during flexion and elongate and become narrow during extension. The eyeballs widen and narrow in accommodation.

The flexion type of sphenobasilar lesion is an exaggeration of the normal flexion position at the sphenobasilar junction. In this type, the front view will show both orbits wider and both eyeballs forward. The zygomatic bones will be turned outward. The greater wings of the sphenoid will be forward, and the petrous portions of both temporal bones will be in external rotation. The lesion may be easily verified by palpation.

The extension type of sphenobasilar lesion is an exaggeration of the normal extension position at the sphenobasilar junction. From the front view, the orbits will be narrow with both eyeballs backward. The zygomatics will be turned inward, the greater wings of the sphenoid will be backward and the petrous portions of the temporal bones will be in internal rotation. The lesion may be easily verified by palpation.

Other cranial lesions come under the head of traumatic types and, in these days of automobile accidents, are frequent. They are described according to the area of traumatic contact.

In the frontoparietal type, the frontal bones have been compressed in between the parietal bones by trauma at the middle areas. The inferior angles of the frontal bones will be found inward, thus locking the normal movement of the greater wings of the sphenoid. The lesion may be unilateral when the trauma occurs either to the right or left of the middle, and in such cases only one inferior angle will be compressed inward at the parietal junction.

In the parietofrontal type, the parietal bones have been compressed downward by trauma at the junction of the sagittal and coronal sutures. There is a consequent lateral position of the anteroinferior angles of the parietals. There is a subsequent malposition of the condyles of the occiput, which have been forced posteriorly within the facets of the atlas. The lesion may be either bilateral or unilateral according to the area of the traumatic contact.

In the parietosquamous type, the parietal bones have been compressed downward between the squamous portions of the temporal bones by trauma occurring at the midway point directly over the sagittal suture. It may be unilateral when the trauma occurs either to the right or left of the sagittal suture. The squamous portions of the temporal bones are forced outward, with consequent external rotation of the petrous portions at the basilar area and with subsequent flexion of the sphenobasilar junction.

In the parieto-occipital type, the parietal bones have been compressed downward by trauma at the junction of the sagittal with the lambdoidal sutures. The trauma tends to force the condyles of the occiput deeply into the facets of the atlas, thus tipping the basilar process upward at the sphenoid. There is a consequent malposition of the petrous portions of the temporal bones into external rotation. The lesion may be either bilateral or unilateral according to the area of contact. These malpositions at the basilar area indicate a rather serious condition in relation to the intracranial membranes that act as channels for the venous flow and which, in my opinion, incite activity of the cerebrospinal fluid.

In the occipitomastoid type, the lateral basilar area of the occiput has been forced upward between the lateral articular areas of the mastoid portions of the temporal bones by trauma at the lower region of the occiput. The basilar process of the occiput has been forced into its junction with the sphenoid, and the petrous portions of the temporals into internal rotation. The lesion may be either bilateral or unilateral according to the area of contact. It is another type indicating serious consequence to the intracranial membranes that act as walls to the venous flow and influence the fluctuation of the cerebrospinal fluid.

The dental traumatic type of lesion opens a field of new possibilities to members of the osteopathic profession. It should interest the dentist as well. Dentists possess special anatomical knowledge and constructive surgical skill in relation to the facial bones, and this type of lesion invites cooperation by the two professions.

It includes a membranous articular strain in relation to the temporal, the sphenoid and the superior and inferior maxillary bones. The temporal bone on the lesion side is found laterally inward with its petrous portion in internal rotation, the pterygoid process of the sphenoid upward and lateral, the superior maxilla downward and the inferior maxilla in malalignment at its temporomandibular articulations.

According to indications, the lesion occurs thus: The patient's occiput rests upon a V-form headrest on the dental chair in such a manner as to cause compression upon the mastoid portion of the temporals immediately anterior to the lambdoidal suture.[18] The dental surgeon chisels around a lower molar or wisdom tooth and applies a specially adapted forceps that extracts the tooth with an inward side leverage movement–that is, not a straight upward lift or pull. This inward side leverage upon the tooth tends to increase the compression upon the temporal bone by way of the temporomandibular articulation. At the same time, the side leverage twists or throws the mandible downward on the opposite side quite forcibly, thereby causing tension upon the sphenomandibular ligament, and swings the pterygoid process on the lesion side upward and laterally.

---

18. The V-shaped headrest is no longer encountered in the modern dental office.

During the extraction of an upper molar, the same side leverage is utilized which twists the superior maxilla laterally downward. In some cases the pterygoid process will be so far lateral as to crowd the coronoid process of the mandible. The crowding of the coronoid process together with the malalignment of the temporomandibular articulation, due to the inward position of the temporal bone, cause overbiting.

This type apparently affects the functioning of the trigeminal and sphenopalatine ganglia, sometimes leading to symptoms of facial neuralgia or tic douloureux. The internal rotation of the petrous portion of the temporal bone affects or twists the cartilaginous portion of the eustachian tube, which explains some of the ear complications that arise. There is tension of the intracranial membranes also, especially upon the lesion side.

The lateral position of the sphenoid bone, as well as the downward position of the superior maxilla, narrows the sphenomaxillary fissure within the orbital cavity, thus disturbing venous drainage from the orbit with consequent eye pathology in some cases. The fixation of the sphenoid is apt to disturb the normal functioning or movement of the orbital cavity, the normal position of the ethmoid with its turbinates, the vomer, the palatine bones, and accounts for many of the irregularities found in the nasal region. The malalignment of the maxillae crowds the turbinates and the palatine bones also. The crowding of the palatines affects the sphenopalatine ganglia.

This type of lesion is not difficult to diagnose. In some cases the removal of an upper dental plate tells the story; the plate being quite irregular in shape, the impression shows the downward position of the maxilla. This position may be verified by observation within the mouth.

The upward and lateral position of the pterygoid process of the sphenoid is diagnosed by inserting an index finger between the upper lip and gums, which travels backward to the posterior area of the maxilla, then turns up under the zygoma and then further posterior until contact is made with the pterygoid process. The pterygoid process upon the lesion side will be found upward and lateral in contrast to the opposite side. In most cases it will be found crowding the mandible upon the lesion side. Palpation of the mastoid portions of the temporal bones will reveal the lesion side as inward in contrast to that of the opposite.

The majority of lesions involving facial bones are found in relation to sphenoidal lesions and usually respond to sphenoidal reduction. However, there are many local injuries occurring to the facial bones that require local attention.

The zygomatic bone is found in malalignment frequently. The lesion is recognized readily by observation, comparing the zygoma on one side with that of the opposite. Its outer and inner borders are found in an outward position with consequent widening of the rim of the orbit and disfigurement of the face. Its semi-oblique articulation with the zygomatic process of the temporal bone will be out of alignment by comparison with the normal. The zygomatic forms part of the articular mechanism relating to the eye.

Malalignments of the maxillae occur frequently through local injuries as well as by dental traumatic initiation and should be given consideration as causative factors in nasal, postnasal and pharyngeal affections. In these cases, the nasal processes will be found crowding the turbinates of the ethmoid bone. The malposition affects the width of the sphenomaxillary fissure within the orbital cavity. In extreme types, the lesion crowds the palatine bone backward to the extent of disturbance to the sphenopalatine ganglion.

Malalignments of the palatines are usually secondary to those of the maxillae and sphenoid. They are readily diagnosed by observation in the mouth.

While the ethmoid belongs to the cranial base, its turbinate processes must be considered with the facial bones. In sinus complaints the turbinates are found in expansion. The frontoethmoidal articulations might be said to be in expansion also, which causes fixation instead of the normal movement of the ethmoid.

There are various types of birth injury cases common to subnormal types of children, but the limit of available space prevents discussing them now.

5. The Hole in the Tree

March 10, 1953.

In our endeavor to interpret Dr. Still's symbolic reference to the progress of the science of osteopathy as a mere grip upon the "squirrel's tail" sticking out from a "hole in a tree," we enter into the prenatal and childhood periods.[19] Herein we are to study, very minutely, skull areas *lacking articular contact* during these eventful periods in a commencement of life on earth. In fact, at this commencement, the skull bones do not even contact one another and have what are known as intermembranous and intercartilaginous unions, perhaps provided by the Creator to accommodate necessary flexibility during entrance into the world. Later on these intermembranous and intercartilaginous unions are replaced by articular surfaces having various mechanical features especially conformative to cranial membranous articular mobility.

In addition to intermembranous and intercartilaginous unions during the prenatal and childhood periods, the occiput and sphenoid possess intraosseous-epiphyseal units that we consider vitally important in study of the cranial concept. These intraosseous-epiphyseal units are subject to frequent luxation and, when not having intelligent skillful reduction, likely become predisposing etiological factors leading to grave disturbances throughout the central nervous system. In our anatomical laboratories, there are multitudinous abnormal skull specimens, or "bent twigs," indicative of abnormal growth/development occurring secondarily from these intraosseous-epiphyseal luxations.[20] There are many X-ray pictures providing indicative evidence

---

19. Dr. A. T. Still presented osteopathy as a science, a philosophy and an art whose potential was not fully realized, much as a squirrel only partially seen within a hole in a tree would not be fully visualized. He stated that only the tail of the squirrel was currently in view.

20. The term "bent twigs" refers to the saying, "As the twig is bent so the tree inclines."

that these types of luxation do occur. Furthermore, clinical records provide encouragement to parents who have been told, "Nothing can be done for your child but to place it in an institution." In fact, this clinical evidence accounts for the following statement made by Harold I. Magoun, D.O.:

> The mind of man will never fully comprehend the possibilities of the osteopathic concept.... When the last great picture is painted it will clearly be seen that a monumental contribution in the unfolding of the osteopathic school of thought and the amelioration of human disease and suffering has been made through the exploration and discovery of the cranial field in osteopathy.[21]

The intraosseous-epiphyseal unions have especial importance in the growth of the occiput. In this growth we find four important units surrounding, or forming, the rim or border of the foramen magnum, this foramen having many indications of being the symbolic hole in the tree to which Dr. Still referred.

The supraocciput, or planum nuchale of the occipital squama, having been formed in cartilage, is beneath the interparietal occiput which was formed in membrane. The supraocciput forms the posterior border of the foramen magnum; the two lateral parts that carry the condyles form the lateral borders; and the basilar part forms the anterior border.

In our study, it is important to note that each unit has lateral-form surfaces with which the intraosseous-epiphyseal facility makes connection. These lateral-form surfaces provide up-and-down as well as forward-and-backward movement as getaway facilities during what is known as *compression of the condylar parts of the occiput.* The mechanism operating with a compression of condylar parts lesion has been described by Drs. Howard A. Lippincott and Rebecca C. Lippincott, in a small booklet published in 1945, as follows:

---

21. Magoun, *Osteopathy in the Cranial Field*, 1st ed., p. 228.

> Due to the convergence of the articular facets of the atlas anteriorly, blows on the vertex or posterior part of the head may cause the anterior portion of one or both of the occipital condyles to be forced medially, narrowing the anterior rim of the foramen magnum. This approximation produces lateral compression of the posterior extremity of the basilar part with a tendency to elevation, lowering or turning on an anteroposterior axis. These stresses on the posterior extremity of the basilar part cause its anterior extremity to be forced downward, upward or turned laterally, respectively. Convergence of the facets of the atlas inferomedially may cause one or both of the condyles to be forced medially at their posterior extremities as the result of trauma to the vertex or anterior part of the vault, narrowing the foramen at its middle portion. Blows lateral to the midline of the vault, according to location of contact and direction of force, affect the two condyles unequally, producing asymmetry of position and compression. Trauma directed to the back of the head exerts a force which is transferred to the atlas, carrying it forward with the occiput. This is due to the posterior facing of the anterior portion of the facets and tends to cause the anterior arch of the atlas to move anteriorly in relation to the odontoid process, increasing the tension of the transverse ligament of the atlas and approximating the posterior arch to the odontoid process. This causes an anteroposterior narrowing of the vertebral canal with disturbance of the medulla oblongata, craniosacral membranes and fluctuation of the cerebrospinal fluid.[22]

These various types of condylar compression are discussed in the text *Osteopathy in the Cranial Field* [1st ed., pp. 197-203], including the

---

22. Howard A. and Rebecca C. Lippincott, *A Manual of Cranial Technique*. This manuscript was often referred to as the "Lippincott Notes" and was prepared from material supplied by Dr. Sutherland. It was later incorporated into Harold I. Magoun's *Osteopathy in the Cranial Field*, 1st ed.

application of technique indicated in reduction.

There are also intraosseous-epiphyseal units present in the growth of the sphenoid bones, requiring special attention because of frequent luxation leading to the development of bent-twig types and having grave indication as predisposing etiological factors. There are two of these union connections: one between the superior area of the body of the sphenoid and its lesser wings, and the other between the lower area of the body of the sphenoid and its greater wing-pterygoid units. The union between the body and lesser wings is somewhat of lateral-form contact surface, allowing a shifting of the lesser wings in their relation to the frontal bones. When this union is malpositioned, the bent-twig type that develops has the indications found in Down's Syndrome children in some occurrences, and in other developments of occurrences, malalignments in the walls of the orbital cavities appear that are common in strabismus. In the various types of strabismus, the cranial diagnostician considers the origin of the extrinsic muscles of the eyeball around the optic foramen in its location within the roots of the lesser wing and on the floor and roof of the orbits. The mechanical factors in the structure of the orbits, as they relate to the muscles of the eyeball, should be considered in conjunction with other problems related to strabismus.

The intraosseous union between the lower area of the body of the sphenoid and the greater wing-pterygoid units is said to possess a tooth and socket mechanical connection, or gomphosis, during prenatal and childhood periods. This connection is later surrounded completely by an osseous formation that leaves the pintle-oval arrangement as a mechanical accommodation feature for normal rotative movement of the unit in relation to the body found in common with sidebending sphenobasilar mobility.[23] This union is also subject to shifting possibilities through traumatic, especially compression, forces. If this has occurred, one may look for disturbances in the pterygoid

---

23. A pintle is a pin or bolt upon which some other part pivots or turns.

relationship with the little palatine bone and consequent irritation to the sphenopalatine ganglion. Also look for disturbances of the pterygoid relationship to the sphenopalatine foramen that should be considered in ear affections.

The possibility of disturbance of the movement of the greater wing with the zygomatic, within the orbital cavity, and the immediately subsequent effect on the zygomatic-maxillary attachment should also be considered by cranial diagnosticians. In fact, compression forces affecting the intraosseous unions of the sphenoid seriously affect the sphenoidal, maxillary and ethmoidal sinuses, and the eustachian tubes.

The temporal bone, known as the "mischief-maker" by cranial technicians, in its prenatal and childhood growth presents problems of an intraosseous nature that provide possible interpretation of the congenital deaf-mute problem. Two units having intraosseous union are indicated as responsible for abnormal twists in the petrous portion found among many bent-twig laboratory specimens. These twists would interfere especially with the delicate ear mechanism. The temporal bone is to be included in our study of traumatic and compression forces upon intraosseous parts.

Although the vault bones originate in membrane, they are subject to various distortions in response to various compression forces, but these will not have detailed mention in the talk today.

We will devote the time on the available recording space to the important realm of the *sacrum between the ilia* which is included in the primary respiratory mechanism and is also subject to intraosseous union luxations during prenatal and childhood life. According to *Gray's Anatomy*, there are variations in the number of units to be considered in its growth development. Sometimes there are six vertebral units and sometimes only four. In some instances, the first and second units fail to unite. This fact of nonunion is of especial importance in those instances, due to the attachment in the area of the second sacral segment of the spinal dura mater acting as the spinal unit of the reciprocal tension membrane. This area is considered as the fulcrum area, affording flexion and extension mobility in conjunction with flexion and extension mobility in the cranium at the sphenobasilar junction.

While the respiratory mobility of the sacrum is considered specifically as *between* the ilia, irregularities in the growth of the ilia frequently restrict sacral respiratory articular mobility. It should be remembered that the pelvic bones have three units to be especially considered in prenatal and childhood periods of growth. One of the units is the ilium, another is the ischium and the third is the pubis. The union of the three occurs through the area of the acetabulum with *intra*osseous-epiphyseal connections which is subject to traumatic or compression forces, like those that the occiput and sphenoid are subject to. These intraosseous-epiphyseal luxations may occur during entrance of the babe into the world, especially in breech presentations. The strain is present during the procedure of drawing first one lower extremity downward and then the other, preceding delivery of the breech. This alternative leg procedure tends to effect movement of the heads of the femurs and strains the epiphyseal unions connecting the heads with the necks, as well as the epiphyseal-*intra*osseous unions connecting the ilium, ischium and pubis units through the acetabulum–thus, in dire consequence, effecting restriction to the respiratory mobility of the sacrum.

The mention of this type of delivery reminds one that it would be wise to pause and during the interval, remind you that though the cranial concept has made great progress in its presentation, the tail of Dr. Still's squirrel is still sticking out from the hole in the tree. The grip on the tail has not gone further than the breech presentation. There still remains a vast undiscovered field for valuable and profitable study in the cranial realm relative to physiological laws "not framed by human hand."[24]

The quotation from the note in *The Cranial Bowl* [1st ed., p. 7] written by the late Dr. C. B. Rowlingson, editor of *The Western Osteopath*,

---

24. "I do not claim to be the author of this science of Osteopathy. No human hand framed its law; I ask no greater honor than to have discovered it." Still, *Autobiography*, p. 302.

will not be amiss: "Osteopathy is a therapeutic gold mine. Many veins of high-grade ore have been found and are now being worked; but others just as valuable are yet to be discovered."

34. The Tour of the Minnow

On various occasions, as a course of instruction in the cranial concept neared its close, Dr. Sutherland gave an extemporaneous talk which he named "A Tour of the Minnow." It never was written down. Consequently, each tour was distinct from the others, although the general idea was the same. As he and his listeners took the tour, the sights within and about the living brain were viewed, concentrated upon, and realized. Requests for repeats proved the efficacy of this unique sightseeing "Tour of the Minnow."

The tour presented here is a composite one put together from notes taken down at the time by Mrs. Sutherland, Rebecca C. Lippincott, D.O. and Marion Howe Wilder, D.O., and from a tape recording transcribed verbatim by Rollin E. Becker, D.O. It has been assembled by Anne L. Wales, D.O.[1] *The talks on which it is based–seven in number–were given in Des Moines, Iowa, Providence, Rhode Island, and Chicago, Illinois on July 1, 1948; October 23, 1948; March 14, 1949; May 19, 1949; October 28, 1949; May 25, 1950 and July 12, 1951. There were other tours of which there is no record, but it is probable that the composite content of these seven includes most of the thought that Dr. Sutherland expressed in this form.*

In childhood days, we frequently demonstrated use of a lively faculty which was ours, the ability to stretch our imagination. The Creator of

---

1. Adah Strand Sutherland (1889-1976) married William G. Sutherland, D.O. in 1924. She acted as a "sounding board" for Dr. Sutherland, listening to his ideas and helping him to express them verbally, while also acting as secretary for early courses in Cranial Osteopathy. Her efforts to compile Dr. Sutherland's writings resulted in this text. She also authored *With Thinking Fingers*, a biography of Dr. Sutherland.

Drs. Lippincott, Becker and Wales were members of Dr. Sutherland's associate faculty. Rebecca C. Lippincott, D.O. (1894-1986: Philadelphia College of Osteopathy, 1923) coauthored *A Manual of Cranial Technique;* Rollin E. Becker, D.O. (1910-1996: Kirksville College of Osteopathic Medicine, 1933) later became president of the Sutherland Cranial Teaching Foundation (1963-80); and Anne L. Wales, D.O. (1904- : Kansas City College of Osteopathy and Surgery, 1926) is the editor of Dr. Sutherland's *Teachings in the Science of Osteopathy*.

the Universe had Imagination–imagination with a capital "I." Without it, no Universe would have been created. I ask you now to make use of this faculty and embark with me on a sightseeing tour; a swim it will be in that great body of potent fluctuant fluid, the cerebrospinal fluid. Spark that imagination of yours and along with me accompany a little minnow, a fluorescent minnow, who can turn his light on or off at will as he explores, searches and reasons. He swims with fins and realizes that his movement fluctuates the cerebrospinal fluid.

The little minnow has learned that the cerebrospinal fluid is distributed within the brain and spinal cord, and outside the brain and spinal cord in the subarachnoid spaces. He reasons that the logical place to embark on his tour is the fourth ventricle, where communication between the ventricles and the cisterna magna is provided so that the cerebrospinal fluid may pass from the ventricles into the body of fluid that surrounds the brain and spinal cord. As he considers this, he recalls what Dr. Still said in the *Philosophy of Osteopathy* [p. 39]: "...the cerebrospinal fluid is the highest known element that is contained in the human body and unless the brain furnishes this fluid in abundance a disabled condition of the body will remain."

Presto! He takes off and finds himself in the fourth ventricle of the living human brain. He looks about and discovers that it narrows toward the central canal of the spinal cord and toward the cerebral aqueduct, as well as into the lateral recesses that have openings into the cisterna magna. This is clearly a strategic center of operation. So he swims along on the floor of the fourth ventricle, noting all the nerve cells and the functions they serve: the physiologic centers of the human body. How all-important that these regulating and control centers be in good working condition. He then swims to the top and sees the living motion of the cerebellum, the anterior part of the roof. He spends considerable time watching and asks himself: What is going on here? He observes the tracts from the pons going around into the cerebellum and the shape of the cerebellum, lying beneath the tent in the posterior fossa of the cranial base and overlying the posterior part of the roof of the fourth ventricle, with its choroid plexuses hanging down from the outside. Why! The cerebellum moves during inhalation and exhalation like a blacksmith's bellows! He sees that the cerebellar lobes have white tissue at their core with the gray matter on the outside. Here the nerve cells look to him like antennae for radio receiving sets. Why, he wonders, is the structure arranged like that?

With all that is located around and about the fourth ventricle fitting so neatly beneath the tentorium cerebelli, inside the curve of the squama of the occiput, above the foramen magnum and the basilar process, and lying up against the posterior surfaces of the petrous portions of the temporal bones, this all begins to look like a natural system for fluctuating the whole body of cerebrospinal fluid. Perhaps one could do exactly that with the squama of the occiput–*how convenient for compressing the cerebellum and the fourth ventricle and fluctuating* the cerebrospinal fluid *up* through the aqueduct to the third ventricle, *down* through the central canal, *out* through the sides to around, under and over the whole brain and spinal cord. Here, in compressing and releasing the fourth ventricle, the tidal movement of the cerebrospinal fluid may be controlled. Think of the fibers of the pons running around from beneath the floor of the fourth ventricle to the cerebellum as not only compressing from above but also drawing together. When you learn to control the tide by compressing the fourth ventricle, you can secure immediately a rhythmic balance interchange between all the fluids of the body, and I mean *all.*

In the floor of the fourth ventricle are all those physiologic centers, especially that of *respiration*, and ten of the cranial nerves (the other two are parts of the brain). You not only fluctuate the fluid, but all this action furnishes nourishment via the "highest known element" that is transmuted along fibers to all tissues: the heart, the lungs, the spleen, the liver. These are *primary* physiologic centers!

Observe that there is expansion and contraction of the aqueduct with the motility of its walls: the midbrain. See the undulation of the flow of cerebrospinal fluid through it into the third ventricle. Note that in this location the minnow is right over the sphenobasilar symphysis. He considers that extreme positions of that joint, in flexion, extension, sidebending-rotation and especially torsion would give a kink in the "hose" that would disturb fluctuation of the fluid from the third to the fourth or the fourth to the third ventricles. *Is* there anything to this skull notion? The little minnow begins to think there is.

See the whole system of the ventricles within the neural tube! The third and the fourth are like the body of a bird: The spinal cord is the tail and the wings are the lateral ventricles surrounded by the motile cerebrum and are attached where all wings would be attached. Wings that rise more posteriorly in flight and fold down in rest. The cerebral hemispheres ride on each ventricle as well as expand. This is why with inhalation there is more widening at the posterior end of the sagittal suture and in the occipitomastoid suture. Everything you study indicates motility of the brain and motion of the bones and all parts of the primary respiration mechanism. I tried to disprove it!

The little minnow now finds himself above a deep chasm at the top of the third ventricle. As he hears a hum along the motor nerve tracts leading down from the cerebral hemispheres, he watches a small cone as it flip-flops on its stem during respiration–a rhythmical function according to mechanical principles. It is the pineal body, tipping backward when the sphenobasilar symphysis is in extension and tipping forward when it is in flexion. Being a curious little fellow, he reaches out and draws it forward and back to see what it will do to that important fulcrum area at the junction of the falx cerebri with the tentorium cerebelli. It feels like a handle that shifts the gears, for it moves back and forth. There must be some connection between the little pineal body and the reciprocal tension membrane! Some philosophers have thought this area to be the seat of the soul. He doubts it. But there does seem to be some mechanical connection because the whole reciprocal tension membrane shifts forward during inhalation and backward during exhalation.

As the little minnow looks forward into the fluid in the third ventricle, he sees a curtain hanging down and the fluid moving. The curtain stretches out during inhalation, and he reasons that the choroid plexus of the third ventricle is changing shape. In fact, the shape of the ventricle changes as the walls move to make a V-shape in inhalation and come together again during exhalation. But these walls are nerve fibers that carry nervous impulses! Then this motility must be another physiologic function, one without which there would be nothing to provide for accommodation of the cerebrospinal fluid from the fourth to the third ventricles and vice versa.

He is very careful where he swims here in the third ventricle, for he hears the hum of the nerve cells in the two thalami, and there seems to be something alive in the walls: the basal ganglia. He's heard something about the electric nerve cells in these walls, and he doesn't care to be electrocuted by contact with electrical force anymore than you would dare to touch one of those high-tension wires that carry the electricity that becomes the 110 volts you use in your home. The potency in that thalamus is so great! Because it receives something from "the highest known element," as Dr. Still referred to it, it is different from the nerve impulses that run along with ordinary messages. It is then transmuted to the characteristic nerve impulses along the nerve pathway that may be compared to the 110-volt current.

The little minnow decides that it would be interesting to see the bottom of this deep chasm and find out what is going on there, so he dives down. The first thing he contacts is the hypothalamus. He spies a small channel and goes through the infundibulum to the pituitary body which is strapped down in its saddle, the sella turcica of the sphenoid, by the diaphragm of the sella. This is really fun–to ride with the pituitary.

The action at the bottom of the third ventricle, when it assumes its V-shape in inhalation, is in contrast to the closing of the V in exhalation. The hypothalamus, including the infundibulum and pituitary body, goes up and down rhythmically as the sphenoid circumrotates back and forth on its transverse axis. In fact, the pituitary is quite mobile, as well as motile, in its moving saddle. The little minnow wonders: does the dilation of the upper walls of the third ventricle lift the infundibulum? Does it lift the pituitary and the sphenoid?

The function of the hypothalamic-pituitary physiology is of fundamental importance to the whole neuroendocrine system. What is of greatest importance to that function? When you look at the whole picture and note all of the blood supply to these tissues, it is not hard to realize that this motion of the pituitary body is more important than any other factor. Could there be a leader of the flock unless there was in him some motility and mobility? He would have to be active in order to be a leader of his flock, the endocrine system.

Dr. Hoover called attention to a statement that was made by a pathologist, an authority in his field, speaking of 40,000 nerve fibers in the infundibulum running between the hypothalamus and the pituitary body with its anterior and posterior lobes. We have the function of secreting necessary fluids that must contact the other glandular systems of the body, but it could not do that work unless it had some mobility and some motility–both.

The little minnow can think. So he reasons: If the sphenoid bone circumrotates, and the little pituitary body rides in the saddle, there is motion. We can see the little pituitary body taking a ride like a trot, or a pace, or perhaps a lady's ride with a foot upon the pommel of the saddle. For it can change its seat according to changes in the position of the saddle. The little minnow has heard of sidebending-rotation and torsion. The sphenoid must be able to turn on its anteroposterior and its vertical axes. All this would go to explain those specimens in the anatomical laboratory where the pituitary has made a depression in its saddle, not in the center but over to one side or forward, or back. All are indications of the positions in which that little pituitary body has been riding other than normally can be found in the laboratory. What would this mean to the functioning of the pituitary and all the systems influenced by it, including the so-called personality of the body?

Let us take a ride with the pituitary and get the view. Look out ahead and see the optic chiasma. See the ethmoid notch widen and narrow. See the optic nerves passing between the roots of the lesser wings of the sphenoid into the orbital cavities which are changing their shape rhythmically. Consider the meaning to the vascular organism of the area, to the shape of the eyeballs in relation to myopia and hyperopia. See the cistern of cerebrospinal fluid above you, the cisterna interpeduncularis, where the fluid lies outside the infundibulum and is part of the "water bed" upon which the brain rests, according to Hilton in *Rest and Pain* [p. 24], often considered an osteopathic text. Realize that here the central part of the brain not only rests but also rocks its cranial articular cradle.

Now we will leave that little pituitary. No, we will do something else. We will have the little minnow reach up and pull on the reciprocal tension membrane and ring the locomotive bell by way of the crista galli. We then see the ethmoid bone rocking forward and backward like the movement of a locomotive bell. Observe the olfactory bulbs above the cribriform plate moving up and down and realize that the cerebrospinal fluid is found along the olfactory nerve tracts that are an extension of the brain–a different formation than the usual nerve system. You read in Speransky about how he blocked off (he called it the circulation) the cerebrospinal fluid along that same nerve tract and began to see little nodules of the color of the ink solutions he used appearing in the cervical lymphatics–by blocking that off.[2]

The little minnow sees how with sidebending-rotation there would be squeezing on the cribriform plate on the concave side that would do the same thing, blocking the transmutation of that cerebrospinal fluid, the protective system of the nasal mucosa to which I called your attention. In a sense, you sprinkle the lawn. When you sneeze, you are not catching cold; you are trying to protect yourself. This is one of the self-corrective actions that shows the possibilities in the science of osteopathy that you can discover by digging. You can use the intrinsic forces within in applications that bring out these healing powers, rather than using something from the outside.

---

2. A.D. Speransky was a Russian scientist who conducted experiments using ink tracers to show the connections between the cerebrospinal fluid, perineural spaces of the nasal cavity and the lymphatic system of the neck. See Speransky, *A Basis for the Theory of Medicine*.

Let us go back now and follow that infundibulum with its 40,000 live wires. Can you see it as a tube, like the copper tube in a coaxial cable, and see that the highest known element transmutes its energy to the copper tube?[3] It gives you something to think about. The master gland does not have nerve fibers going to it from the brain. See the pituitary body functioning, without any connection with the hypothalamus, by way of nerve fibers. There is some other means of control by the central nervous system. If it is found, it will lead to the correction of many disturbances in man's nervous system. Swim around in your imagination and see the pineal body in the positions it assumes when the sphenobasilar symphysis is in flexion and extension, when the whole neural tube is in inhalation and exhalation.

Let us ride up to the top of the third ventricle and see the curtain that stretches. That is what I want you to see–the real stretch of the roof of the third ventricle during inhalation, and I want you to see that choroid plexus bunching up during exhalation. Then you will begin to understand something about what the authorities on the cerebrospinal fluid mean when they say there is an *interchange* between the chemicals in the blood and the cerebrospinal fluid *within* the choroid plexuses. They don't know what it is. There is your mechanism, your mechanical principle, for the interchange between the chemicals of the blood and the cerebrospinal fluid.

The choroid arteries branch from the internal carotid arteries and pass up through the transverse fissure of the brain to become the choroid plexuses of the third ventricles and the two lateral ventricles. The tela choroidea is outside the ventricles but projects into them with the ependyma. Cerebrospinal fluid surrounds them in the subarachnoid distribution and in the ventricles. The choroid veins empty

---

3. A coaxial cable is composed of an insulated central conductor with tubular stranded copper conductors laid over it concentrically and separated by layers of insulation. This arrangement allows the cable to simultaneously transmit thousands of telephone, radio or television signals while preventing a loss of signal strength from outside electrical interference.

eventually into the straight sinus through the great cerebral vein. In fact, this area is called the cistern of the great cerebral vein.

The choroid plexus proper is in the arterial stream in the pia mater and not in the venous system. In principle, the same arrangement is found in the choroid plexus in the roof of the fourth ventricle. Thus, this system in the blood stream is surrounded by cerebrospinal fluid within the neural tube and without it. The motility of the brain alters the shape of the ventricles and produces rhythmical changes in the walls where the choroid plexuses are located, stretching them out and relaxing them. The plexuses of the lateral ventricles curve with each cerebral hemisphere down into the inferior horn. They are not located in the anterior or posterior horns. As the cerebrum is free to move from its base on the lamina terminalis above the tent on each side of the falx, the spiral curve gives you the mental picture of the pattern the motion of each hemisphere makes. Do you see why I liken the cerebral hemispheres to the wings of a bird? Do you see why the mastoid angles of the parietal bones move anterolaterally in inhalation and the spiral curve stretches out?

Listen to this from Dr. Still: "The brain is God's drugstore, having within all drugs, lubricating oils, opiates, acids, and every quality of drug that the wisdom of God found necessary for human happiness [*Happiness*] and health."[4] You, as one of the mechanics of the cranium, become a pharmacist in your art of knowing this mechanism–not merely the articular mechanism and that little fulcrum of the falx and the tent, but the fulcrum in the fluctuation of the cerebrospinal fluid, *its still point.*

Bring the fluctuation of the cerebrospinal fluid down to its rhythmic balance where all the fluids have that immediate interchange between the cerebrospinal fluid and the blood. Do you get the picture? An interchange from the chemicals in the blood with those in the cerebrospinal fluid.

Now let's take a little journey from the third ventricle. Up at the top

---

4. Still, *Autobiography*, p. 182. Note that in the 1908 revised ed., Dr. Still changed the word "brain" to "body;" cf. the original 1897 ed., p. 219. The bracketed form of "happiness" is thought to have been added by the original editors, probably to indicate the strong emphasis that Dr. Sutherland placed upon that word in his spoken presentations.

of the front wall, you will find little entrances that go out into the lateral ventricles. You decide to go out the one on the right side. If you don't make a little mark there so that you will know where you are when you come back, you may get lost because the ventricle curls around like a ram's horn, with a little horn off this way and another way back there.

First we go into this anterior lake that is surrounded by what some call the center of intelligence, the frontal lobe of the cerebrum. Here the frontal bones lie closer to the brain than any other cranial bones. The frontal bones turn out and in as the ethmoid notch widens and narrows, the olfactory bulbs rocking in the crib with pulsating motility and riding mobility.

The little minnow begins to see the simplicity of the neural tube. The anterior area has become the superior area because the cerebrum curls back down and around to the tip of the temporal lobe that is now under. Thus, the transverse fissure comes to hang over the midsection. The little minnow swims on in the lakes inside the parietal lobe, the temporal lobe, where he again hears the hum of the motor tracts, and back into the posterior horn where the visual cortex lies up against the reciprocal tension membrane, where the falx cerebri is the wall and the tentorium cerebelli is the floor. If the angle between the wall and the floor should be reduced, the visual cortex would get pinched.

The little minnow wishes himself back in the fourth ventricle. Presto! he is there. The choice between a trip down the inside of the spinal cord or the outside is made in favor of the outside. Through a lateral recess, he swims and finds himself in the cisterna magna that surrounds the medulla just above the foramen magnum. This is the area where things are big: the big cistern and the big hole. Could this be the hole in the tree that Dr. Still referred to? It is certainly a good-sized hole in the occiput.[5]

---

5. Dr. A.T. Still presented osteopathy as a science, a philosophy and an art whose potential was not fully realized, much as a squirrel only partially seen within a hole in a tree would not be fully visualized. He stated that only the tail of the squirrel was currently in view.

The little minnow has heard that the occiput has four parts at birth with cartilage between them. It sits on top of the spine and has little condyles that rock in the pits of the atlas when the head is nodded. The four parts go into the formation of the foramen magnum. It is clear that the shape of the foramen is directly related to the arrangement of the four parts that make its margin.

Resting here in the cisterna magna, the little minnow can see the pyramidal tracts on the under surface of the medulla oblongata. Right under them is the basilar process of the occiput. What could happen, he wonders, if a person had a fall landing hard on the feet and this drove the basilar process up and shook those pyramidal tracts? Or if through another of the traumas that may create strain here, the basilar process pressed on the pyramidal tracts or the medulla was pushed too tightly into the foramen? Perhaps such possibilities were implied in Dr. Still's reference to the body of the squirrel that was still in the hole in the tree.

At rest here, the tiny minnow feels a little quiver in the cerebrospinal fluid coming right up to the center. It doesn't spill off to one side or the other, and waves do not dash up here or there. The quiver comes right up to the center. He then begins to realize what we mean by bringing that fluctuation of the fluid right down to that short rhythmic period where we have balance; everything is balance, interchange; complete interchange between all the fluids in the body. That is enough to see the picture of the possibilities.

The little minnow swims down around the spinal cord which begins to resemble a tadpole's tail moving up and down during inhalation and exhalation. Then he sees the filaments called a "horse's tail" [cauda equina] going down, clear down to the bottom of that spinal mechanism: nerves and pia mater and the arachnoid membrane all within the spinal dura mater. This dural tube, a continuation of the inner layer of the cranial dura mater, is a reciprocal tension membrane. I want you to see this little mechanism between the occiput and the sacrum. This is the core-link between the cranial bowl and the pelvic bowl.

The spinal dura mater is firmly attached around the foramen magnum and the body of the second cervical vertebra. It has no other firm attachment to bone until it reaches the sacrum. As the occiput circumrotates on its transverse axis to its inhalation position, the foramen magnum changes from a lower level to a higher level. The pull of the membrane draws the base of the sacrum up and back and the apex moves anteriorly. When the occiput turns back to its exhalation position, the foramen magnum returns to its lower level and the sacrum drops into its extension position with the base forward and the apex back. As the occiput is part of the cranial mechanism, the mechanical principle of the spinal dura mater functioning as a reciprocal tension membrane makes this little mechanism a part of the primary respiratory mechanism. The outer surface of the cranial base participates in the secondary respiratory mechanism.

These are the mechanical principles you do not see in the anatomical laboratory. You have to observe them in living human bodies. As you begin to look at the individuals you see, you wonder about the significance of what you see. You can become so expert in diagnosis that you can point your finger and name the lesion, believe it or not.

Back in the cisterna magna, the little minnow goes forward under the brain through the cisterna pontis to the cisterna basalis. The arachnoid membrane spans the inequalities of the surface of the brain while the pia mater, carrying the arterial stream, adheres closely to it. As the cerebrospinal fluid occupies the space between them, there are many places where there is an accumulation of fluid. The cisterna basalis is divided into two parts: the cisterna interpeduncularis and the cisterna chiasmatis. There is a cistern around the optic tract and one in the lateral fissure of the cerebrum, as well as the distribution up through the transverse fissure to the cistern of the great cerebral vein. In fact, all the sulci are little cisterns of cerebrospinal fluid because the arachnoid membrane bridges over them, too, while the pia mater clings to the depths.

The whole picture begins to appear: The neural tube as a whole is like a house in an ocean, and there are open doorways between the rooms of the house. This ocean is a constant body of fluid contained within the arachnoid membrane and within the neural tube. The movement of the fluid within its natural cavity is a tidal movement, a fluctuation. The motility of the brain and the fluctuation of the cerebrospinal fluid shift the fulcrum of the reciprocal tension membrane that moves the cranial bones in relation to each other and the sacrum between the ilia. This is how the brain not only rests on its water bed but also rocks its articular cradle through the gear mechanism in the joints between the cranial bones.

The reciprocal tension membrane of the cranium is a reduplication of the inner layer of the cranial dura mater, called the falx cerebri and the tentorium cerebelli. In the vertical posture, the two sickle-shaped halves of the tent are suspended from the falx cerebri. If you stand on your head, the falx is suspended from the tent. If lying on the side, the falx and half of the tent are suspended from the other half of the tent. In terms of mechanical function, the membranous articular mechanism of the cranium is moved and regulated by the automatic-shifting-suspended fulcrum of the reciprocal tension membrane, located in the area of the straight sinus where the falx adjoins the tent.

This suspended fulcrum is comparable to the one in the old scales that I saw suspended from the ceiling in a replica of the first trading post on Cape Cod. The fulcrum around which the balance worked was the still point, the point of power in the function of the mechanism. It took hardly a touch to shift it, the balance was so sensitive.

Through the art of knowing the mechanism, and observing and palpating the living cranium, you can learn to understand the normal action of the primary respiratory mechanism. Through knowledge of the normal, you can diagnose the abnormal. The swing of the reciprocal tension membrane and the fluctuation of the cerebrospinal fluid tell you the diagnosis, and they can be utilized for the reduction of membranous articular strains of the mechanism.

There are patterns of adaptation in the articulations of the cranial base, and there are particular traumatic effects that need to be understood. We discuss them in terms of what happens at the sphenobasilar symphysis or, in the case of trauma, in terms of the point of impact and the local joints affected. Let's join the tiny minnow on a trip to see some of these.

As he goes sightseeing again in the great pond of cerebrospinal fluid, the little minnow realizes the presence of the light, the light which lights up the field. It is like the beam that goes out from the lighthouse: It lights up the ocean but does not touch it. Sometimes I call it a "fluid within a fluid," or the "liquid light"–something that you turn on in this dark room and the darkness disappears. Where does it go? It is something that is invisible: the Potency, the Breath of Life, or Dr. Still's highest known element.[6] We can utilize it when we get in trouble, not knowing what to do. As we seek to get the real picture of what goes on in the primary respiratory mechanism, we find more and more; everything *but* the liquid light.

In the cisterna magna, you look upon that cerebellum, you see where it has tipped backward, perhaps because of a punch on the back of the head, perhaps following a lumbar puncture to withdraw cerebrospinal fluid.

In the cisterna interpeduncularis, you can see where a compression force from the top of the head, or in a cranial lesion pattern, in pressing down on that cistern would press forward on the cistern above it. Such pressure around the optic tract could give an effect in the eye like that caused by an enlargement of the pituitary body or a growth. Not all indications mean a pituitary abnormality or a growth. The osteopathic application of the sense of touch over that cranium will tell you much. If you have a sensation like the feel of a rotten tomato, look for some pathology, such as a growth in that mechanism. You can make a differential diagnosis through the combined art of knowing

---

6. For a fuller discussion of Dr. Sutherland's use of the Breath of Life see article 23, "Untitled Talk 1944." Cf. "And the Lord God formed man of the dust of the ground, and breathed into his nostrils the breath of life; and man became a living soul." Gen. 2:7, King James Version.

the mechanics and the application of your skilled sense of touch in your thinking-feeling-seeing fingers.

These factors, such as compression forces that create disturbances in the normal fluctuation of the cerebrospinal fluid–or restrict it in one cistern–disturb or restrict it throughout the entire ocean area that surrounds the brain. Not only surrounds the brain, but is within its ventricles, its chambers, and all around the spinal cord, within the spinal cord and out on the nerve tracts a certain distance. The *magnitude* of it!

As you ride up here on the cerebral hemispheres, you find little fissures and you look down into them. You see the pia mater carrying the arterial circulation in the bottom of these fissures and the cerebrospinal fluid right down over the pia. You see the arachnoid membrane above *not* going down into those fissures but stretched across. Then you begin to realize what had happened to the young men returning from the war, emerging from planes and battleships with gray hair.

Through fear and vibrations, the membranes had locked down on the mechanism right over these fissures and sulci. Do you get the point? It is like the man we called your attention to in *The Cranial Bowl* [p. 54] who received a meningeal shock by mixing bad liquor with cold water; not internally, but through the chill of one and the influence of the other, a meningeal shock that locked his membranes down upon the cerebral hemispheres. There was no fluctuation of the cerebrospinal fluid, no pulse beat, no respiration. I don't know how long that liquid light remains, but it happened that we were fortunate in being able to "crank the car" at that time, and with the appearance of the Breath of Life, the patient began to breathe with the breath of air and to continue his walkabout on earth.

I want you to get that picture. When a meningeal shock occurs, I want you also to get the importance of the fulcrum, not only the one in the membranous articular mechanism, but especially the *fulcrum point*, the *still point* in the fluctuation of the cerebrospinal fluid where you come closer in your understanding of what Dr. Still meant when he referred to the highest known element in the living human body.

Let's go down to the area of the lateral fissure of the brain, between the frontal lobe and the temporal lobe that lies in the middle cranial fossa. The middle cerebral artery courses through the lateral or Sylvian fissure; the free border of the lesser wing of the sphenoid fits into the stem of it. You think of what happens after some little child has had a bump on the frontal bone that has driven the sphenoid backward. You begin to see a compression between those two lobes upon the middle cerebral artery, somewhat like the compression that the cuff of a sphygmomanometer makes when the blood pressure is measured, something that temporarily restricts the pulse beat. Such a compression between the two lobes could happen. Then think about the so-called "light" strokes. If you look into the history of your patients who have had light strokes, you may find an event of that kind. You have a possibility, one of many possibilities in diagnosis, through the art of knowing the mechanism and looking into the history of some little bump.

When the sphenobasilar symphysis is in a sidebending-rotation position we have one side of the head less convex than the other. The concave side is higher than the convex side. If the little minnow were to swim around in the lakes of the lateral ventricles, he would find a larger body of fluid on the side of the convexity, the lower side. We visualized the kink in the hose that would occur in the cerebral aqueduct in instances of marked sidebending-rotation or torsion or in extreme flexion or extension. Now visualize the same effect, the same kink, in the infundibulum disturbing the flow of cerebrospinal fluid. We saw that the little pituitary body may change its seat when its saddle tips, and we saw that the olfactory bulbs at the front and the visual cortex at the back may get pinched. All of these are considerations to take into account when you take hold of cases. Observe, diagnose, and reason out your data. Then use the intrinsic powers within for the reduction of the lesion. Hold the reciprocal tension membrane and the fluctuation of the fluid at the *balance point.* You can feel them tug-tug-tug.

At the sides of the sphenoid body, there is another fluid channel. The cavernous sinuses pass down from the ophthalmic veins through the dura mater to the superior and inferior petrosal sinuses. Realize that restriction in the flow of venous blood through the petrosal sinuses could influence the fluids in the orbital cavities. There are lots of "why's" as we go along. Osteopathy is a science with possibilities as great as the magnitude of the heavens.

If the cerebrospinal fluid locks down on the olfactory bulbs, the motion of the ethmoid bone is locked. Congested turbinates in the nose can also restrict the motion of the ethmoid.

When the situation in the cranial mechanism has resulted in protrusion of the eyeballs, exophthalmos, you may be able to get them to recede by changing the mechanism. When they have receded, the dilation of the pupils has also changed.

Suppose the patient has had a fall, landing hard on his ischial tuberosities. Or suppose he has had a blow on the superior angle of the occiput. Such events not only produce cranial articular lesions but also "plop" the cerebellum down over the cisterna magna. What a dull feeling one has when there is a lesion of the occipitomastoid and the cerebellum is pushed down. Many mentally ill people are so afflicted. An anterior plop of the sacrum, perhaps during childbirth, can have the same effect through the core-link between the cranial bowl and the pelvic bowl and fascial drag. Release of the articular mechanism and a fluid lift of the cerebellum corrects the situation. If you are going to reseat the sacrum with a technique for pushing back the sacral base, be sure to spread the ilia so as to permit success. This will take the drag off the reciprocal tension membrane and the fascia so that the cerebellum can lift.

Swim around in your imagination and see the pineal body in inhalation and exhalation. See the pituitary body functioning without any connection with the hypothalamus by way of nerve fibers. The master gland does not have nerve fibers going to it from the brain. There is some other means of control by the central nervous system. If it is found, it will lead to the correction of many disturbances of man's nervous system. See the infundibulum as a tube, like the copper tube in a coaxial cable, and see that the highest known element transmutes its energy to the copper tube. It gives you something to think about. With all these sights and thoughts, the minnow considers that he has enough to think about for years. So he dives to the very bottom, makes a lumbar puncture and departs.

Dr. Still could not speak of all the things he understood about the living human body. We were not ready to hear him. If you read between the lines in his *Philosophy of Osteopathy*, you will see that this is so.

Bibliography

Books Cited

Berchtold. *To Teach, To Heal, To Serve! A History of the Chicago College of Osteopathic Medicine*. Chicago College of Osteopathic Medicine, 1975.

Carson, Rachel. *The Sea Around Us*. New York: Oxford University Press, 1951.

Cunningham, Daniel J. *Textbook of Anatomy*. New York: William Wood, 1907.

Davis, Gwilym G. *Applied Anatomy: The Construction of the Human Body Considered in Relation to Its Functions, Diseases and Injuries*. Philadelphia: Lippincott, 1913.

Gaskell. *Involuntary Nervous System*. London: Longman, Green & Company, 1916.

Gerrish, Frederick H. *A Textbook of Anatomy*. Philadelphia: Lea Brothers, 1899.

Gray, Henry. *Anatomy of the Human Body*, 26th ed. Charles Mayo Goss, ed. Philadelphia: Lea and Fabiger, 1954.

Halladay, H. Virgil. *Applied Anatomy of the Spine*. Kirksville, Mo.: Journal Printing Company, 1920.

Hazzard, Charles. *The Practice and Applied Therapeutics of Osteopathy*. American School of Osteopathy, 1901.

Hilton, John. *Rest and Pain*, E.W. Walls et al., eds. Philadelphia: J. B. Lippincott Company, 1950. (Originally published in London in 1863.)

+Lippincott, Howard A. and Rebecca C. *A Manual of Cranial Technique*. 1943. Reprint, The Cranial Academy, 1995.

*Magoun, Harold I., Sr., ed., *Osteopathy in the Cranial Field*. 1st ed. 1951. Reprint, Sutherland Cranial Teaching Foundation, 1997.

*+Magoun, Harold I., Sr., *Osteopathy in the Cranial Field.* 3rd ed. 1966. Reprint, Sutherland Cranial Teaching Foundation and The Cranial Academy, 1997.

#Millard, Frederick P. *Lymphatics: The Third Circulation; A Brief Popular Discussion of the Circulation Involved in All Disease Conditions.* American Osteopathic Association, 1922.

Speransky, A. D. *A Basis for the Theory of Medicine.* C. P. Dutt, ed. and trans. New York: International Publishers, 1943.

#Still, Andrew T. *Autobiography of A. T. Still.* Revised ed. 1908. Reprint, American Academy of Osteopathy, 1989.

____. *Autobiography of A. T. Still.* 1st ed. Kirksville, Mo.: published by the author, 1897.

#____. *Osteopathy Research and Practice.* 1910. Reprint, Seattle: Eastland Press, 1992.

#____. *Philosophy of Osteopathy.* 1899. Reprint, The American Academy of Osteopathy, 1986.

#____. *The Philosophy and Mechanical Principles of Osteopathy.* 1902. Reprint, Kirksville, Mo.: Osteopathic Enterprises, 1986.

+Sutherland, Adah Strand. *With Thinking Fingers: The Story of William Garner Sutherland, D.O.* The Cranial Academy, 1962.

*Sutherland, William G. *Teachings in the Science of Osteopathy.* Portland, Ore.: Rudra Press, 1990.

+____. *The Cranial Bowl.* 1939. Reprint, The Cranial Academy, 1986.

#Trowbridge, Carol. *Andrew Taylor Still.* Kirksville, Mo.: The Thomas Jefferson University Press, 1991.

Vernier, Phillipe. *With the Master: Short Devotional Studies.* London: Lutterworth, 1942.

Wright, Samson. *Applied Physiology.* London: Oxford University Press, 1928.

Books available from:

The American Academy of Osteopathy, 3500 DePauw Blvd., Indianapolis, Indiana 46268. Phone: (317) 879-1881.
* The Sutherland Cranial Teaching Foundation, Inc., 4116 Hartwood Dr., Fort Worth, Texas 76109. Phone: (817) 926-7705.
+ The Cranial Academy, 8202 Clearvista Parkway #9-D, Indianapolis, Indiana 46256. Phone: (317) 594-0411.

About The Sutherland Cranial Teaching Foundation, Inc.

The Sutherland Cranial Teaching Foundation, Inc. is a not-for-profit organization established in 1953 by Dr. Sutherland and senior members of his teaching faculty. Dr. Sutherland conceived of the foundation as a way of providing a continuity for his teaching.

Dr. Sutherland was the first president of the foundation, and since his death in 1954, there have been just four subsequent presidents, which has provided for a continuity in the organization's teaching program. The presidents who followed Dr. Sutherland were Howard Lippincott, D.O., Rollin E. Becker, D.O., John H. Harakal, D.O., F.A.A.O., and Michael P. Burruano, D.O., who has served as president since 1993.

The charter of the Sutherland Cranial Teaching Foundation calls for the organization to dedicate itself to educational activities. It specifically states its objective as using its resources to establish the principles of osteopathy in the cranial field as conceived and developed by William Garner Sutherland, to disseminate a general knowledge of these principles and the therapeutic indication for this approach to treatment, to encourage and assist physicians in osteopathy, and to stimulate continued study and greater proficiency on the part of those practicing osteopathy in the cranial field.

In its endeavor to carry out these objectives, the Sutherland Cranial Teaching Foundation supports research, produces publications, and offers both basic and continuing studies courses. As a not-for-profit educational foundation, it accepts charitable contributions to support its work of perpetuating and disseminating the teachings in the science of osteopathy as expanded by William Garner Sutherland, D.O. The current address of the Sutherland Cranial Teaching Foundation is 4116 Hartwood Dr., Fort Worth, Texas 76109.

Index